PRIMARY NURSING

Contributors

Joyce Bloom, R.N., M.S.N.
Assistant Professor, Graduate Program
in Administration of Nursing Services
Boston University School of Nursing
Boston, Massachusetts

Delores Bournazos, R.N., A.D.
Staff Nurse
Tufts-New England Medical Center
Hospital
Boston, Massachusetts

Joan Gluck, R.N., M.S.N., C.N.P.
Education Coordinator
Harvard Community Health Plan
Boston, Massachusetts

Patricia A. Miodonka, R.N., B.S.N.
Community Health Nurse
Visiting Nurse Association of Greater
Lynn, Inc.
Lynn, Massachusetts

Arlene Schiro, R.N., M.A.,
C.C.R.N.
Critical Care Instructor
Staff Education
Tufts-New England Medical Center
Hospital
Boston, Massachusetts

PRIMARY NURSING

Development and Management

Karen S. Zander, R.N., M.S.N.

Nurse Leader, Psychiatry
Tufts-New England Medical Center Hospital
Boston, Massachusetts

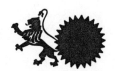

AN ASPEN PUBLICATION®

Aspen Systems Corporation
Germantown, Maryland
London, England
1980

Library of Congress Cataloging in Publication Data

Zander, Karen S.
Primary Nursing, development and management.

Includes bibliographical references and index.
1. Nursing service administration.   2. Nurse and
patient.   3. Nursing—Practice.   I. Title.   [DNLM:
1. Primary nursing care.   WY101 Z27p]
RT89.Z36   610.73   79-28837
ISBN: 0-89443-170-6

Library of Congress Catalog Card Number: 79-28837
ISBN: 0-89443-170-6

Printed in the United States of America

1 2 3 4 5

To my parents,
Hazel and Edward Zander,
Park Ridge, Illinois

Table of Contents

Preface

Primary nursing permits nurses to make the broad concept of professional commitment to patients and their families a functional reality. A health care delivery system based on primary nursing involves a complex but exciting process in which nurses perform at their highest developmental level for the benefit of persons requiring their expertise. Primary nursing provides a realistic vehicle through which to define, plan, deliver, and evaluate quality health care. However, the purpose of this volume is to present a useful overview of the many elements involved in managing good primary nursing care, not to sell it as the only kind of nursing.

Because primary nursing is a dynamic process requiring increased authority for qualified nurses, both the positive and the negative aspects of the nursing profession are intensified and, therefore, demand thoughtful action. This action begins with a planned, gradual restructuring of a nursing department from the bottom up, so that "a stable pattern of work flow and person-to-person interaction" is established (Miller, 1972, p. 23). Thus, the role of the primary nurse must be understood, integrated, and supported at every level of a nursing organization. Primary nurses must be assured that the values and behavior expected of each primary nurse-patient relationship will be supported in the unit's nursing station and the department's administrative offices.

Some aspects of primary nursing can be incorporated into a staff's daily routine —which is probably the state of the art nationally. The difference between what occurs in many institutions and what occurs with primary nursing is the concept of a professional commitment that is promoted by a responsive managerial and administrative structure. A great deal of confidence and skill is required for a staff nurse to say: "Hello, I'm your primary nurse. I will be responsible for the outcomes of the nursing care you receive while here. I will work with the rest of the staff on your behalf, and I will use my experience with you to evaluate the consequences of primary nursing." This commitment of primary nursing requires constant care and monitoring by leadership personnel at all levels of the organization.

The phrase *managing toward* which begins many chapters indicates that there are goals in primary nursing that can only be attained by the continual assertive action of nurse-managers. To manage toward a goal also means that mastery of a series of skills must be achieved so that staff and unit leadership personnel can succeed with primary nursing. A larger scope of management skills is required for primary nursing due to the increased professionalism of the staff (Elpern, 1977).

This book is written for those who are contemplating or are already involved in primary nursing. The emphasis is on managing toward specific professional qualities and behaviors, because management makes the difference in the clinical area. Even the best primary nurse cannot achieve consistent excellence or satisfaction without the support and follow-through of management. Therefore, primary nurses should be aware that:

- Empathy expands your data base
- Education expands your repertoire
- Common sense expands your credibility
- Collaboration expands your professionalism
- Mentors expand your confidence
- But only responsive managers can expand your potential for effectiveness and satisfaction

The decision to become committed to primary nursing as the vehicle for professional behavior has many repercussions. Every change generates a need for new support systems to reinforce that change. Thus, the goal of primary nursing sets an evolutionary chain into motion. Professional development cannot take place without concomitant organizational development. Therefore, the management framework is described in this book before guidelines for implementation of primary nursing are addressed.

Beyond the obvious goal of optimum care delivered by competent primary nurses, the consequences of this avenue of professional development are also explored. For this purpose, "Managing Toward a Viable Identity for Professional Nursing" is offered both as a summary and as an indicator of investigations that primary nursing has stimulated.

Karen Zander
March 1980

REFERENCES

Elpern, E. Structural and organizational supports for primary nursing. *Nursing Clinics of North America, 12*(2), 205-219.

Miller, D. Organization is a process. *Journal of Nursing Administration,* March/April 1972, pp. 19-24.

Acknowledgments

I implemented primary nursing in 1973 after the staff for whom I was nurse-manager requested that we try it to see if it was a better approach to giving care. As a result, primary nursing has stimulated my growth as a manager, and the staff primary nurses continue to excite and challenge my teaching and leadership potentials. They, together with Ellen McTiernan, RN; MaryLou Etheredge, RN, MSN, and Susan Alperin, RN, BSN, have taught me a great deal and I am very grateful to them. I have found many mentors in the process of researching and writing this book. My husband, Bernhard Metzger, and Joan Gluck have always been there when I needed them—my very own primary nurses! I would also like to thank Sandra Twyon, chairman, Tufts-New England Medical Center, Department of Nursing, Dr. Stephen Bernstein, chief, Tufts-New England Medical Center, Inpatient Psychiatry, and my colleagues on the Primary Nursing Committee for their daily contributions to my thoughts and actions. Finally, I would like to acknowledge you, the reader, for your interest in primary nursing. I hope that this book answers your questions and encourages your creativity as managers and nurses.

Part I

"Hello, I'm Your Primary Nurse"

INTRODUCTION

"Hello, I'm your primary nurse" is the most difficult introduction that any nurse can make, because it requires a commitment to the complex role of a primary nurse. The strength behind this statement is directly proportional to the quality of leadership that is provided to primary nurses who need this to support the nursing process. Nursing leadership must *enable* the primary nurse to work and live with the implications that follow this introduction.

Primary nursing is a professional commitment made by a registered nurse to direct and provide comprehensive nursing care to specifically assigned patients and their families during their contact with the health care unit or agency. The primary nurse follows all the steps of the nursing process and uses this position of authority and autonomy to assess, plan, administer, and evaluate nursing interventions on behalf of patients and families. Because primary nurses collaborate with other nursing and health practitioners about the needs of their primary patients, primary nurses become patient advocates within the health care delivery system.

Before primary nursing, the nurse-manager was expected to carry out all of these activities for each and every patient — a superhuman task! Even today, the public, as well as many nurses, believe that a nurse-manager can actually keep track of and meet the infinite needs of all patients and staff members involved with a unit or agency. However, primary nursing by its nature acknowledges the impossibility of one nurse in a managerial position doing absolutely everything, and it returns to individual nurses the authority and autonomy to give and direct nursing care for the patients with whom they have the most contact. At the same time primary nursing allows the nurse-manager to function at a high level of clinical and managerial expertise. Primary nurses need skillful managers:

1

Primary nursing is a sophisticated form of health care delivery, requiring maturity, a certain level of expertise, and a sense of professionalism. Not every nurse is capable, not to mention willing to deal with all the responsibilities involved. It is no surprise then that the success or failure of the approach on any unit depends not only on the nurses providing the care, but also on the strength of leadership they have (Norton, 1978, p. 72).

Nursing leadership at the unit or first-line level is the focus of this book because the effectiveness of such leadership is the critical ingredient in primary nursing. "The first-line manager works close to the actual steps of production, being responsible for turning out the desired product through effective use of personnel, materials, and systems" (Stevens, 1976, p. 3).

For each primary nurse to be useful in working with each primary patient, staff nurses need a realistic role description within a well-defined administrative structure. The interpreter of what is expected of the primary nurse is the nurse-manager. A nurse-manager's skill in management and staff development is the greatest contribution to the long-term, lasting success of primary nursing.

Who is the nurse-manager?

The nurse-manager in primary nursing is the first-line manager whose major responsibility is to provide patient care through primary nurses and their colleagues. In addition, the nurse-manager must formally evaluate the primary nurse's performance. Thus, the nurse-manager is delegated by the institutional administration, the responsibility of holding primary nurses accountable for their actions. No matter how autonomously a staff of primary nurses function, there must be a designated nurse-manager working "at the juncture between administration and creation of the desired product" (Stevens, 1976, p. 3) who daily enables primary nurses to carry out their complex roles with the accountability of a true professional.

The management task of the nurse-manager is distinct from that which other nurses assume for limited periods of time (shift charge nurse) or for limited groups of patients (primary nurse).

The difference between being a *nurse* manager and a nurse *manager* is more than a matter of semantics. A primary nurse working with a limited number of patients uses the management process in providing and managing the care of those patients. The emphasis is on a personal application of the nursing process while providing guidelines and leadership to other members of the patient care team as a secondary responsibility. A head nurse, however, or a patient care coordinator responsible for several units, necessarily has to place major emphasis on the personnel management aspects of the work. Clinical skills are still necessary and important, but the management skills must at the very least be of equal importance (Ganong & Ganong, 1976, pp. 20-1).[1]

A nurse-manager has 24-hour accountability for getting the "product" of patient care delivered safely and therapeutically by all levels of nursing staff within a defined territory. Generally, this distinction is given to the head nurse of hospital inpatient units and to the first-line supervisors of more ambulatory or preventive health services.

Primary nursing requires decentralization of what has traditionally been the nurse-manager's role. Nurse-managers who are committed to primary nursing find that they must adjust their leadership style from a directive to an interactional one. The nurse-manager must have the qualities of a growth-enhancing mother as well as the qualities of a primary nurse. The nurse-manager of primary nurses walks the fine line between providing structure without stifling creativity, allowing autonomy without abandoning, teaching without telling, and fostering growth without undermining confidence. No easy task!

Reportedly, some units or agencies implementing primary nursing have experimented with no head nurse and other concomitant changes in an attempt to give primary nurses complete autonomy and to enforce peer support (Mealy et al., 1976, p. 81). In these situations one or several people ultimately pick up the tasks of clinical management. The role and accountability of the nurse-manager becomes fragmented, victim to another onslaught of the "misplaced idealism" (Ciske, Note 1) prevalent in primary nursing. In effect the primary nurses lose their primary nurse—the nurse-manager! Whatever new titles emerge from these experiments, it is essential that one person be identified as the nurse-manager of a defined area, accountable to both administration and to the primary nursing staff.

The nurse-manager has both the formal authority and the informal influence to support or to sabotage primary nurses in their work. This places the nurse-manager in the key position to ensure that individual primary nurses are effective, as well as to ensure the national success of the primary nursing concept. For the nurse-manager's own professional development as well as for the growth of the primary nursing staff, the nurse-manager must know the major implications of saying, "Hello, I'm your primary nurse." To do this the nurse-manager must formulate an operational, or working, definition of primary nursing and of the professional commitment to patients that primary nursing entails.

---

[1]Ganong, J.M., & Ganong, W.L. *Nursing Management* (Germantown, Md.: Aspen Systems Corp., 1976). This quote and others in the text citing this source are reprinted with permission of the publisher.

REFERENCE NOTE

1. Ciske, K. Comments presented at the Primary Nursing Annual Research Conference, North Central Regional Medical Education Center, Minneapolis Veterans Administration Hospital Nursing Service, October 1978.

REFERENCES

Ganong, J., and Ganong, W. *Nursing management*. Germantown, Md.: Aspen Systems Corp., 1976.

Mealy, S., Mann, J., Simandi, G., and Kiener, M. Shared leadership—No head nurse! *Nursing Administration Quarterly*, Fall 1976, 1 (1), pp. 81-93.

Norton, C. What's primary in primary nursing? *American Journal of Maternal-Child Nursing*, March-April, 1978, p. 72.

Stevens, B. *First-line patient care management*. Wakefield, Mass.: Contemporary Publishing, 1976.

Chapter 1

Managing Toward an Operational Definition

There are as many definitions of primary nursing as there are nurses, yet some core elements must remain constant or the essence of primary nursing is lost. Certainly, different patients and institutions will require primary nurses to perform differently, but certain principles cannot be sacrificed to the convenience or pressures of the nursing profession.

Twelve key elements have been identified in order to formulate an operational definition—which defines a concept by prescribing actions—for primary nursing:

1. Accountability
2. Advocacy
3. Assertiveness
4. Authority
5. Autonomy
6. Continuity
7. Commitment
8. Collaboration
9. Contracting
10. Coordination
11. Communication
12. Decentralization

Making these concepts function in reality is the task of the nurse-manager and the nursing service department. In order to define primary nursing in a reasonable and workable way for each setting, they need to understand the history behind the concepts. An operational definition stated without using any of the 12 concepts would be similar to this example.

Primary nursing is a series of nursing activities performed on behalf of a patient and/or the patient's family by the same, specifically assigned registered nurse who is answerable both to the patient and to the administration of the institution for the outcomes of those activities. Patient outcomes, as delineated by the Joint Commission on Accreditation of Hospitals for retrospective nursing audits, are health status, activity level, and knowledge (Jacobs and Jacobs, 1975). The primary nurse is the consistent representative of the whole nursing staff to the patient and the patient's family throughout the length of their contact with the health care unit or agency. To be most effective, the primary nurse must deliver hands-on care to the primary patient when on duty. This includes assessing, planning, intervening, and evaluating nursing care. Even when off duty, the primary nurse is responsible for the nursing care that others have been directed to give. By talking with peers, physicians, and other members of the health care team on behalf of a primary patient, the primary nurse becomes the patient's spokesman within the system.

The nurse-manager of a primary nursing unit has the complex job of insuring that all the work of patient care is completed, regardless of shifts and staffing. There are many maintenance operations, from giving medications to distributing water pitchers, that must be done on a regular basis. These routine functions must go hand-in-hand with primary nursing functions, neither at the expense of the other.

It is useful for a nurse-manager to know and be able to define the ideal way the staff should function. With the 12 concepts of primary nursing in mind, the nurse-manager will find that there are specific management techniques which help most nurses to practice quality nursing. By using primary nursing as the vehicle for providing professional nursing care, the nurse-manager will find that accomplishment of routine tasks improves.

The seeds of good nursing care through primary nursing need to be planted and continuously nurtured in order to produce viable, productive results. Like any good garden, growth takes time! A nurse-manager is constantly managing toward an ideal which acts as a yardstick for evaluation.

In order to evaluate personal progress, as well as the performance of primary nurses, the nurse-manager needs to understand how the basic tenets of primary nursing originated and how they relate to the unit or agency. Because the nurse-manager has the all-important task of structuring primary nursing, the nurse-manager's role must be assessed to see if the nurse-manager's energies are being spent on the daily functions that contribute to an operational primary nursing system.

THE PRIMARY NURSING LEGACY

To understand the trend toward primary nursing and its problems, the nurse-manager should view primary nursing as a group legacy. A legacy is that which is passed along from generation to generation within a specific group. Every legacy contains a powerful mixture of fact and fiction, which is believed to be fact. Thus, any legacy combines knowledge with prescribed attitudes. The knowledge and attitudes, or norms, of a group "may be transmitted through an interactive process between the leader and the group members or independently by old members to new members." Legacies tend to "stabilize the group in spite of its instability of membership" (Bailis, Lambert, & Bernstein, 1978, p. 417).

Primary nursing is a legacy of the nursing profession. The mention of the phrase elicits certain reactions and behaviors from nurses and the professional staff groupings to which they belong. For primary nursing to reach the position that it has today in nursing literature and practice took years of legacy building and passing, resisting and refining within the profession. For nurse-managers and administrators to analyze the validity of primary nursing for their institutions, some background on the legacy of primary nursing is invaluable.

As a philosophy of nursing practice, primary nursing is the accumulation of the best legacies contributed over the years. Marram, Schlegel, and Bevis (1974) compare nursing's history to Erikson's developmental tasks and claim that primary nursing is a step toward professional maturity. If maturity means taking responsibility for one's actions and being accountable for the results, then primary nursing is indeed an affirmation of professional nursing practice.

The current debate is whether primary nursing is a return to an old pattern of nursing with a new name or whether it is a truly new idea. Primary nursing, as described in this text, is a new idea. It is an integration of attitudes, knowledge, and skills, of which some have been part of the nursing profession since its inception and some are relatively modern and even futuristic.

> [Primary nursing] is not merely old wine in new bottles, however, since there have been numerous changes, particularly in the scope of nursing practice and in the setting in which care is delivered. So, while the concepts of continuity and a one-to-one relationship build on the past, the expression of primary nursing as a philosophy and an organizational style is a relatively recent innovation (Hegyvary cited in Pryma, 1978, p. 7).

Primary nursing is as old as the laying-on of hands and as new as consumer rights. Because of this paradox, primary nursing is potentially the most powerful force in the health care delivery system. The task of the nurse-manager, with the solid backing of the nursing administration, is to maximize the potential of primary nursing by enhancing each primary nurse's performance.

The History of Primary Nursing

Nursing in the Early 1900s

Before World War I, most patients received medical treatment in their homes, and those who needed extensive care hired live-in nurses to assume nursing duties as well as household chores. "While private duty nurses gave intense individualized attention to patient's needs, they were not prepared to meet the many psychological needs of their patients" (Pryma, 1978, p. 4). Although the foundations of individual responsibility and continuity of care were laid during this period, the nurses who administered this one-to-one care were limited in the depth and scope of what they could offer patients.

However, nurses began proving their technical competence and usefulness between 1873 and 1900. When the hospital boom occurred between 1900 and 1910, the physicians who started them needed nurses to staff them. These were small, specialty hospitals such as tuberculosis and mental hospitals. "Medicine was scarcely developed to the point of having many services to offer, especially in hospital wards, but nursing was . . . . It was from the sale of nursing services that revenue was produced" (Ashley, 1977, p. 6).

Public health nursing came the closest to providing a prototype for primary nursing because of its basis in scientific principles and the higher educational level (Hegyvary, 1977). Although public health nurses followed the case method of assignment, they lacked concepts such as the nursing process.

After World War I, patients were treated in hospitals more often than in private homes, and nurses became a small group (often only student nurses) caring for many patients. This was not primary nursing; rather, there was perhaps one registered (RN) or licensed practical nurse (LPN) working as the only skilled person on a shift. Working conditions were not conducive to safe and therapeutic nursing care nor to the professional development of nurses. Nursing became focused on tasks in order to take care of large numbers of patients. As a result, the patient's "humanism was mechanized; his organic whole was fractured into parts, his basic physiological and technical needs were reduced to a checklist on paper. Thus he became an automated patient" (Marram et al., 1974, p. 15).

Nurses owed allegiance to the institution that trained and hired them rather than to the patients and their families. Beginning with this period, nurses fell into the authoritarian, task-oriented modality of the institution largely because that role was the natural extension of their low status and religious or military educational background. Their practice as nurses within a bureaucracy was merely a reflection of their general position in society as women from a working class background (Hegyvary, 1977).

Many nurses today paint an idealized picture of what nursing must have been like during the early 1900's and mistakenly equate it with primary nursing.

> It is said that in "the good old days" nurses were warm, comforting, and intimately concerned with the welfare of their patients. This is true: my recollection of private duty nurses in the 1930's coincides with this judgement. But, and I think unfortunately, these nurses operated intuitively, and sometimes they were autocratic and overprotective of their patients (Peplau, 1964, p. 29).[1]

---

[1] Peplau, H. Professional closeness. Nursing Forum, 1979, 8(4). This and other quotes in the text citing this source are reprinted with permission of author and publisher.

The problems of nurses working in institutions stemmed from numerous, complex professional difficulties. Many of the issues confronting primary nursing today are leftover from this era. For instance, institution-based care still shelters nurses from setting fees for their own services or facing legal implications of serious malpractice. Because nursing care has always been included in the room rate, nurses are not aware of the real price of health care or what proportion goes to nursing services. Worse, this custom allows the public to take nurses for granted, much as the price of police and fire protection which is included in the property tax bill. Thus, in many ways, the institution has and still can interfere with the nurse-patient relationship.

Functional Nursing

Functional nursing, the most common modality for the delivery of nursing care, came into great use after World War II. The war produced large numbers of underskilled health care workers who were available for minimal pay. As LPNs/ licensed vocational nurses (LVN), nurses' aides, and orderlies became the main source of inexpensive hospital labor, registered nurses were removed from the bedsides of all but the most acute patients. Patient care was divided functionally, so that the task requiring the least skill would be done by the least skilled worker. Thus, no one person integrated a patient's total needs into a whole picture.

The head nurse assigned tasks, not patients, to personnel and inevitably filled in as one of the few registered nurses available for complex needs. The role of nursing was to follow the physicians' orders, which were also written with a task focus.

With the advent of functional nursing, the uniqueness of nursing was nearly lost in the hope that larger numbers of cheaper help would provide more efficient health care. Even today, a nursing staff may feel falsely secure because of the number of ancillary staff rather than because of the quality of work provided.

Some functions, such as housekeeping and secretarial duties, were a relief to lose. New departments sprung up to help the nurses get back to the bedside. However, even in the late 1970s, these departments insist on doing this work during the convenient daytime hours, Monday through Friday and refuse to staff personnel around the clock. The proliferation of new departments in health care institutions has also added a confused legacy to primary nursing.

Unfortunately, while nonclinical departments were starting to provide support services, nurses were giving away parts of their clinical roles. New nonprofessional positions developed during this period to alleviate the stresses on the nurses, but this only diluted the registered nurse's power base and influence. Clinical responsibilities seemed to slip away without much attention or planning from registered nurses. Erosion of the profession continues today, such as medications administered to inpatients by the pharmacy and registered nurses replaced by technicians in intensive care units.

Eventually the problems of functional nursing were felt: "There were not enough nurses to do the job and not enough supervisors and head nurses to provide adequate supervision to poorly-trained personnel. Team nursing seemed an answer to a profession in a care delivery crisis" (Marram et al., 1974, p. 15).

Team Nursing

For team nursing the whole nursing staff of a shift is divided into teams that care for a limited group of patients — the divide and conquer approach. Each team is led by a registered nurse who directs the work assigned to the team by the head nurse. The patients to be covered by each team are also assigned by the head nurse, who takes unit geography and acuity of patients' status into account. Each member of the team is assigned specific patients by the team leader and is expected to assist other team members when the work is finished.

The team modality introduced improvements over functional nursing:

- For at least eight hours at a time, the patient has fewer staff members to get to know, and the team members can focus attention on individual needs.
- The use of a team leader signifies some decentralization of the head nurse's authority.
- The chance for high morale is increased by staff subgroups.
- The patient care conference provides continuing education for the staff and unites each team by group problem solving.
- The written nursing care plan is developed as a communication tool between team members and between shifts.
- Dividing a unit into smaller sections (a forerunner of district/modular nursing) increases manageability.

There were also several expectations for team nursing that never worked out, such as "The head nurse has more time to carry out her own functions" and "non-professional workers receive close help and guidance from a 'professional' person" (Williams, 1964, pp. 66-67). The team leaders on whom the team modality relied had a position of status on one hand and impossible demands on the other. In fact, many a team leader found "the demands of managing groups and staff overwhelming and often are not equipped with the skills necessary to be both good clinical managers and effective administrators" (Pryma, 1978, p. 5).

Essentially, team nursing yielded no change in methods of delivery. Patient conferences rarely took place and because team assignments could be changed often, continuity of care was impractical. Team nursing merely provided the illusion of better organization, but actually there were more chiefs than Indians. Sadly, the one head nurse and two team leaders in a unit were almost automatically removed from most direct care, and aides were left to do more than their jobs required at the bedside. The most unfortunate legacy of functional and team nursing is that patients often call aides "nurses," because they are the caring people with whom the patient has the most contact.

Overall, team nursing has not withstood the test of time. In many ways, it has become the *wordfact* that Williams (1964) warned about — wordfact being John Kenneth Galbraith's term for pretending something exists solely because it has been given a name. Team nursing failed because it arose from a lack of identity within the profession rather than from its strength. Team nursing was perhaps bureaucratically sound, but lacked soundness in nursing theory. Work was defined by the tasks that needed to be completed within eight hours rather than by the process of providing responsive care over an extended period of time. Finally, the team nursing model could not be transferred easily to non-inpatient settings.

As team nursing was being tested in practice, some in the nursing profession began pushing for greater professionalism in nursing. Action was taken toward "increasing the educational requirements for nursing, defining the theoretical basis of nursing practice, and establishing a code of ethics for nurses" (Hegyvary, 1977, p. 191). These trends served to promote the evolution toward primary nursing.

Nursing Education

As nursing education has evolved, it has woven its own web of positive and negative legacies. Three trends in current nursing education have helped build a foundation for primary nursing: (1) incorporation of basic level nursing education into university programs; (2) emphasis on understanding and caring for people holistically in the context of the patient's illness and psychosocial background; and (3) use of the one-to-one case model for combining theoretical material with clinical realities.

The development of colleges of nursing set a standard by which primary nursing can only benefit. Philosophies stating the role of the nurse in relation to patients, their families, and their communities guided nursing educators in curriculum development in the 1960s. After that the nurse was educated to assist patients in utilizing all potential physical and mental strengths while helping to minimize any elements that could disrupt health.

That registered nurses can be thoughtfully intelligent and interpersonally adept at assisting people is reinforced by the presence of collegiate schools of nursing in American society. It indicates that those entering nursing are committing themselves to a career, not just a means to earn a living until marriage and motherhood.

A career in nursing requires learning a distinct and growing body of knowledge, separate but equal to that of other professions. Nurses entering the profession at the college level can more easily proceed through master's and doctoral programs, which establishes nursing expertise in the education, research, and administrative arenas as well as specific clinical areas of practice. With this trend, nursing can become self-reliant and thus retain autonomy while functioning interdependently with other professions. So in many ways, the collegiate schools of nursing have contributed a positive legacy for primary nursing.

The curriculum of basic nursing education has increasingly incorporated the theory and skills of how to meet patients' comprehensive needs, another legacy crucial to primary nursing. The idea that patients, and their families, should be approached as more than a collection of symptoms goes a long way toward setting a climate for primary nursing. When tasks geared to symptom relief are viewed within the larger framework of total patient care, functional nursing suddenly looks like a chaotic, impersonal method of care.

The nurse-patient relationship is the backbone of primary nursing. Introduction of principles of nurse-patient relationships into a curriculum can only aid primary nursing. If a nurse accepts that "the nurse-patient interaction — the verbal and non-verbal exchanges in a nursing situation — can influence recovery" (Peplau, 1964, p. 32) (or comfort or strength to endure), the nurse will gain confidence in dealing with patients and will seek the chance to help heal through a relationship.

The clinical model of nursing education is the paradigm of primary nursing:

> The professional commitment is very similar to that made by a student nurse to her patients and is indeed the model of nursing education. Students assume basic care for one or two patients for a limited period of time, concentrating very much on the patients' individual needs and often caring for the patient more than once. To accomplish her assignment, the student nurse needs close supervision, time to prepare, and time to evaluate the care given. The most effective evaluation can be obtained by returning for a second day with the same patient. As a result of the consistency and the personalized approach, the student and her patient often feel a great deal of satisfaction about their experience together, regardless of the patient's health status. Primary nursing is an extension of the student nurse-patient relationship. The model of professional commitment remains the same even though the nurse has additional responsibilities along with two to five primary patients (Zander, 1977, p. 20).[2]

Another influence from the educational system was the identification of the clinical nursing approach by Frances Reiter in 1966 which proposed putting skilled nurses with the patients: "The primary responsibility of nursing education is to prepare clinical nursing practitioners, that of nursing service is to utilize these practitioners in such a way that professional standards of patient-side practice are maintained" (p. 43). She also made a strong argument for faculties in schools of

---

[2]Zander, K. Primary nursing won't work unless the head nurse lets it. *Journal of Nursing Administration,* October 1977. This and other quotes in the text citing this source are reprinted with permission.

nursing to become actively involved in clinical practice and research, thus contributing directly to patient services.

Whenever the value of placing a registered nurse in a pivotal position with a patient is taught, a contribution is made to the primary nursing legacy. Without adequately educated nurses, primary nursing would be an impossibility. Without the continued influence of nursing education, the skills and attitudes needed by primary nurses would have to be developed from scratch.

The Nursing Process

Definition of the nursing process arose as the most precise tool with which to strengthen the nursing profession and hence primary nursing. Simply stated, the nursing process is assessing, planning, intervening, and evaluating patient or family needs and their responses to nursing care. The nursing process can be universally applied and individually used. In effect, as nursing synthesized the knowledge from other disciplines, it wisely claimed the common-sense but scientific problem-solving process as its own tool — the nursing process. At last, something useful and original that would give identity and structure to nursing practice and intelligent care to patients!

The nursing process joins primary nursing in bridging the gap between education and practice. The nursing process links systematic problem solving with daily patient care, whether the nurse works in an agency or inpatient unit. Although any nurse can and should apply the nursing process to each patient, the nursing process is most effective when used by a primary nurse.

The nursing process begins with either a predetermined, initial assessment or a situational crisis assessment

> which results in the identification of needs, their analysis, and their
> logical arrangement according to priorities. Subsequently, decisions are
> made regarding those needs which fall within the nurse's competence
> and which can be met within the context of the nurse-patient relation-
> ship. This is followed by goal-setting, accomplished, when at all possi-
> ble, jointly between nurse, client, and family (Mauksch and David,
> 1972, p. 2190).[3]

Goals become realities through actions suggested, written, or ordered by a nurse and carried out by the entire nursing staff. The nursing care and its outcomes in terms of goal accomplishment should be continually evaluated by the assigned nurse and staff colleagues. The nursing process and primary nursing are made for

---

[3]Mauksch, I., & David, M. Prescription for survival. *American Journal of Nursing*, December 1972. This and other quotes in the text citing this source are reprinted with permission of the authors and publisher.

each other, because the best use of the nursing process occurs when it is systematically applied to the individual patient's situation by the designated primary nurse.

The nursing process is the strongest legacy upon which primary nursing can be developed, because it gives each primary nurse a meaningful, useful basis of practice. In fact the intervention phase of the nursing process "is the one within which nurses can really make a significant change in the delivery of healthcare. It is at this point — while carrying out the care plan — that nurses can shift their emphasis from performing daily routine chores to a goal-oriented focus on meeting individual needs and helping to resolve individual patient problems" (Ganong and Ganong, 1976, p. 53).

The evaluation of goal achievement can be difficult, but it is the most crucial element in planning nursing because it implies accountability. Assessing and care planning are merely a beginning, a guide to action. It is the continual evaluation of the primary nurse's plans and actions that indicates the degree of personal and professional responsibility. Finally, the measurement of goal achievement holds the primary nurse professionally accountable for practice. Clearly, the nursing process exists separately from primary nursing, however, primary nursing requires full utilization of the nursing process. In fact, Mauksch and David (1972) state that the nursing process is the best and last chance for the nursing profession to respond to the patient as a consumer in the competitive health care fields. They list six tenets to substantiate this:

1. The nursing process is a means of unifying the occupation, now sadly divided. It will bridge the distances between the greatly varying ideologies of nursing in hospitals and in other settings, and it will span the wide range between nurses with different kinds of education. . . .

2. The nursing process demonstrates nursing's function through the use of science, art, humanity, and skills, a combination that is unique and unreplicated.

3. The nursing process restores nursing to its primary commitment, delivering care to people on a one-to-one basis, and thereby eliminates our present tendency to relinquish this overall function to those who are not prepared to fulfill it.

4. The nursing process promotes consumer satisfaction. By making the patient the undisputed focus of the endeavor, a nurse brings forth a one-to-one relationship in which the patient is an active partner and participates in crucial decisionmaking. The current much deplored anonymity and impersonality of health and illness care will finally be replaced by this personalized and individualized approach.

5. The nursing process provides a means of assessing nursing's economic contribution to the totality of patient care. Because evaluation is an integral

component of the nursing process, both the effectiveness and the amount of nursing performance can be determined and economically valued.

6. The nursing process enables a nurse to realize her potential as an independent decision-maker who has command over competencies which heretofore were not used in carrying out predominantly assistance-type functions (p. 2190).

Nursing and the Family

Nurses and the families of patients have been working together for a century, but not until the 1960s was this interaction studied, formalized, and encouraged in a way that contributed to primary nursing. The increase of the nurse's involvement and responsibility to families is finely intermeshed with changes in nursing education and delivery systems.

The decade of the 1960s brought the family progressively into focus. A comparison of the 1960 and 1970 editions of the *Cumulative Index to Nursing Literature* (Granbois, 1964, 1971), illustrates the types and number of changes in topics on issues of family life in relation to nursing practice, for both generalist and specialist, and the interaction of nurses with patients' families in a variety of settings.

Of the 38 entries under "Family" in the 1960 index, 28 are from periodicals other than basic nursing publications. The majority of titles revolve around subjects such as family size and child welfare. Only a few could be considered contributions to theory building. Almost all of the 38 articles are child oriented; 2 exceptions cover family planning clinics and admissions of schizophrenic patients and their families (Kvarnes, 1959).

Although there are only 42 entries under "Family" in the 1970 index, an increase of 4 articles, 34 were from basic nursing periodicals, and many covered subjects in more depth than earlier articles. The 1969 Clinical Conference of the American Nurses' Association alone contributed nine articles about the family with titles such as "Utilization of Behavior of Science Concepts for a Family in Crisis" and "Development of an Interdisciplinary Team to Care for Dying Patients and Their Families."

The scope of articles expanded into all nursing areas: 19 general articles; 6 on maternal-child health; 7 on medical-surgical topics; 2 on public health; and 8 on psychiatry. Only a few articles had the informational quality of the 1960 titles. The articles seem action oriented both in terms of theory and clinical practice. Significantly, several broad categories accompany "Family" in the 1970 edition including "Parents," "Grandparents," "Family Planning," and "Family Nurse Practitioner" (under "Public Health and Nursing"). The parent category alone has 29 entries.

Several of the articles listed in 1970 in the basic nursing periodicals are written by nonnurses, usually social workers. A good example of this is Costello's highly sophisticated article (1969), which discusses interactional patterns in family communication systems.

Work with families has traditionally belonged to social work, while the nurse has worked with the individual patient. Yet as early as 1954, M. Roberts (cited in Lipeles, 1959) in *American Nursing: History and Interpretation* stated: "Through teamwork in giving patient-centered care, the encapsulation of the several professions in their immediate interests is being broken down" (p. 343).

The "separate but equal" relationship of nursing and social work has continued since the teamwork approach was initiated to respond to the totality of the patient's welfare. Both professions have unique functions that were helpfully delineated by Church:

> The nurse has understanding of disease process and treatment of the individual, but also as a member of a family and of a community, she recognizes the emotional and social factors that affect him in his particular situation.
>
> Social work's unique function is helping people individually and in groups, with problems which interfere with social functioning— problems that they cannot cope with unaided (Church, 1956, pp. 201-202).

In their 1968 text Trick and Obcarskas extended nursing's role by offering family theory on the dynamics of anxiety and guilt, stating that the nurse's relationship with a family not only helps in prevention and treatment but also in education and public relations. Black's study of graduate students at the Catholic University of America in 1970 showed that students "perceive the family, whether or not it is a unit in the biological sense, as a system of interacting persons, with anything that affects part of the system likewise affecting the whole" (p. 58).

The changing focus of nursing education in regard to the family has impact on all areas of clinical practice. The 1970 cumulative index (Granbois, 1971) reflects this trend through articles listed on family therapy in hemodialysis and transplantation, child distress and the family, and family-centered care in public health nursing. In practice there are many support mechanisms for families, including increased home visits, well-baby clinics, family participation units, and utilization of family health-teaching concepts.

The 1960s reflected increasing attention to the work that nurses do with families and other professionals. As nurses became increasingly concerned with the total patient and increasingly skilled at intervention to promote wellness, the family became a legitimate concern for all areas of nursing. Working with families can be an integral part of any nursing practice, and the concepts that evolved in the 1960s set the stage for primary nursing in the 1970s.

Nursing and the Institution

As the nursing curriculum became more sophisticated, incorporating nursing process, family dynamics, and other progressive ideas, nurses working in an institutional setting had fewer opportunities to use these theories and skills directly. The nurse is often placed in conflict between the hospital administration's idea of efficiency and the quality of professional nursing care. Because of nursing's long, dependent ties with hospitals, "the nurses' image of themselves had too long been as providers of services to institutions, rather than providers of care to clients within the context of family and community" (Rutledge, 1974, p. 78).

In 1964 Mary Malone clearly identified the dilemma of nurses in a bureaucracy as the expectation that nurses respond to three hierarchies simultaneously: nursing administration, hospital administration, and physicians. "There is a basic conflict between the nurse's concept of a nurse and that held by other important groups within the hospital" (Malone, 1964, p. 51). In contrast, primary nursing implies that the nurse works for and with the patient, yet within the context of the bureaucracy. Primary nursing responds to the plight of the patient and is consistent with a professional conscience that dictates adherence to standards and the priority of individualized attention to patient needs. However, before primary nursing was clinically tested, the opposite situation was nearly universal:

> In view of the circumstances where the nurse does not know the patients as individuals, where she is not permitted to use her range of professional knowledge and skills, where she is not caring for patients but just doing things to them, where she merely carries out procedures on a series of patients, and where she must be the policeman on the unit, she believes she is justified in being dissatisfied and in continuing her search for a setting which will permit her to be a professional nurse. Unfortunately, moving from one hospital to another rarely solves her dilemma since the organization of all these facilities is essentially the same (Malone, 1964, p. 52).

Aware that something was missing from institutional nursing care, some nurses tried to combat fragmentation by care-delivery methods such as "continuity," "total patient care," and "following" of selected patients. Such personal selection methods were superimposed on team and functional organizations and offered a degree of satisfaction to the patients fortunate enough to be chosen and to the well-meaning nurses able to follow through with their continuity of care.

Problems with this custom arise, however, because one-to-one continuity is not administratively supported (although it may be verbally sanctioned) and therefore is given low priority in situations of stress. A selection system is also conducive to overinvolvement with patients and families, and nurses can become exhausted quickly and bitter due to lack of support. Even worse, a nurse may feel isolated by a hidden fear that others will view involvement as the sign of a goodie-goodie, an apple polisher, or candidate for the "super nurse" award. Without meaning to, a nurse who tries to live up to ideals also may induce guilt in fellow staff members by such actions as staying overtime to chart or discuss a patient's therapy program. Further problems may result when an important multidisciplinary conference is scheduled about a selected patient, but the nurse is needed to give medications and cannot attend. Often after this happens a few times, nurses think of leaving because the system's rewards do not compare with the investment. Being the only role model in a system with no support from management and administration is lonely at best and devastating at worst.

In 1974 Marlene Kramer termed the frustrations experienced by newly-graduated nurses as "reality shock":

> Reality Shock is a term used to describe the phenomenon and the specific shocklike reactions of new workers when they find themselves in a work situation for which they have spent several years preparing and for which they thought they were going to be prepared, and then suddenly find that they are not. [There are] shocklike reactions that follow when the aspirant professional perceives that many professional ideals and values are not operational and go unrewarded in the work setting (p. vii-viii).

Reality shock has provided some of the impetus for primary nursing and, thus, forms part of its legacy. Primary nursing is the middle ground between necessary bureaucratic demands and patient well-being. There is a way to practice professional ideals in a complex organization, and that way is through primary nursing. However, one nurse alone cannot carry out primary nursing, and similarly, a single pilot unit will find it extremely difficult to carry out primary nursing over an extended period of time without the total support of the nursing administration both philosophically and operationally.

Burnover is another legacy that can either add support to the rationale for primary nursing or can work against it. Burnover is a term derived from the professional hazard of burnout (Shubin, 1978) and the institutional problem of turnover. When nurses cannot balance their ideals with reality, they burnout and join the astounding number of nurses who leave positions every year. If a nursing department has a firm commitment to primary nursing, including specific, built-in resources, primary nursing can potentially decrease burnover.

One very positive legacy has been the advent of the psychiatric nurse consultant. Ideally, this role is filled by a nurse prepared at the master's level who is adept at using the consultative process and is interested in helping staff nurses to gain knowledge and skill in their nurse-patient relationships. The psychiatric nurse consultant can help prevent severe reality shock and intractable burnover by being available to individuals or staff groups for consultation about problem patients. Coming from outside a given unit or agency, the psychiatric nurse consultant is an adjunct to the nurse-manager and is able to lend objectivity to stressful and confusing patient care situations which facilitates learning, problem solving, and confidence. Although any department of nursing benefits from such a role, a psychiatric nurse consultant is essential for the development of primary nursing.

Nursing and Society

Because it takes place within a highly social, people-to-people context, nursing and society are intimately related. Of the trends in American society in the 1970s, three have formed direct legacies for primary nursing: the women's movement, expanded roles for nurses in health care systems, and consumer pressure for quality assurance.

Because most nurses are women, the historical role of women in general can be applied to nursing and should be understood in the context of primary nursing. It is not surprising that the need for women to have pride in themselves as women and to assert themselves to be effective, is being raised simultaneously with the primary nursing movement. In essence, primary nursing combines the exciting prospect of women working at their highest personal and professional level together with the optimal aspects of health care delivery. Thus, primary nursing benefits both nurse and patient.

To become an effective primary nurse, each nurse must consciously strive to resolve ingrained conflicts about power. These conflicts are most vividly typified by male-doctor — female-nurse struggles. Although these conflicts are everywhere, "Most nurses think they are powerless. Many nurses see themselves as objects of the power of others, and have internalized the attitudes of subordination projected by those in positions of authority and by other health professionals" (Bowman & Culpepper, 1974, p. 1054).

There are historical reasons why nurses have developed a negative self-image; why they have "often let themselves be manipulated and eliminated from significant decision-making roles regarding health care" (Bowman & Culpepper, 1974, p. 1054). The women's movement encouraged nurses to step back and understand their own history so that changes could be made for the future: ". . . the strength of the women's liberation movement provides a backdrop for the development of group consciousness among nurses. In contrast to their predecessors, those nurses are developing and projecting a positive self-image" (Bowman & Culpepper, 1974, p. 1055).

The women's movement gives positive reinforcement to assertiveness and also to the role of women in management. Training programs for both assertiveness and management skills are becoming increasingly available to nurses. These are valuable resources to a nurse-manager of primary nursing as well as to individual primary nurses. Assertiveness is an essential skill for primary nurses and for the managers who guide them.

The second positive influence on primary nursing was the advent of expanded nursing roles in response to society's need for more health services. Expanded roles, such as the nurse midwife, nurse anesthetist, nurse practitioner, and the psychiatric-mental health nurse clinician and consultant, set several key examples for the primary nursing role.

One model of the expanded role asserts that nurses can and should have specific caseloads of patients to whom they are identifiable and accountable. By saying, "I am your nurse," the nurse is no longer hidden in the team:

> The team enforces group decision making; the nurse need not assume individual responsibility and, in fact, is prevented from doing so. Shared responsibility is dilute responsibility because it is not identifiable with an individual. Responsibility under this system is temporal, is dependent on the nurse's presence on the unit, and is not based on a protracted individualized relationship. It is responsibility of this type to which most nurses have become accustomed (Manthey et al., 1970, p. 77).

These expanded roles imply that nurses are not tied to specific institutions nor to a physician's minute-to-minute supervision. They set an example for nurses as independent decision makers who collaborate with members of other health disciplines at various stages of the nursing process. That nurses are considered skilled colleagues by other professions is an important trend for primary nursing.

Closely entwined with expanded roles is the concept of primary care, which is often confused with primary nursing because both involve nurses who have direct access to patients, work at the highest level of skill, and take responsibility for their actions. However, primary care refers to care given by nurses in expanded roles or other health professionals when the patient needs immediate assessment and treatment at the borders of the health care system. Primary care is longitudinal, that is, responsive to the multiple situations that arise in a person's health life. The nurse giving primary care is a primary care nurse. However, primary nursing is episodic, that is, given and directed by a qualified registered nurse during one episode in a person's health life. Although the terms are confusing, an important aspect here is that nurses working in primary care settings provide a realistic model of autonomous, collaborative practice for primary nurses working in other settings.

The third societal trend that directly influences primary nursing is the increased attention to quality of care and cost-effectiveness. "The Patient has now become the Consumer and must be satisfied; he is the main reason that costs, quality, and accountability are woven together. The patient's frustrations have created the demands that are forced on health care agencies, and hence on us (nursing)" (Nodal, 1978, p. 58).

Regulatory agencies such as the Professional Standards Review Organization (PSRO) and the Joint Commission on Accreditation of Hospitals are making it necessary for nursing to identify standards, outcomes of care, and accountability for practice. These and other pressures to prove quality and cost-effectiveness are now felt at the administrative levels of nursing services, and it should not be long before accountability is traced to individual primary nurses. Primary nursing puts nurses on the line; their actions can be studied, audited, and evaluated according to the priorities of the times.

A related and very important contribution to the primary nursing legacy is certification for competence and/or excellence by the American Nurses' Association. The certification program was designed in 1973 primarily to identify members of the profession "who practice on a level higher and more sophisticated than that determined by state licensure examinations. The development of these programs has been greatly influenced by the emergence of a more enlightened consumer who demands quality in modern health care" (Mauksch, 1978, p. 4).

To be certified in a specialty, a nurse must meet certain criteria, including written descriptions of interventions with identified patients. The nurse must prove that a certain number of hours are spent in direct care (to an individual, family, and/or community). The nurse applying for certification must also prove that personal responsibility for the outcomes of nursing actions was taken for the person(s) receiving services.

In general practice, only a primary nurse qualifies for these criteria because only a primary nurse has direct care responsibilities to specific patients or families over a period of time. Only a primary nurse can claim responsibility for the outcomes of care which that nurse has directed. To expect nonprimary nurses to meet the criteria would be unfair to them and also would be contrary to the purposes of certification.

Each of the three major social movements can either threaten the legitimacy of the nursing profession or bolster the status of individual primary nurses. A positive eventual outcome lies in the ability of nurse-managers and their support systems to enhance the role of the primary nurse.

THE ROLE OF A PRIMARY NURSE

"Primary nursing is a philosophy, not a staffing pattern or different patient assignment regime" (Bolder, 1977, p. 79). For primary nursing to become a coherent philosophy, the threads of many ideas had to be pulled together in real life institutions. The nurse-manager should know why, when, and how the legacies of nursing finally emerged as primary nursing.

Rationale for Primary Nursing

1. Nurses are in business to provide some degree of satisfaction of patients' needs for safety, comfort, and growth.
2. Meeting these needs is most easily accomplished if there is a specific task associated with the need, i.e., safety through isolation precautions, comfort through pain relief or listening to a person's fear of surgery, and growth through birth control and other forms of counseling.
3. Both preexisting and new needs which are secondary to a change in condition are most easily assessed if the same nurse has daily or frequent contact with the patient/family. Continuity of care is optimal.
4. Because the same nurse has frequent contact with the same patient/family, the nurse begins to know the patient/family as an individual for whom the completion of nursing tasks is only one aspect of life.
5. The nurse also begins to see directly the consequences of care given personally or by others to that patient over the course of hours, days, or weeks.
6. As the same nurse begins to see the patient holistically, in totality, the nurse makes judgments about what to do in light of present health status and future needs. This mental activity requires problem solving, which is the root of the nursing process.
7. When problem solving, the nurse talks with others in the work setting who can offer objectivity, suggestions, validation, and other support.
8. The nurse may become aware that some of the problems which the patient/family is experiencing are due to elements in the health care system. At this point, the nurse becomes the patient/family advocate.
9. With each new patient/family, the nurse applies the nursing process, which is reflected in increasingly sophisticated verbal and written presentations.

The logical chain of events in a nurse's role forms the essence of primary nursing. The model for primary nursing was established at the Loeb Center for Nursing and Rehabilitation at Montefiore Hospital in the Bronx section of New York in the early 1960s. The model was based on the ideas of Lydia Hall, who believed that nurses could have a greater role in nurturing and healing. "Because the nurse is giving the care, she is in the position of most closely helping the patient work with the cure, as well as using aspects of the cure to help her modify the care, and she can help the self [patient] use the caring and the curing to grow and become, which is the core" (Bower-Ferres, 1975, p. 811).

Patients come to hospitals almost exclusively for nursing care, otherwise they would be treated in another setting (many of which are also staffed predominantly with nurses). The Loeb model, which was implemented in 1963, concretely acknowledged the importance of registered nurses: "Loeb is run by nurses; its service is primarily nurses, and only nurses can determine nursing" (Bower-Ferres, 1975, p. 810).

The Loeb Center reversed the trends that had taken nurses out of direct contact with patients because of the belief that "It is in relinquishing direct care to others that nursing has been most self-destructive" (p. 811). If nurses assign feeding, bathing, toileting, dressing, and ambulating to other care takers, they miss the chance to intimately know and work with patients. Thus, they have no basis on which to use the nursing process. As a result, the nurse's communication with the patient becomes intellectualized "with the patient trying to tell the nurse what she wants to know and the nurse telling the patient what she wants him to hear" (Bower-Ferres, 1975, p. 812).

Each registered nurse at the Loeb Center had a caseload of eight patients, divided into districts, for whom the nurse directed all care and gave a great deal of it personally. This was possible because the same number of registered nurses staffed days and evenings and because two-nurse groups shared a messenger-attendant to do nonpatient activities (set up equipment, make beds, test urine).

In 1969 the term *primary nursing* was given to a new pattern of nursing care that was used in one medical unit at the University of Minnesota Hospitals. The word *primary* reflected the principle that a nurse's relationship with specific patients would transcend shifts and remain primary in priorities and interactions.

> Under the new system, each RN and each LPN has primary responsibility for the total nursing care of an assigned group of from three to six patients. She performs all the daily care tasks for her patients, taking their vital signs, giving them morning care, administering their medications, performing their treatments, preparing them for tests, and so on. The nurse's aides are used primarily for non-nursing activities such as housekeeping, dietary, and transportation functions. When they have time available for patient care, they are assigned to assist an RN or LPN (Manthey et al., 1970, p. 70).

This new primary nursing proved to be successful and has spurred almost a decade of experimentation. Researchers have studied various aspects of primary nursing, including patient satisfaction, nurse satisfaction, quality of care, and cost-effectiveness.

Difficulties in implementation and research have arisen due to the lack of consistent definition and practice. Overall, however, clinicians, managers, and administrators who have worked with primary nursing over a period of years have found it to be a viable concept which, when applied in the real world, results in quality patient care given by satisfied registered nurses.

Job Description for the Primary Nurse

When a nurse says, "Hello, I'm your primary nurse," both the nurse and the nurse-manager must understand exactly what that statement means. It is essential that there is consensus between the nurse-manager and each primary nurse about what the role of the primary nurse is. The definition of the primary nurse must be clear to all levels of the nursing hierarchy and must be as closed to individual interpretation as possible. There can and should be a great deal of flexibility in how a nurse works with each primary patient, but the broad structure within which the work is performed must be crystal clear. A job description may be used by the nurse-manager and others to provide the structure or guidelines for the primary nurse's practice.

Responsibilities

Each primary nurse is responsible for

1. Discussing assignments of primary patients with the nurse-manager.
2. Introducing of self as the primary nurse to the patient and the patient's family.
3. Explaining the role of the primary nurse in terms of what the patient can expect from the nurse in regard to direct and indirect services.
4. Assessing the patient/family's nursing care and education needs initially using all data, including an interview, at the nurse's disposal.
5. Developing short- and long-term goals (outcomes) for problems needing nursing care and including the patient and family in the planning process whenever possible.
6. Designing a plan of care through nursing orders, including nursing treatments, approaches, and protocols which will help the patient to reach the designated outcomes.
7. Revising the plan of care according to continual assessments, which are performed when the primary nurse is giving direct care to the patient/family.
8. Conveying verbal and written information and plans about nursing care to the nurse-manager and other members of the nursing staff.
9. Evaluating the patient's response to planned care through discussions with the patient/family, peers, and other members of the health care team.
10. Planning a discharge or transfer that provides continuing attention to needs with the patient/family.
11. Providing appropriate documentation for each phase of the nursing process.
12. Delegating another registered nurse (sometimes referred to as the associate primary nurse) to follow through on high priority care when the primary nurse is absent.

13. Supervising aides, technicians, and LPN's when they have contact with the nurse's primary patients.
14. Presenting reports, documentation, and seminars of work with specific primary patients for peer review (audit, primary nurse conferences, forums).
15. Attending, arranging, or conducting multidisciplinary conferences concerning the primary patient when necessary.
16. Seeking out educational resources that will enhance the understanding of a patient/family's needs and the expertise to meet those needs (consultation, seminars, journals, inservice).
17. Responding to audit reports which reflect accountability for outcomes of the nurse's practice with identified primary patients.
18. Completing a self-evaluation of activities on behalf of primary patients/ families at predetermined intervals.

Who Can Be a Primary Nurse?

A primary nurse must be a registered professional nurse who has the education and legal sanction to consistently and confidently carry out each of the complex responsibilities listed. Even with the professional socialization that schools of nursing offer, not every registered nurse is willing or able to be a primary nurse. However, in time an effective nurse-manager can enable most RNs to function at least minimally in the role of primary nurse.

The nursing profession and agencies employing nurses must begin to determine who is qualified to provide knowledgeable, comprehensive care. The bottom line is, of course, the registered nurse, who cannot be replaced by other levels of nursing staff. Such an interchange is unfair to the public and a devaluation of the professional registered nurse.

The public deserves to have contact with the best-prepared nursing personnel available. To achieve the visibility and accessibility that primary nursing requires, staffing ratios and patterns must be adjusted so that there is a high proportion of RNs.

> Primary nursing does not necessarily call for more people than team or functional nursing, but it does require a higher percentage of RN staff. Many hospitals make extensive use of LPN's and nursing aides working under the direction of an RN to provide nursing care. Primary nursing means that nurses plan *and give* the care. A criterion of a professional is that he/she *provides* a service, not that he/she directs a service. Until nurses are doing the nursing; it is questionable whether a professional service is offered (Mundinger, 1977, pp. 70-1).

A nursing service that has relied heavily on LPNs and aides will experience an identity crisis and conflict when the decision is made to implement primary nursing. The tension may be heightened if the nonprofessional staff members feel that their jobs are threatened by changing priorities. Primary nursing brings into question many policies that have been left carefully untouched for years.

The group that is most threatened by primary nursing, other than RNs who feel unprepared for the new role, are the LPNs who for years have been used as nurse-extenders and interchanged with RNs when convenient or economical for the institution. The nurse-manager is often forced to allow especially talented LPNs to do tasks that are legally and educationally beyond their scope of practice, due to poor staffing ratios.

Unfortunately, the nursing profession has allowed the inappropriate use of LPNs, because RNs have begun to feel that some care-taking activities are too menial for a professionally prepared nurse. When menial activities are constantly delegated, the line between menial and valued activities becomes blurred, and eventually there is no distinction of roles. Primary nursing creates definite boundaries between professional and nonprofessional nursing practice. "Primary nursing lifts the lid from RN practice and clamps it down on LPN practice; what is liberating for the RN is confining to the LPN. . . . When diagnosis and treatment of unhealthful responses is added to the role, as it is in primary nursing, the LPN cannot do the same job as an RN" (Mundinger, 1977, p. 76).

Similarly, any RN cannot and should not be a primary nurse. The nurse-manager will need to review the primary nurse's responsibilities, which were presented earlier, to determine what is essential for a particular unit or agency. Interviewing and hiring will be discussed in Chapter 3. However, the nurse-manager should know that no RN enters a new setting completely prepared to be a primary nurse. No matter how competent and confident, how mature and assertive, how ethical and motivated an RN is, the nurse-manager still has the major role of enabling that nurse to use knowledge and experience creatively in a new area of practice.

Associate Primary Nurse

The associate primary nurse role is the least carefully defined in primary nursing. The associate role attempts to formalize the relationship of a primary nurse to a member of the nursing staff who is designated to follow through on the care plan during the primary nurse's absence or periods of unavailability. The term *associate primary nurse* is often used but seldom fully implemented for realistic reasons.

Because the primary nurse has round-the-clock (or time-unlimited, in ambulatory services) responsibility for the outcomes of each patient's nursing care, the primary nurse must feel certain that the care which has been authorized will be either accomplished or changed with newly assessed needs. In this light, the associate primary nurse should be someone prepared to pick up any of the primary nurse's responsibilities. Consequently, the associate primary nurse must be an RN.

If permanently assigned, professional coverage of primary patients by specific associates is impossible around-the-clock or unwieldy in terms of scheduling, the term associate primary nurse should be dropped by that unit or agency. Designation of associate primary nurses in this circumstance confuses the nursing staff, sets up false expectations, and adds built-in frustration because it is technically unworkable.

However, rather than abolishing this role, units and agencies have allowed LPNs and aides to be associates. This practice has added to the confusion about how to manage primary nursing, largely because of the premise that someone who can be an associate primary nurse can also be a primary nurse.

In reality a primary nurse cannot be available whenever needed by a primary patient. However, there must be a means of insuring that an RN directly assesses each patient's needs on each shift or each day a patient comes to a clinic. Provision of patient monitoring by an RN each shift or each day is the responsibility of the nurse-manager who may achieve this through policies, protocols, and staffing patterns.

When a primary nurse expects to be absent from work, there must be a system that guarantees that the primary nurse's patients will be appropriately cared for. The associate system does not necessarily guarantee this because the associate may also be off, and if there are three shifts each day, there is always at least one shift without an associate. This has implications for peer support systems and the structure set up by the nurse-manager.

When planning for vacations or rotation to the night shift, the primary nurse should talk with the nurse-manager about which staff RNs could cover for that nurse's patients. The covering nurse may be the same nurse for each primary patient or a different one, depending on each patient's predicted needs. ·The nurse covering for a primary nurse over an extended period is in the valid role of associate primary nurse.

In most instances the term *associate primary nurse* should be dropped because it is impossible to implement. The formal designation of an associate may need to be made in three situations:

1. when the needs of a patient are so complex or demanding that it is felt that two RNs are necessary to handle the case
2. when the primary nurse is going on vacation for more than two or three days
3. when the primary nurse is going on an extended night rotation

In each of these situations, the associate, or colleague, should be a registered nurse.

The point of distinguishing roles is to make primary nursing realistic and workable. Primary nursing must be easy to apply if it is to succeed. Therefore, terms and roles should have consistent definitions based on clear concepts. Once the nurse-manager is familiar with the legacy and roles of primary nursing, the next step is familiarity with the patient advocate philosophy.

THE PATIENT ADVOCATE PHILOSOPHY

Advocate, ombudsman, lawyer — all are roles that entail one person representing the interests of another. In the health care setting, the patient is the person needing an advocate and the primary nurse is in the best position to offer that service. Patient advocacy is a natural extension of nursing's role and should be a major part of every primary nurse's daily practice.

Anytime a nurse intervenes in the patient's behalf, the nurse is being an advocate. Advocacy occurs when the nurse promotes the patient's safety (enforces seizure precautions), physical comfort (arranges rest periods between painful procedures), psychological comfort (encourages the family to bring in a favorite toy), or autonomy (teaches self-catheterization to a rehabilitation patient). Nurses do all of these things without necessarily being a patient's primary nurse.

Advocacy differs in primary nursing, because the primary nurse is better prepared and more obligated to be active as the patient's advocate due to accountability for the outcomes of health care. Errors of omission are less likely to occur if a specific nurse handles a case. A primary nurse is more likely than a shift nurse to catch things from a forgotten birthday to a subtle but significant change in condition. The primary nurse becomes involved, which makes it more difficult to pass the buck to other nurses or physicians or to blame the system. Consequently, a primary nurse has both a formal and an emotional investment in seeing that the patient gets the best care on every shift or visit.

Historical Role of the Patient

The Patient Patient

Who traditionally make the worst patients? Doctors and nurses.

Why? Probably because doctors and nurses are vividly aware of the helpless position in which patients are placed, even when they have the most skilled and well-meaning personnel assigned to their cases. If doctors and nurses were put on the other side of the bedrail, they would see firsthand what they usually overlook: fragmentation of care and information to the patient; exclusion of the patient in decision making about the body; the defensiveness of health care personnel when the patient disagrees about the cause of illness and treatment; and, most of all, the expectation of health care personnel that the patient will be patient.

The traditional role of the patient is one of passivity and submission to the authority of health care providers. Sick quickly turns into defective; something is wrong with the person that needs setting right through variations of physical or psychological exorcism.

When a person feels weak, vulnerable, and fearful, it can be comforting initially to turn oneself over to stronger, caring, more confident individuals. Some people make this a way of life (Lipsitt, 1970). However, most people do this only when they need help from members of the helping professions.

Nurses are as guilty as other professionals for the high expectations they have about patients. Good patients are those who comply, have insight, allow nurses to help them help themselves; they are a nurse's dream. Grateful patients are those who thank nurses because they know that the painful treatments will help, whose families bring candy, who come back to visit; they can turn a frustrating day into a rewarding one. There is nothing wrong with liking the good and grateful patient. However, there is something wrong with rejecting or neglecting the patients who are not or cannot be obviously appreciative.

Patients are the low men on the institutional totem pole, who are often considered to be just one rung below the nursing staff. Unfortunately, patients are sometimes the only people that nurses can control. Logically it would seem that if nurses are at the mercy of a doctor's directives, then the patients must unquestionably follow the nurse's directives. This is the health care institution's pecking order. An analogy with the family puts the patient in the child's position, the nurse as mother, and the doctor as father.

Until nurses realize that they are equal partners with physicians, they will not be able to allow patients to be equal partners in their own health care and will tend to unite with physicians for fear of disapproval or with patients as stalemated and victimized. Neither of these positions are objective or workable.

There are circumstances, such as, protecting a patient in a life-threatening situation, in which nurses have to take extreme positions as patient advocates. However, a middle ground aimed to avoid standoffs is usually the best place from which to negotiate.

The advocate role is easier when the nurse is familiar and comfortable with patient's rights, the channels for advocacy issues, and the knowledge that nobody is all knowing, all caring, or all powerful. A beginning model for advocacy is presented in Figure 1-1.

The Consumer Patient

Nurses are beginning to gain awareness of the rewards of treating patients as clients whose lives revolve around more than just their need for health care. Patients are being viewed as consumers with rights as well as needs (American Hospital Association, 1975). Similarly, patients have responsibilities when receiving health care. Statements of patients' rights and responsibilities have serious

Figure 1-1 The Patient Advocacy Model

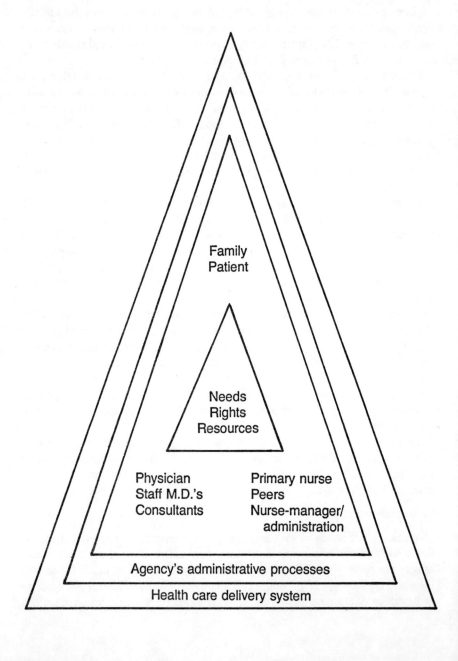

implications for nursing, and the primary nurse is in the best position to deal with these issues.

Patients have the right to know not only what is being done to them, but also what is being planned or prescribed for them. Patient teaching is rightfully being considered as within the scope of nursing (Zander et al., 1978). Poorly informed consumers are potential health hazards to themselves and others in their environment. Patient education in the areas of prevention and health maintenance further expand the nurse's opportunities to be a patient's advocate.

Advocacy Process

The advocacy process is an extension of the third step of the nursing process, intervention. The difference between intervention as a result of the care plan and as the result of advocacy is that advocacy implies activities done for the patient or family, but not directly with the patient or family. Whenever problem solving leads to discussion of the patient or family's needs with others, the primary nurse begins the advocacy process which is diagramed in Figure 1-2.

The middle phase of the process includes the one-time or multiple times that the primary nurse meets with others to present, explain, negotiate, bargain, plan, and even plead on behalf of the patient/family. This is the most difficult phase for nurses, because it requires a confidence in one's own assessment, logic, and collaborating skills. It means that the primary nurse is on the line, individually concerned about some aspect of patient care, and willing to follow the concerns through to some resolution.

Resolution is the final phase of the advocacy process. It does not always involve the solution that the primary nurse initially hoped for, but it usually means that all sides of a situation are understood well enough that the proposed solution is tolerable to most of the participants. If the resolution is unacceptable, the primary nurse may repeat the process in a new way. When the advocacy process is

---

Figure 1-2 The Advocacy Loop

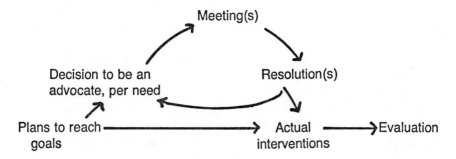

successful, the resolution leads to new and different interventions by nurses and others in regard to a patient/family.

Here are two examples of the advocacy process in action.

The primary nurse assesses that a young male is denying his precarious cardiac status, because he is refusing to have a cardiac catheterization. The primary nurse knows that the procedure is scheduled in six weeks and spends time matter-of-factly discussing the patient's perception of his condition. The patient tentatively agrees to the test as a result of the primary nurse's explanation. Two days before the catheterization the patient is arbitrarily bumped off the schedule for another month. The primary nurse believes that postponement will threaten the patient's tenuous agreement to the procedure and speaks with the patient's physician (who is unaware of the delay) and the lab to reinstate the patient on the schedule. After the primary nurse explains the problem, the patient is put back on the schedule and goes through with the catheterization. The primary nurse was the patient's advocate by accurately assessing his denial of condition and ambivalence about the procedure; establishing an accepting, trusting relationship in which the patient felt that his concerns and decisions were accepted; giving the patient information about the test; and insuring that the test would take place without further anxiety. The primary nurse decided to be an advocate, met with the key people, and worked for a resolution.

The primary nurse assesses that Mrs. C , a 66-year-old woman, her husband, and children are very downhearted about her diagnosis of organic brain syndrome. Mrs. C is able to do daily activities with reminding and is able to converse about her past, though not recent, life. She knows she has lost some of her capabilities, but her family is angry with her at times, as if she is pretending to be confused. The primary nurse talks with the family about their frustrations, sadness, and plans for their mother, emphasizing how they can help make full use of her remaining areas of functioning. A neurology physician consultant has recommended that Mrs. C have a pneumoencephalogram to rule out the one percent chance that her condition is operable. The primary nurse informs the family of this recommendation and encourages them to question the physician about such a risky procedure, which probably would not have been ordered outside of a medical center. Mrs. C continues to say she wants to go home. The primary nurse attends the meeting with the neurologist, Mrs. C , and her daughter. When the daughter expresses Mrs. C's wishes, the neurologist says, "Her death will be on your shoulders." The primary nurse helps the daughter reconsider her mother's and her own position, eventually deciding to again refuse the pneumoencephalogram. Mrs. C goes home with her daughter.

In this case, the primary nurse became the patient advocate by reinforcing family involvement for a patient who was questionably incompetent, encouraging well informed consent, and supporting the daughter's right to decide against the procedure by separating objective risks from the intimidation of the neurologist.

The primary nurse made a plan to help the family based on initial and continuing assessments of Mrs. C's status. When the primary nurse realized that active participation would be necessary to help this family reach its own resolution, the primary nurse made it a priority to be objectively involved. The resolution was one that the family could live with, regardless of the nurse's or physician's personal opinions.

Levels of Advocacy

The primary nurse will find that there are several kinds of intervention that fall under the category of advocacy: interventions with other nursing staff, other units/agencies, nonnursing staff, and the nursing/hospital administration. Traditionally, the nurse has defended patients against pain, anxiety, and disease. Advocacy implies that the primary nurse may need to defend the patient from the health care system itself.

Advocacy with other members of the nursing staff may include: explaining the context in which the primary patient views hospitalization so that the nursing staff can empathize and approach the patient more positively; reminding the nursing staff that they are not allowing a primary patient to do enough personal hygiene even though the primary nurse and patient have reached an agreement about self-help; or leaving a message with the nurse covering the clinic for the day that a certain patient is due for an appointment and should be contacted if the patient does not show up.

Advocacy with other units or agencies may include: giving a call to the inpatient unit to alert the staff (hopefully the future primary nurse) about a child's current hematologic status and the parent's responses to a repeat admission; inviting the primary nurse of another agency to a case conference about a patient they have in common; or visiting a future primary patient in the surgical intensive care unit and discussing care with the current primary nurse.

Advocacy with nonnursing staff may include: arranging for a rabbi to visit a primary patient in a Catholic hospital; disagreeing with a certain treatment approach for an interdisciplinary psychiatric patient because there is good reason to believe that the patient will regress; or contacting the continuing care office to speed up discharge plans, presenting the particular situation clearly, and learning about an agency newly available in the patient's community.

Advocacy with the nursing/hospital administration may include: volunteering to be on the pharmacy committee after noticing adverse medication reactions; requesting that a psychiatric nurse consultant be available in the oncology unit on a regular basis to help the nursing staff deal with the patients' feelings about death and dying; working with the nurse-manager and admitting office to have a patient in critical condition placed in a room close to the nursing station; or sending a letter to the hospital director explaining the implications of unclear policies on terminal care for several primary patients and their families.

Techniques of Advocacy

"Assertive nurses can change the whole health-care system (Donnelly, 1978, p. 68). How? By not trying to change the whole system, but by working on the parts that directly affect each individual primary patient.

Although advocacy is a developing function that lacks substantial documentation or conscious practice, it is a role that involves skills which nurses have aways used with patients and now must apply to the people and policies that make up systems.

Anticipation. The primary nurse is usually the person in the best position to predict the kinds of conflicts that may arise due to a patient's personality, socio-economic background, or health status. Being able to anticipate difficulties is the first step to minimizing them. Anticipation also allows the primary nurse more time to plan strategies to avoid unnecessary problems.

Gaining Objectivity. The primary nurse must gather enough facts to see a situation as clearly as possible. Gathering facts includes reading a patient's past medical record, talking to significant health care personnel, and sorting out strong emotions that have little to do with the real dilemma at hand. Although motivated by ideas about what is right, the primary nurse must integrate ideals with an understanding of the facts. Objectivity can often be gained through discussing the situation with a third party, such as a spouse or friend who is not afraid to disagree.

Timing. Timing is a crucial part of advocacy because something said too early or too late may make a situation worse. A sense of dramatic but prime moments is useful. A sense of when to make a point, loudly or calmly, is a good quality to have. Subtlety should be saved for matters that are less crisis oriented.

Preparedness. Being prepared for a conference or meeting is the best way to facilitate resolutions to difficult situations. When a primary nurse has drawn up a list or written a proposal, it adds weight to the point. Documented facts, written telephone numbers, and names of resources establish the primary nurse as a serious professional who is prepared to do business with other professionals.

Active Participation. Follow-through on ideas and alternatives requires active participation, even when the primary nurse gets weary or frightened by the advocacy process. Being active entails asking key questions that clarify or high-light issues. It also means listening carefully to answers and to the assumptions that others have about rights, health, patients, and the current situation.

Cognitive Dissonance. Cognitive dissonance is the discomfort that arises when two or more perceptions about the same situation do not correlate, but instead, conflict (Labovitz, 1975). Cognitive dissonance is so common in health care and nursing that it is not usually recognized by the participants. Conscious identification of cognitive dissonance can help the primary nurse to facilitate a resolution. For instance, the primary nurse may notice possible side effects of a medication and may call the physician's attention to the concern. The physician may have great faith in the medication and the diagnosis and not want to hear about problems in what seemed to be an easy case. Both primary nurse and physician are experiencing cognitive dissonance at this point because what was hoped to be helpful may even be harmful. The internal dissonance will be compounded if they try to get rid of it by disregarding each other or entering into a standoff. Advocacy entails working with the conflict until it is worked out and cognitive dissonance is relieved.

In regard to cognitive dissonance, advocacy and collaboration have much in common. The primary nurse is often the first person to experience the initial discomfort of cognitive dissonance. Advocacy forces the primary nurse to pursue a resolution, which necessitates collaboration with other professionals. The primary nurse often has to make others feel the same level of discomfort in order to motivate them to a resolution.

Evaluation of Resolution. The primary nurse needs to know when a problem that has required advocacy is resolved and when it requires further action. Even when a satisfactory resolution is reached, evaluation of the results of new approaches or policies is necessary. The advocacy process does not end until the patient is discharged.

Involving Patient and Family. The primary nurse will have to decide to what degree the patient and family should be informed during each step of complex advocacy problems. They should be told enough to help them feel that their concerns are being attended to, and they should definitely be informed of the final resolution. How much more is said should be discussed between the primary nurse and the other professionals involved. If information is requested or given in a concerned, professional way, the patient and family usually appreciate an honest communication without mixed messages.

Issues in Advocacy

There is some philosophical debate about whether a person who is working for a system can be an advocate for someone in the same system (Annas, 1975). Is it better for patients to have primary nurses as their advocates or should they have a representative from outside the health care agency? Without question, the primary nurse is the only person who is qualified and available to be the patient's advocate. Patient advocacy is a full-time job, needed as much (if not more) in a patient's everyday contact with health care agencies as in the acute crisis of impending death. Often patients are unaware that they need an advocate, and by the time they or their families do know, the situation may be irreversible or unworkable. Undoubtedly, the public does not realize how often professional nurses have been their advocate.

> Do people know how often RNs intervene in their behalf with everything from recognizing subtle changes in condition to maintaining a safe environment? If the public does not acknowledge (these) basic nursing functions, how can they understand primary nursing with its added responsibilities for patient advocacy, assessing movement toward outcome criteria, collaboration with other health care disciplines, and growth of professional knowledge (Zander, 1978, p. 52).

With patient advocacy by primary nurses, the professional nurse is more visible and identifiable than ever before. Unfortunately, it is just this visibility that nurses back away from:

> Nurses keep saying and writing that we are accountable to the patient and we tell the physicians that we are not accountable to them but to the patient. And we tell hospital administrators that we are not accountable to them but to the patient. But has anybody told the patient this? When was the last time a patient asked a nurse to be accountable? (Shorr, 1977, p. 1787)

Patients need to know that primary nurses are their advocates and that nurses can have the objectivity to represent their needs to others in the helping professions. Primary nurses need to explain this role clearly to each patient so that they can feel free to ask their primary nurse to initiate advocacy when needed. Likewise, the primary nurse needs to assess how and when to inform a patient about activities that have been undertaken.

Informing patients and families about what they can expect from primary nurses begins with the introduction, "Hello, I'm your primary nurse." To feel comfortable with the introduction, each staff primary nurse must feel confident of support from the nurse-manager and nursing administration. When the going gets rough and advocacy gets difficult, the primary nurse must not feel alone or abandoned. Both the primary nurse and the nurse-manager must be able to check out assumptions, policies, and advocate strategies. The nurse-manager must believe in the value of advocacy and be able to assist primary nurses. Competent advocacy results from solid application of the nursing process, well thought out plans of action, and the guidance of the nurse-manager within the framework of the nursing administration. Each part of the system must recognize that patient advocacy is the distinct function of the primary nurse.

STRUCTURING PRIMARY NURSING

Even with a highly motivated, intelligent, and professional nursing staff, the nurse-manager must be active in structuring primary nursing. Structuring, when applied to primary nursing, is the nurse-manager's major role. It is the active direction of the staff's energies to the areas needed, within a well-defined boundary of clinical practice.

In short, structuring means "putting your money where your mouth is," by constantly reinforcing values about good patient care and by enabling the staff to put these values into action. If all patients need a written nursing assessment, the nurse-manager must structure the workday to allow assessments to be done as a rule and not an exception.

The true test of good structuring is whether these activities and attitudes prevail even in the nurse-manager's absence. Therefore, structuring entails more than organizing and delegating; the nurse-manager must help the staff to act upon values, as well as set up policies and procedures to motivate the staff to carry them out.

Structuring is goal-oriented management. It allows no-fault nursing in that a nurse-manager's activities are always directed toward helping staff primary nurses accomplish their roles. Structuring is the most creative and rewarding activity a nurse-manager can do, because it involves coordinating needs and manpower, politics, and potentials.

Structuring effective primary nursing includes making sure that maintenance care is delivered within acceptable standards. To get the work done, a nurse-manager first must accept the position of authority personally and then utilize the organization's standards to direct and enforce optimal patient care through primary nursing.

Authority of the Nurse-Manager

If the goal is quality patient care then the head nurse must be out in the area where this care is given. Both as a role model and by working closely with the staff and patients, she can more effectively determine the standards under which patient care will be delivered. Her own practice, expectations, and priorities have an important influence on staff performance. Patient care must be constantly held as first priority and staff energies directed towards use of the nursing process in pertinent observations, assessment of patient needs, care planning, intervention and evaluation. It is our experience that individuals will most often excel in those areas consistent with the indicated expectations and rewards (Bartels, Good, & Lampe, 1977, p. 27).

The nurse-manager has the authority to set expectations and build in rewards when the work is completed. The nurse-manager organizes the primary nursing unit daily and must accept the invested authority "otherwise, she is likely to be directed by the environment" (Stevens, 1976, p. 10). To avert the tendency to become drowned in the details of daily business, the nurse-manager needs a clear focus on what is happening. The repetitious aspects of nursing must be recognized and accepted as well as preestablished landmarks that staff at all levels of a department can cite as progress. There must be clear performance descriptions, as well as continual evaluation of activities and the delegation of them to the most appropriate staff members. The nurse-manager is the orchestrator of energies.

Every day, the nurse-manager has a chance to provide top quality nursing care based on the minute-to-minute decisions that are made. The power and freedom to direct priorities belong to the nurse-manager. Contrary to popular belief, a nurse-manager manages the constant conflict of time and task, rather than people. No nurse-manager can directly control each staff member's nursing; it is priorities and energies which are managed. Indeed, the nurse-manager who attempts to control everything done by each staff member is in effect being controlled by everyone else. Rigid control, which is no real control at all, is contraindicated in primary nursing.

Interactional Leadership Style

The nurse-manager of primary nursing needs to integrate the traditional functions of management — organizing, planning, directing, controlling, coordinating — with the interactional leadership style which fosters professional growth in the staff. "Thus, leadership involves a working relationship between the group members and the leader, who acquires leadership status through active participation and demonstration of his capabilities for completing, or helping the group to complete cooperative tasks" (Heimann, 1976, p. 23).

In regard to primary nursing, an interactional leadership style requires agreement between the staff and nurse-manager about the definition and operationalism of primary nursing. Together they must strive for consistency in philosophy and action. Only with a mutual working framework can there be enough energy left for true responsibility, independence, and calculated risk taking by primary nurses. Only when the nurse-manager is sure that safe and therapeutic nursing care will be given at all times can the nurse-manager relinquish and redefine control.

Nurse-managers have the authority to adjust leadership style and decisions to the situations at hand. However, authority must not be abdicated, but rather it must be used appropriately and consciously with the goal in sight at every moment.

Why Must There Be a Nurse-Manager?

The question of whether a nurse-manager is needed at all in primary nursing is often raised. It is feared that any person designated as leader will not be conducive to the autonomy, independence, and group cohesion necessary in primary nursing, regardless of the manager's leadership style. Although philosophically this is an interesting hypothesis, it disregards important realities about group dynamics and, if put into operation, may do more to hinder than to help effective primary nursing.

Why?

The nursing staff is a group which like any other group, seeks cohesion (commonality of view) by fending off individual differences that tend to split the group apart. The person who can best work for the beliefs and goals of the group is viewed as the leader.

Because of the highly pressured and complex environment in which a nursing staff works, it is essential that a high level of consensus exists. If a staff group does not have a leader, it will make one.

Especially during periods of transition (such as to primary nursing) and rapid growth, a designated leader is necessary for the survival of the group, because by nature the group responds to stress by increased dependency needs. These needs are not bad, but they must be acknowledged. There is usually some regression in preparation for major developmental growth.

Even with a stable, mature, and professional nursing staff, the ambivalence about work (the tendency to be lazy or to be selfish) is ever present. Only within a group that feels gratification from task completion and social bonds will the tendency toward regression be willingly put aside. An interactional leader will make the difference.

Contrary to popular belief, the autonomy often referred to in primary nursing was never meant to mean "alone." Autonomy is self-directedness in which the individual makes multiple decisions about where to put time and energies. This is done within the context of broad expectations and individual expectations (professional ideals). At this phase of autonomy, the nurse-manager is a powerful influence. The nurse-manager is needed to define an overall structure within which primary nurses can be self-directed and will request the nurse-manager's knowledge or support when necessary.

The nurse-manager sets a crucial example for attitudes toward authority and responsibility. As primary nurses watch the way a nurse-manager handles authority and responsibility for a nursing staff's outcomes every day, week, and month, they learn a powerful lesson about how such functions are handled.

Authority is not a negative or fearful quality, and it is an essential part of the primary nursing role. There must be room in a nursing staff for every RN to have specific areas of authority. Just as each primary nurse has authority for the nursing care of each primary patient, someone must have authority for the smooth running and overall outcomes of the total unit. The best person is a unit-based manager, although when such a position is not feasible, authority should be placed with the nurse-manager who is organizationally closest to the primary nurses.

Especially in primary nursing, a specific person, the nurse-manager, must have the responsibility and authority to monitor and define staff development needs. This role includes the formal evaluation of staff primary nurses and the establishment of resources to help the staff meet professional goals. Handling formal evaluation is a fine art. However, the role of evaluator cannot be given up or given away, because primary nurses cannot work in a vacuum without any checks and balances. Professional nursing involves putting one's own work in the focus of professional review. Peer review is a good goal, but most primary nurses need encouragement and guidance in evaluating their own work, let alone the work of others.

Even in an experiment where leadership was shared among staff nurses with no head nurse, the nurses found a need for certain leadership tasks to be taken on by designated people. Two separate roles were developed, resource nurse and contact nurse, and were filled by different nurses every two weeks with a stable clinical director overseeing the system (Mealy et al., 1976). The new roles together approximated that of nurse-manager. However, splitting the roles and putting them on a temporary basis dilutes the authority and thus the effectiveness of the persons carrying them out. The constructive influence of a full-time, full-fledged nurse-manager is lost. For long-range staff development, as well as frequent analysis of the agency's nursing care delivery system, reliance on the clinical director would probably have to increase or these important activities would be lost in the shuffle.

Agencies need not and should not eliminate the nurse-manager position in hope of instilling values like accountability, autonomy, and motivation in primary nurses. Mature, motivated, professional nurses and nurse-managers are not mutually exclusive. There must be room for competent managers and competent primary nurses sharing the same territory but not the same roles. Ironically, the nurse-manager is most effective when each primary nurse becomes the nurse-manager for each primary patient.

The concept of structuring offers the nurse-manager an alternative to the ironclad managing that stifles development and creativity, including that of the nurse-manager. As upholder of the structure, the nurse-manager cannot be arbitrary. Instead, the manager role becomes that of reminding primary nurses of the expectations by which they have agreed to work and then of working with them to determine how to best fulfill these expectations every day.

Standards of Care

The structure that a nurse-manager sets for a unit of care delivery must be consistent with the nursing administration's stated standards of care regarding the basic service that patients can expect from each representative of the nursing department. The standards are a guarantee that the patient as health care consumer will receive definite kinds of nursing services. They are the nursing department's portion of the promise of quality that the agency makes to the public. The standards of care from one agency (Twyon, 1979)[4] are the following:

1. Every patient will be assigned a primary nurse.
2. Every patient will have a written nursing assessment.
3. A written plan of nursing care will be maintained by the primary nurse.
4. Patient teaching will be included in the nursing plan of care.
5. Patient care will be delivered by utilizing the problem solving method.
6. Plans for the patient's health care after discharge will be included in the written plan of nursing care.
7. Documentation of nursing care will be recorded by utilizing the problem oriented method of charting.

A nurse-manager should view these as structural standards, the baseline mechanisms for delivering nursing care. They do not necessarily designate who is responsible for carrying out the service or the quality with which the service is provided. Thus, structural standards give the nurse-manager a framework within which to work, but do not specifically address primary nursing.

Primary nursing requires its own set of standards, firmly rooted in the structural standards of care of the nursing department. These standards are a further description of how the nursing department intends to provide its services on a daily basis. In other words, standards, or structure, for primary nursing provide the basic rules and regulations, or mechanisms, without which primary nursing will not take place.

The Structure of Primary Nursing

The primary nursing structure delineated here is a compilation of the essential elements required for primary nursing to occur in a unit. The rationale for each point is also discussed. This model was developed through several years of trial and error without any written structure, or protocol. The establishment of such a structure is tantamount to the successful implementation and continuation of primary nursing (Twyon, 1979).

1. *Each patient is assigned a primary nurse who will complete a written assessment and a plan of care within 24 hours of the patient's admission.*

When left to their own direction, nurses will not choose to be primary nurses for every patient. The ambivalence about caring for a less than desirable patient is only human. This can be seen over and over again in every nursing setting, no matter how professional, mature, and motivated the staff. The idea that primary patients

---

[4]This and other quotes in the text citing this source are reprinted with permission of Ms. Sandra Twyon, Chairman, Department of Nursing, Tufts New England Medical Center.

should be selected by nurses has done a disservice to the primary nursing movement, because the selection system does not work and is not professional. Primary nursing should not be a system of adoption. Rather, it should assure that every patient's needs will be at least adequately met.

In one pediatric unit there were four admissions in one day. Two patients were chosen as primaries and two were not. Which ones?

- the battered baby of a young couple
- a baby admitted for cleft lip/palate repair
- a baby with FUO (fever of undetermined origin)
- a baby known to the staff, dying of leukemia

The battered baby and the dying baby were readily selected as primary patients. This, and similar phenomena, may be explained by a nurse's tendency to pick patients whom they feel adequately skilled and useful to care for. When questioned the staff revealed that the baby admitted for cleft lip/palate repair seemed routine and uninteresting, and the baby with FUO presented an undefined, potentially dull or difficult problem.

Every unit or agency has certain patients who would never be selected as primary patients. Even when patients are selected, it can often take several days for a primary nurse to work directly with a primary patient. Once again, the selection procedure does a disservice to primary nurses and primary nursing, because if patients can do without a primary nurse for several days, they can do without having them at all!

The nurse-manager needs to assign patients to primary nurses as a routine procedure at each patient's admission. Staff primary nurses should have the option to request a certain patient, but the nurse-manager must make the final decision.

2. *Assignment of a primary nurse will be made by the nurse-manager or, in the nurse-manager's absence, by the senior staff nurse in charge or a day charge nurse.*

As the first-line manager of a unit of nurses, the nurse-manager answers to patients and supervisors for the quality of care delivered by all of the nursing staff. Because primary nursing requires the delegation of much decisionmaking about nursing management to staff primary nurses, the nurse-manager must feel confident about making assignments.

The nurse-manager is the only person in the unit with the scope and responsibility to know the capabilities and interests of each nurse and the extenuating circumstances surrounding time scheduling, and with the expertise to assess the needs and priorities of a group of patients. It is absolutely essential that the nurse-manager control the assignment of patients to primary nurses.

In the nurse-manager's absence there must be a responsible person who can see situations with a perspective similar to that of the nurse-manager. A senior staff nurse or assistant head nurse is usually that level of personnel and may have the advantage of being in charge on off shifts when patients are admitted. For instance, a permanent evening charge nurse may be the best person to assign new patients to primary nurses on the evening shift, but the assignments would need to be coordinated with the nurse-manager. Thus, the nurse-manager and other nurses in leadership positions must agree on how to make primary nursing assignments.

Primary nursing assignments should be distinguished from assignments done on a shift-to-shift basis that insure completion of the nursing care plan, treatments, medications, and crisis intervention. These shift assignments are crucial to safe, therapeutic care and can be made by whoever the nurse-manager has designated for charge responsibilities. This is very different from the cross-shift commitment that a primary nurse is asked to make when informed of the admission of a new primary patient.

The only other person with the authority to make primary nursing assignments should be a staff nurse acting as charge nurse in the nurse-manager's absence. For instance, a day charge nurse would have the nursing supervisor and other resources available in case of questions or conflicts about assignments. The nurse-manager must hold accountable for the decisions regarding assignments of patients to primary nurses those persons to whom charge responsibilities are delegated.

3. *The person who makes the primary nursing assignments must notify the primary nurse as soon as the assignment is made. The primary nurse must be notified verbally or in writing.*

All nurses must be notified as soon as they are assigned to a primary patient so that the primary nurse can assess the new patient immediately and determine time priorities. The primary nurse must not be put in the embarrassing position of learning hours into a shift that a new primary patient has been assigned. Unfortunately, primary nurses who have not been informed usually find out by seeing their names on a bulletin board, chart, or Kardex next to patients' names. This catches them off guard and often makes them so angry that they never really adjust to the new patients.

By personally informing a nurse of a new primary assignment, the nurse-manager opens an opportunity for teaching through anticipatory guidance. The nurse-manager and the new primary nurse can share information about the patient and make tentative plans. The primary nurse can ask for theoretical or physical assistance if needed. The attitude that the nurse-manager has about the patient and the road ahead will directly influence the primary nurse's attitude toward the patient.

The nurse-manager can never assume that staff nurses should or will be as aware of the total functioning of a unit or agency in the same way the nurse-manager must be. It simply is not their responsibility to do so.

4. *Assignments of primary nurses will be based upon the nurse's time schedule and ability to independently carry out the nursing process with the patient.*

Assignments of patients to primary nurses should rarely be unilateral decisions of the nurse-manager. The primary nursing structure is based on an interactive leadership style. It is the nurse-manager's responsibility to know the developmental levels of each staff nurse and make assignments accordingly.

The best way to facilitate a primary nurse's interest in a new patient is to appeal to the nurse's curiosity and, occasionally, the need for a challenge or a change. If the patient presents a new experience, the nurse-manager should let the primary nurse verbalize any apprehensions and then offer support.

> *NM:* Remember last week you told me you hadn't worked with a burned patient? One is being admitted today and you're next for a primary patient.
> *PN:* I didn't mean I wanted one this soon!
> *NM:* Why not?
> *PN:* I don't know enough about burns yet.
> *NM:* You showed in your work with Mr. K that you are thorough and remain calm under stress. That's what this patient will need. Jan and Sue can help you with the details about a burn patient's special needs.
> *PN:* Okay. What room is he going into?

A sense of humor is sometimes indicated in assignment making:

> *NM:* Now that you're off night rotation, I bet you can't wait to get involved with another colostomy patient?

Informing a nurse about a primary patient assignment immediately allows for changes to be made before things go too far:

> *NM:* I assigned you to Ms. B because she needs good diabetic teaching.
> *PN:* I already have two diabetics and my other two patients need a lot of discharge planning. Isn't there anyone else?
> *NM:* I think maybe Carol could take her. I didn't realize you were that busy.

Or

> *NM:* I've looked over the schedule and you're the only person who is here now who will be here all week. If you take Ms. B, I'll try to give you a non-diabetic next time. Maybe you could save time now by getting the diabetic patients together in a group to teach them.
> *PN:* I hadn't thought of a group. How do you do that?

A belief shared by most new nurse-managers is that to get good care for patients nurses must be happy and to make nurses happy means giving them whatever they want. This is an unworkable outlook for a nurse-manager because it can interfere with getting the work done.

Sometimes it will be necessary for the nurse-manager to insist that a nurse fulfill a primary patient assignment. This is the nurse-manager's prerogative, and the nurse-manager has the right to expect that nurses will do their best with the assignments, even if at times they get angry or discouraged.

Assignments should be presented unapologetically because there is no need to apologize for asking people to do the work for which they were hired. The nurse-manager should not have to cajole people to work with patients. Nurses who are not willing to accept the responsibility for a primary patient should not be working on primary nursing units.

5. *Assignment of a primary nurse for orientation or professional development purposes will occur only when adequate supervision and support can be provided to the nurse.*

Assignments always need to be considered carefully, but especially when made to nurses who are new to a particular primary nursing experience. When patients are used as learning experiences, the nurse must be adequately supported. Frequent discussions, consultations, bedside instructions on new techniques and equipment, and other planned sessions with the nurse-manager or designated nursing staff serve this purpose. As with many aspects of primary nursing, the nurse-manager's control by planning ahead is crucial to make the concept operational.

6. *The names of the primary nurse assigned to each patient will appear in a central location on the unit as well as in other specific key locations.*

Posting the names of primary nurses with their assigned patients facilitates identification and association of the patient with nurse. Secretaries, physicians, and other non-RNs can easily identify which nurse has the overall responsibility for which patients and can then put their energies into contacting that nurse. Visual display of assignments on a large central board also helps the nurse-manager to determine an individual nurse's caseload and thus to plan for future staffing arrangements.

Any other places that the names of primary nurses can appear helps to identify the responsible primary nurse. This could be done on the nursing assessment, care plan, patient's chart cover, clipboard, room door, and information pamphlets.

7. *Nurses who work permanent nights or less than four shifts per week will not be assigned to primary patients except in extenuating circumstances approved by the nurse-manager.*

Primary nurses need frequent contact with their patients. In most cases, nurses who work less than four shifts per week are not available enough to be consistently responsible for a patient's round-the-clock care. An exception to this may be part-time nurses working several consecutive days on a unit with planned, short-term admissions, such as dental surgery or prediagnostic tests. It is also feasible for a part-time nurse in an ambulatory clinic to be assigned a caseload of primary patients. Ambulatory patient visits can usually be arranged according to the nurse's time schedule, and the contact hours with patients can be spread over time.

In most instances nurses who work permanent night shifts also find it difficult to fulfill the role of primary nurse. Expecting night nurses to function as well as nurses who have more contact with patients and families is neither fair to the patient nor to the nurse. Some exceptions are the nurse who works in an intensive care unit where day and night are indistinguishable or the nurse who is available to a family or physician who visit only during the night hours. The arrangements made for primary nurses doing a temporary rotation to nights need to be carefully coordinated between the primary nurses and the nurse-manager.

8. *Daily patient assignments will be based upon each patient's individual requirements for varying levels of nursing care. Primary nurses will be responsible for the direct care of their primary patients whenever possible, especially if it facilitates successful completion of a nursing plan of care.*

"The strength of the nursing profession is in combining the use of our bodies with an intellect that can assess problems and compassionately, creatively, and sensibly move patients to an improved health status" (Zander, 1978, p. 52). RNs cannot be above giving direct care, no matter what role they take in relation to nursing service. PN should never stand for "paper nurse," the primary nurse who coordinates and directs but never gets physically close enough to be identified as primary nurse by the patient. Whenever possible, primary nurses should give direct care to their patients.

The nurse-manager will need to make different decisions every day about where to guide each primary nurse's energies. Planning is of the essence in daily assignments. To help organize a day, each primary nurse should present a plan for the day to the nurse-manager. Staffing and other concerns need to be taken into consideration as the nurse-manager coordinates the day's activities. The consistency of primary nursing assignments makes it possible to plan ahead, unlike the crisis-orientation of many nursing staffs.

As the primary nurses discuss their plans for the shift, the nurse-manager may assist them or may ask for alterations based on a managerial assessment of the nursing needs of the total unit. Give-and-take between staff nurses and the nurse-manager is as necessary, if not more so, in primary nursing as in team nursing. The difference in primary nursing is that the nurse-manager is the catalyst for bringing the staff together when and where needed. The nurse-manager makes the desired team spirit a reality by encouraging primary nurses to discuss priorities and share resources.

At times the nurse-manager will need to interrupt one primary nurse's plans because another primary nurse's patient needs immediate intervention. The nurse-manager cannot let primary nurses get so nearsighted that they can see only the needs of their own primary patients. Such isolation creates an unworkable situation in any agency where patient's needs demand attention immediately.

Appropriate utilization of non-RNs is also critical to the smooth running of primary nursing. Nurse aides, LPNs, mental health workers, and part-time personnel should fulfill their own job descriptions but not be expected to be mini-primary nurses. Their roles should be organized around tasks and treatments which are directed by primary nurses. In this way, primary nurses can really be responsible for 24-hour nursing management and its outcomes.

Asking or allowing non-RN or part-time staff to do more than their job descriptions require neither helps their self-esteem nor solves the problem of inadequate staffing for primary nursing. However, it is essential that part-time and ancillary staff be taken into consideration and given the respect due to working colleagues. The nurse-manager and professional staff need to work out systems of care delivery and patterns of communication with the non-RN staff members. Decisions need to be made about their inclusion in shift reports, walk rounds, conferences, and other formal meetings of the nursing staff.

Regardless of the way the nurse-manager and staff utilize non-RNs, daily assignments for them should be very specific. For example, if they are paired with a primary nurse for a certain shift, the primary nurse will need to give them specific instructions for what should be done, recorded, and reported back to the primary nurse. By listening carefully to the non-RNs, registered nurses can help define and meet the ancillary staff's learning needs. In all cases, non-RNs' input into discussions about patients is invaluable, and the nurse-manager sets the model for acknowledgment and respect for their viewpoints.

9. *Primary nurses will communicate with colleagues, physicians, and other professionals involved in patient care through vehicles such as change of shift report, physicians' walk rounds, multi-disciplinary conferences, discharge planning meetings, and formal documentation.*

The nurse-manager needs to study the flow of information to, from, and within the nursing staff before deciding where the best expenditure of nursing time will be. Is it more important for primary nurses to regularly attend walk rounds or sit-down rounds with physicians? Or both? How do you decide which primary nurses come to shift report and which ones cover the floor during the report? Such questions are difficult but necessary to answer. A good rule of thumb is that a primary nurse must attend any nursing-oriented conferences or meetings about a primary patient.

Being a primary nurse should also be a ticket to physician-run discussions which may have implications for the nursing care of specific primary patients. A primary nurse needs to know why decisions are made about patients and, in fact, is obligated to give professional input before major decisions are made. Often the primary nurse will have data that other health care professionals do not because of their limited perspective on a patient's total needs. Participation in conferences, rounds, and meetings can help the primary nurse more easily support decisions during contacts with primary patients.

It is absolutely essential that the nurse-manager work politically to have primary nurses invited and accepted at interdisciplinary meetings. Planning and structuring are required to get the right nurse to the right event. When in doubt, the nurse-manager should always send the primary nurse, and may elect to go also if the primary nurse needs moral support.

The nurse-manager will often have to help primary nurses prepare for public presentations. The nurse-manager therefore needs to help a primary nurse to be ready to be a patient advocate.

When a primary nurse's attendance at an important meeting is impossible, the nurse-manager must make sure that a nursing staff representative goes prepared for the agenda. The representative then has the obligation of telling the primary nurse what happened at the meeting.

10. *Each unit/agency will establish consistent times for weekly patient care presentations designed as both problem-solving and educational sessions focused on the nursing care of an individual patient. The nurse-manager will assign to specific nurses the responsibility for presenting at the primary nursing conference.*

The tone set by primary nursing presentations is critical to the staff's attitudes toward their role. Primary nursing presentations are the central core of primary nursing and must take priority over just about anything except a cardiac arrest! Even when the nurse-manager and a primary nurse sit down for a few minutes to discuss a case, the opportunity provided for thinking rather than doing sets an important example.

The nurse-manager must be in attendance at the presentation for several reasons:

- to encourage group problem solving, which is more efficient and stimulating
- to offer perspective and clinical expertise
- to evaluate a primary nurse's ability to think through a patient's nursing needs from problems to outcomes
- to show firm belief in the value of peer supervision and nursing care based on the nursing process

The aim of the presentation should always be constructive and should give the primary nurse a new opinion, an approach, or different way of working with peers for a primary patient. A format facilitates presentations and leads to constructive results. Either the nursing care plan or a format similar to that offered below (Twyon, 1979) can be used for presentations. With structure a great deal of thought and work can be accomplished in a short period of time.

Primary Patient Presentation

Presentation of a primary patient can be made to serve different purposes and focus on one or more aspects of nursing care. For example, the presentation may be an information-relating conference or a problem-solving session. Unique or interesting medical diagnoses may be discussed; however, presentations should primarily focus on nursing care issues such as teaching, discharge planning, or utilization of resources.

The following form should be followed for each presentation. Once the focus of the presentation is decided, any one part of the format may be more fully developed. This should be done in terms of the nursing process, providing appropriate information about the assessment of the specific area of concern, identification of needs, plan, implementation of the plan, documentation and evaluation of the plan.

Patient name (or initials):   Diagnosis:
Pertinent medical therapy:
Nursing history: (use nursing assessment form)
Patient's nursing needs:
Long-term goals signifying resolution of needs: ("The patient will . . .")
Short-term goals for immediate needs: ("The patient will . . .")
Nursing intervention measures: (in use or proposed)
Evaluation of care plan:

If the presentation times are consistent each week (i.e., Tuesdays, 11 or 11:30 a.m.), nurses can usually plan their day's schedule around the session. A half-hour weekly conference is the bare minimum for primary nursing. A primary nursing presentation session is as crucial as shift report. In fact, if shift report can last 45 minutes, the nurse-manager may opt to shorten report to 30 minutes and use the other 15 minutes every day for primary nursing presentations. No matter how sessions are organized, the primary nursing presentations are a necessary mechanism for thoughtful, careful, and competent primary nursing. The nurse-manager may even want to keep a log about who presented and what was discussed.

The nurse-manager will initially need to assign primary nurses to present cases. Arrangements must be made for coverage of the clinic or agency while some of the nurses are meeting together. The presentation should occur ideally without interruptions by the phone, call lights, or people. (Ever notice how nurses are always interrupted?) A new date in the same week should be set if the session becomes impossible.

There will always be some nurses who are too shy or unsure about presenting without an encouraging push. The nurse-manager needs to make the sessions as unthreatening as possible by beginning with a statement such as "What would you like us to do for your patient?'' The primary nurses will need to perceive the sessions as informative and helpful to them, rather than a test of their capabilities. The sessions can also be used as practice grounds for the more formal presentations that primary nurses need to make in public, outside the protection of the nursing staff.

Eventually, the nurse-manager can expect that most primary nurses will autonomously request that they present particular patient care situations. When such volunteering begins, or when primary nurses are complimented by other professionals on their public presentations, the nurse-manager will know that support and structuring have paid off.

REFERENCES

American Hospital Association. A patient's bill of rights. Chicago: American Hospital Association, 1975.

Annas, G.J. The rights of hospital patients.: Avon Books, 1975.

Ashley, J. Hospitals, paternalism, and the role of the nurse. New York: Teachers College Press, 1977.

Bailis, S., Lambert, S. & Bernstein, S. The legacy of the group: A study of group therapy with a transient membership. *Social Work in Health Care,* Summer 1978, *3* (4), pp. 405-418.

Bartels, D., Good, V. & Lampe, S. The role of the head nurse in primary nursing. *Canadian Nurse,* March 1977, *73*(3), pp. 26-30.

Black, K. Teaching family process and intervention. *Nursing Outlook,* June 1970, *18* (6), pp. 54-8.

Bolder, J. Primary nursing: Why not? *Nursing Administration Quarterly,* Winter 1977, *1* (2), pp. 79-87.

Bower-Ferres, S. Loeb center and its philosophy of nursing. *American Journal of Nursing,* May 1975, *75*(5), pp. 810-5.

Bowman, R. & Culpepper, R. Power: Rx for change. *American Journal of Nursing,* June 1974, *74* (6), pp. 1053-6.

Church, G. Understanding each other to achieve a common goal. *American Journal of Nursing,* February 1956, *56* (2), pp. 201-4.

Costello, D. Communication patterns in family systems. *Nursing Clinics of North America,* December 1969, *4,* pp. 721-9.

Donnelly, G. The assertive nurse. *Nursing 78,* January 1978, *8* (1), pp. 65-9.

Elpern, E.H. Structural and organizational supports for primary nursing. *Nursing Clinics of North America,* June 1977, *12* (2), pp. 205-19.

Ganong, J. & Ganong W. *Nursing management.* Germantown, Md.: Aspen Systems, 1976.

Granbois, M. (Ed.). *Cumulative index to nursing literature* 1-5 Glendale, Calif.: Glendale Adventist Hospital, 1964.

Granbois, M. (Ed.). *Cumulative index to nursing literature,* 15. Glendale, California: Glendale Adventist Hospital, 1971.

Hegyvary, S.T. Foundations of primary nursing. *Nursing Clinics of North America,* June 1977, *12* (2), pp. 187-96.

Heimann, C. Four theories of leadership. *Journal of Nursing Administration,* June 1976, *6* (5), pp. 18-24.

Jacobs, C. & Jacobs, N., *The PEP primer*. Chicago: Joint Commission on Accreditation of Hospitals, 1975.

Kramer, M. *Reality shock*. St. Louis: C.V. Mosby, 1974.

Kvarnes, M. The patient is the family. *Nursing Outlook*, March 1959, *7* (3), pp. 142-4.

Labovitz, G. Perceptions and attitudes. In *Motivational dynamics*. Minneapolis, Minn: Control Data, 1975, pp. 4-5-4-11.

Lipeles, J., Case material — Meeting ground for nurses and social workers. *Nursing Outlook*, June 1959, *7* (6), pp. 343-5.

Lipsitt, D., Medical and psychological characteristics of crocks. *Psychiatry in Medicine*, January 1970, *1*, pp. 15-25.

Malone, M., The dilemma of a professional in a bureaucracy. *Nursing Forum*, 1964, *3* (4), pp. 36-60.

Manthey, M., Ciske, K., Robertson, P., and Harris, I. Primary nursing — A return to the concept of "my nurse" and "my patient." *Nursing Forum*, 1970, *9* (1), pp. 65-83.

Marram, G., Schlegel, M., & Bevis, E. Primary nursing: A model for individualized care. St. Louis: C.V. Mosby, 1974.

Mauksch, I., Certification — Assurance of quality. *American Nurse*, March 15, 1978, p. 4.

Mauksch, I., & David M. Prescription for survival. *American Journal of Nursing*, December 1972, *72* (12), 2189-2193.

Mealy, S. et al. Shared leadership — No head nurse! *Nursing Administration Quarterly*, Fall 1976, *1* (1), pp. 81-93.

Miller, D. Organization is a process. *Journal of Nursing Administration*, March-April 1972, *2* (2), pp. 19-24.

Mundinger, M. Primary nursing: Impact on the education department. *Nursing Administration Quarterly*, Winter 1977, *1* (2), pp. 69-77.

Nodal, M. Facets of retrospective chart audit. *Supervisor Nurse*, May 1978, *9* (5), pp. 58-9.

Norton, C. What's primary in primary nursing? *The American Journal of Maternal – Child Nursing*, March/April 1978, p. 72.

Peplau, H. Psychiatric nursing skills and the general hospital patient. *Nursing Forum*, 1964, *3* (2), pp. 28-37.

Pryma, R. Primary nursing: A working philosophy — An organizational style. *Magazine of Rush-Presbyterian – St. Luke's Medical Center*, Spring 1978, *2* (2), pp. 3-17.

Reiter, F. The clinical nursing approach. *Nursing Forum*, 1966, *5* (1), pp. 39-44.

Rutledge, K. The professional nurse as primary therapist: Background, perspective, and opinion. *Journal of Operational Psychiatry*, Spring-Summer 1974, *5* (2), pp. 76-83.

Shorr, T. Let's hear it for primary nursing. *American Journal of Nursing*, November 1977, *77* (11), p. 1787.

Shubin, S. Burnout: The professional hazard you face in nursing. *Nursing 78*, July 1978, *8* (7), pp. 22-7.

Stevens, B. *First-line patient care management*. Wakefield, Mass.: Contemporary Publishing, 1976.

Trick, K. & Obcarskas, S. *Understanding mental illness and its nursing*. London: Pitman Publishing, 1968.

Twyon, S.: Basic standards of nursing care. Boston: TNEMCH, 1978.: *Primary nursing structure*. Boston: TNEMCH, 1978.: *Primary Patient Presentation*. Boston: TNEMCH, 1978.: Adapted from *Primary Nurse Role Description*. Boston: TNEMCH, 1979.

Williams, M. The myths and assumptions about team nursing. *Nursing Forum*, 1964, *3* (4), pp. 61-73.

Zander, K. Primary nursing won't work . . . unless the head nurse lets it. *Journal of Nursing Administration,* October 1977, *7* (8), pp. 19-23.

Zander, K. Reactions to Donna McCarthy and Marita MacKinnon Schifalacqua, Primary nursing: Its implementation and six month outcome. *Journal of Nursing Administration,* August 1978, *8* (8), pp. 52, 54.

Zander, K., Bower, K., Foster, S., Towson, M., Wermuth, M.R., & Woldum, K. (Eds.). *Practical manual for patient-teaching.* St. Louis: C.V. Mosby, 1978.

Chapter 2

Managing Toward a Professional Commitment

The nurse-manager can help each primary nurse to say, "Hello, I'm your primary nurse," and stand behind that statement by imparting the concept of professional commitment.

> Professional commitment is an unwritten contract in which a nurse promises that she will give every patient assigned to her the best nursing care she can give, depending on her level of expertise. She will find other resources to fulfill those areas of the patient's care plan that she cannot carry out herself. Whether her patient comes into her care on an ambulatory basis or due to a prolonged illness, she will try her utmost to empathize with his situation. She will remain responsive to his needs regardless of her personal feelings about him, his family, or his diagnosis. Most significantly, the primary nurse assumes first-line accountability for whatever nursing care is done and/or is not completed. Her role includes health-teaching, working with families, and documentation of the patient's physical and emotional responses to treatment. In carrying out her responsibilities, the primary nurse becomes her patient's advocate in the health care system. Ultimately, nursing based on a professional commitment gives more to patients because more is required of each nurse (Zander, 1977, p. 20).

A professional commitment from a primary nurse to a primary patient must be built on the principles of professional closeness (Peplau, 1969), which begins with empathy. The nurse-manager's analysis of the empathy process in each primary nurse's practice can be invaluable for the quality of care given.

Once the empathy process is started, the primary nurse needs to be aware of the specific role(s) that a primary patient may unknowingly seek. After gaining this awareness of what is happening in the nurse-patient relationship, the primary nurse can use the relationship to move a patient toward the desired outcomes of care with the numerous alternatives available to both the nurse and the patient. The level of professional nursing in the unit/agency will be determined by the nurse-manager's understanding of the awareness and alternatives aspects of making a professional commitment.

While striving to foster professional commitment through leadership, the nurse-manager will need direction and support. Nurse-managers need realistic and dependable resources at the unit level which are built into the agency's formal structure. Top-level nursing administrators must structure primary nursing for the nurse-manager as firmly as the nurse-manager structures the system for primary nurses. Nurse-managers must be given the same authority and autonomy that they are expected to give to the staff primary nurses. The mutual goal of the nursing administration and nurse-managers must be the professional commitment of all primary nurses to their patients.

PROFESSIONAL CLOSENESS: A MODEL FOR PRIMARY NURSES

What does it feel like to be a primary nurse? How should I act? What is the nature of my relationship with my primary patients?

The best answer to these difficult questions which face nurses daily in every clinical area is Hildegard Peplau's concept of professional closeness. Professional closeness is the balance between over- and underinvolvement that a primary nurse should maintain with patients. It is a workable model for primary nursing practice, because it encourages sensible and responsive involvement and allows a reasonable level of concern and activity that can extend as long as the nurse has contact with the patient.

Professional closeness and primary nursing are almost synonymous because both demand that the needs, concerns, and experiences of patients and their families are the focus of the primary nurse's energies. Actually, professional closeness is a description of an ideal primary nurse-patient relationship in which the nurse uses positive elements from other relationships to establish an interpersonal framework in which to deal with each new primary patient. To establish each primary nurse-patient duet takes a great deal of energy, so the primary nurse must put personal needs aside, except the need to do the job well. Primary nursing requires fine tuning to the patient's situation while retaining the objectivity necessary to collect data, analyze it, and skillfully intervene on the patient's behalf.

The nurse-manager has the role of forming the attitudes which are essential for each primary nurse on the staff to establish professional closeness. Professional closeness can be attained and maintained by primary nurses if they adhere to three principal stages, or bases: empathy, awareness, and alternatives. This model is a fine guide for the nurse-manager and staff primary nurses who are striving to practice effective primary nursing.

Base One: The Empathy Process

Empathy is the first step to achieving professional closeness. It is feeling with someone rather than feeling for them (sympathizing). It is trying to understand the position of another by temporarily viewing a situation from that person's frame of reference.

Empathy occurs in two phases. First, people almost instantly identify aspects of their own personalities with those of another; and second, sometimes immediately, people will sort out their own uniqueness from that of the other. Thus, there is an immediate identification and then a gradual separation of identities as an empathizer gets to know the other person.

The two phases of empathy are clearly evident when a nurse deals with a patient who is in pain. It is natural for the nurse to identify with the feeling of pain—perhaps remembering dental pain, the frustration of getting a fast appointment, the fear of what it might take to relieve the pain, or the strange feeling produced by the prescribed codeine. Though pain is particularly difficult to recall, the nurse is quickly flooded with memories and develops immediate empathy for the patient. As if one with the patient for an instant, the nurse makes a purely emotional connection with the patient. Presumably, the more experiences that a nurse has had in life, the more chance that the patient's experiences will identify with the nurse's. Furthermore, a nurse does not have to have had exactly the same experience to identify briefly with the patient.

The nurse then begins to sort out the response objectively by remembering that only the patient is in pain and that the pain is not in the teeth. Realizing that the patient needs a response, the nurse quickly refocuses energies on the individual.

Model of the Empathy Process

A drawing of the empathy process may help the nurse-manager clarify expectations of the primary nurse-patient relationship (Figure 2-1).

Figure 2-1 The Empathy Process

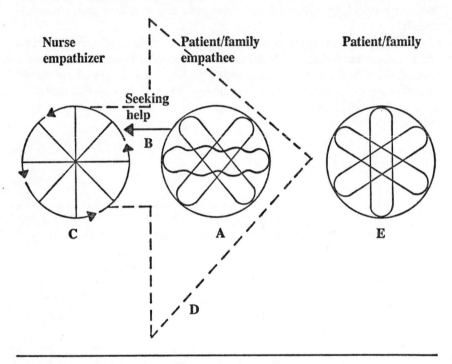

The person, A, is seeking help, which in the nursing world could be in the areas of crisis in physical or mental health, adaptation to change, need for specific tasks, information, or support, and nonmedical problems. A has attributes shown by several interlocking orbits, one, some, or all of which A wants to change or modify. A approaches the source of desired help by presenting the situation in an individual fashion, shown by arrow B.

A's approach strikes C in a very personal way. Like A, C has many attributes, but because the relationship is professional, the attributes that C uses to respond to A come from a repertoire of learned skills. Each new A will strike C in a slightly different way, as shown by the revolving arrows. C responds by refocusing the attributes which are stimulated onto A's attributes. A is viewed in totality with special attention to those segments which require C's help. The output of empathy is shown by D, which is outlined by a dashed line because the amount of empathy can expand and contract. Output is in the shape of an arrow to indicate a process with a direction.

E is the empathee with some modification of one or more attributes. The change is not necessarily good or bad and may be very difficult to measure. If there is no change, E will look the same as A.

The expectations that the nurse-manager has of primary nurses will be based on attitudes about why patients need help and what kind of nursing care will make them well or more comfortable. Before primary nursing, nurses could administer task-focused care without being very involved in the empathy process. However, because the professional commitment of primary nursing to patients is based on empathy, the nurse-manager needs to include empathy among daily expectations from primary nurses.

Disturbances in the Empathy Process

The model can be used by a nurse-manager to locate where the empathy process is breaking down for certain individuals or among the staff group. There can be disturbances in the empathy process at any stage of nurse-patient interactions. Some of the most common disturbances are discussed below.

Physical Avoidance. This can be seen in many situations, such as when the assigned primary nurse does not get around to a nursing assessment, forgets to do some treatments, or delegates direct care of certain patients regularly to another staff member and the nurse-manager who is never able to be a primary nurse. When an assignment is made, the nurse-manager may fairly expect the primary nurse to have as much personal contact with the patient as possible. Furthermore, it is the nurse-manager's responsibility to arrange a unit or agency's care delivery to ensure that patients have direct access to their primary nurses.

Poor Listening. Careful listening is definitely a skill that every primary nurse should have, a skill which can be accentuated by an alert nurse-manager. When with a patient, the primary nurse must hear the patient's message. Initially, primary nurses will hear only the spoken words and their tone, such as urgent, hopeless, frightened, defensive. However, after listening to a primary patient over a period of time, the primary nurse will learn to distinguish the message between the lines as well as hearing the words. The primary nurse will also learn when and how to ask questions that reach beyond daily business to feelings and responses and when to just listen to the silence. Such interpersonal learning can be encouraged by a nurse-manager who believes that listening is as important as doing. "Care-full" listening is a large part of the work of a primary nurse.

Minimum Life Repertoire. The primary nurse needs to identify, at least minimally, with the requests, complaints, or attitudes of a patient. The primary nurse who has limited life experience or imagination will have extreme difficulty with the identification step of the empathy process. An active imagination ("how would I feel in a full-body cast?") is sometimes even better than identical life experience. However, without imagination or experience, the nurse has no personal repertoire to respond to the patient with, even for a second. Primary nurses in their early twenties lack many of the life experiences that adult patients have lived through, and a nurse-manager who is older or relates easily to adult problems, such as sexual habits, divorce, and parenting, can be a useful translator for young primary nurses.

Conflictual Mothering. One of the biggest disturbances in empathy is difficulty with the role of nurturer. Young primary nurses who are not yet parents may not have explored and defined the nurturing side of their personalities. They usually respond to the empathizer role by being too mothering and sometimes smothering. Unfamiliarity with the nurturer role can be seen when:

- the primary nurse in pediatrics competes with a child's mother
- the nurse angrily scolds a patient
- the nurse is unable to tolerate a patient's temporary regression during a crisis
- the nurse feels lonesome when certain primary patients die or are discharged
- the nurse unintentionally fosters dependency by doubting the patient's proven capabilities
- the nurse cannot set caring limits or expectations for a patient

The nurse-manager must acknowledge the parenting aspects of primary nursing by helping primary nurses regain the balance provided by professional closeness.

Memory Blockades. The nurse-manager may need to help primary nurses remember experiences that could help them to empathize with primary patients. A nurse may block against remembering certain events. For example, the nurse who has lived through adolescence but does not remember much from that period may find it difficult to be empathetic or even tolerant of a teenager's situation. This disturbance in identification and objectification could severely limit the nurse's ability to compassionately or effectively treat and teach a teenager. While a nurse-manager cannot and should not be a staff nurse's therapist, there may be something that can be done to decrease the nurse's emotional interference.

Overidentification. Another disturbance in the empathy process occurs when nurses spend too long in the identification phase. Progression to the objectification phase is impeded because nurses cannot sort out the difference between the patient and themselves. "The nurse who makes the focus of the nurse-patient situation the description, analysis, and validation of meaning of the personal experience of both nurse and patient is putting the patient into the role of chum instead of treating him as a client" (Peplau, 1969, p. 344). When the primary nurse loses objectivity, it often means that the nurse, the patient, or both are expecting more from the relationship than is possible or professional. Such relationships are a special hazard for nurses "because of the tendency of physically ill people to regress to more childlike modes of behavior, thinking, and feeling as part of the usual adaptation to illness" (Schwartz & Schwartz, 1972, p. 13).

The alert nurse-manager will recognize signs of overidentification, usually shown by extreme emotions of persistent duration, at shift reports, primary nursing presentations, or informal discussions around the coffee pot. Sometimes a group of nurses or the whole nursing staff will become overidentified with a patient or family. Special staff meetings are often helpful to regain perspective, and the primary nurse is usually grateful for the chance to discuss difficult situations with peers. Especially when the entire staff is overidentified, the nurse-manager should request an outside consultant, such as a nurse-manager from another unit or a psychiatric nurse consultant.

Facilitating Empathy

There are several ways a nurse-manager can expedite the identification and objectivity needed for empathy. The nurse-manager can cut down on possible disturbances in empathy as well as encourage the desire of nurses to be empathetic.

One of the most important things a nurse-manager can do is direct the system of reinforcements to the nursing staff so that each primary nurse can use staff interactions, not patients, to meet personal needs. When staff members can look to each other for praise and growth, they have more energy to get involved with patients. This is positive peer review.

Staff interactions should be constructive and noncritical with the aim of helping primary nurses to succeed in their work and receive credit for their efforts. Professionals need as much praise and positive support as any other group of workers. Indeed, when assured that overall good work will be noticed and acknowledged, the primary nurse will be emotionally free to function on a highly professional, patient-focused level.

How much can a primary nurse "give" to a patient? Every nurse, whether primary or not, has experienced failures in being empathetic, and sometimes, the best a nurse-manager can do is to acknowledge the ebb and flow of a primary nurse's ability to be empathetic. The nurse-manager must be careful not to say or do things that will increase a primary nurse's guilt about not giving enough to patients. By determining if the primary nurse has gone through the phases of identification and objectification, the nurse-manager can help the primary nurse define what the patient is really asking for and if basic needs are being met. If the primary nurse feels accepted by the nurse-manager during a slump, chances are that this in itself will give the primary nurse more energy to become committed.

The nurse-manager also needs to assess the specific learning needs in order to set up classes or to send staff members to seminars. This can help because sometimes lack of knowledge can close a person to learning things on a spontaneous basis. The more obsessive or compulsive nurses will need a lot of theory before they can relax enough to be professionally close to patients.

Further knowledge may help in situations such as the admittance of a hemophiliac to a unit not accustomed to treating hemophilia. For the primary nurse and the staff to be comfortable enough to be empathic, they need to be familiar with the pathophysiology of hemophilia and its treatment, especially protocols for bleeding. Once the nurses know the facts and the regimen, they can see the patient as a person and not a chapter from a medical textbook. When the nurse-manager urges the primary nurse to find details and teach them to the rest of the staff, the empathy process is greatly facilitated.

Another activity for a nurse-manager is the determination of the end product of the empathy process. What are the realistic expectations for the primary patient? Although a model for change is more realistic than a model for cure, change is still considered of great value among health professionals. To empathize with a patient or family, the primary nurse must be as free as possible of the hope that patients will change in some way. Otherwise, the primary nurse may make an unconscious deal with the patient: "I'll empathize with you as long as you get better." The nurse-manager may need to remind primary nurses often that all a nurse can really change in a relationship with a patient is "awareness of her own behavior. . . . The nurse cannot change the patient's responses, nor can she demand responses that are different from those obtained. What she can do is to manage her own behavior as the stimulus to which the patient's behavior is a response" (Peplau, 1969, p. 349).

When trying to facilitate empathy, the nurse-manager would do well to remember that empathy requires a fine balance between personal humility ("I have no impact in the world") and professional competence ("I am an effective nurse"). Primary nurses need to feel competent enough to be useful but humble enough to know that they do not control all the solutions to the patient's problems. If the nurse-manager's attitude displays this, it will be easier for staff primary nurses to incorporate it in their work.

Base Two: Awareness

What happens after the empathy process is set in motion? How can the nurse-manager enhance professional closeness between staff primary nurses and patients?

The second principle of professional closeness is the primary nurse's awareness of the quality and style of relationship that has been established with each primary patient and family. Because patients put nurses in roles and nurses put patients in roles, primary nurses must be aware of these roles to increase endurance and effectiveness. Some of these roles may need to be modified. In situations such as psychiatric nursing or working with patients for behavioral change, nurses may need to make patients aware of the role that they themselves are playing.

When nurses become involved with patients as primary nurses, the nurse-patient relationship is activated beyond mere acquaintance. Primary nursing is analogous to dating someone steadily, while nonprimary nursing is like an occasional date. Primary nursing is serious and often intense. If the nurses and the nurse-manager believe that effective nursing occurs within a relationship, that relationship must be clearly understood to be used appropriately.

Not only does the nurse-manager's position provide the objectivity needed to facilitate awareness, the nurse-manager also has the power to require that primary nurses do what is needed to gain awareness of the relationships that they establish with certain kinds of patients.

Common Reactions of Patients to Nurses

1. When patients regress to childlike modes, "Nurses are often expected to be all-giving mothers, and if they do not fulfill these expectations, certain patients will react as though they have been rejected or mistreated in spite of objective evidence to the contrary. In the hospital setting, the patients' seeing doctor and nurse as father and mother is to some extent based on an unconscious reenactment of childhood illness" (Schwartz & Schwartz, 1972, p. 13).

2. Patients can be jealous or envious of nurses, depending on their background and current life situations. Jealousy implies that someone wants something that belongs to another but knows that it may be possible to obtain. Envy is closer to hatred, and implies that the person who does not possess the desired object believes or knows that it can never be attained. Envy is a difficult feeling to cope with on either the giving or receiving end. A patient may be jealous of a nurse's health or looks, but knows or hopes to return to health himself. However, the paraplegic envies the nurse who walks, the postmastectomy patient envies the female nurse who has both breasts, and the welfare patient envies the modern, expensive hospital and everyone working in it.

3. Entitlement is the sense that you are entitled to something and deserve special privileges or services. Entitlement may occur among any social class and is often expressed in terms of rights and obligations. Nurses tolerate patients who feel entitled if they agree that, indeed, these patients deserve specific treatment, such as the post-op patient who deserves pain medication and the child who deserves a home without physical abuse. However, entitlement is relative and often causes strong disagreements between members of the nursing staff and great conflicts between nurses and patients. Does an alcoholic deserve equal treatment in an emergency room? Does a terminally ill child deserve to see siblings even though visiting rules prevent it? Because primary nursing promotes individualized care, the questions of entitlement are personal and difficult. Nurses do not want to be arbitrary or rigid in decisions concerning appropriateness of care. Yet there are human and professional limits, such as the recently discharged elderly woman who asked the nurse on a home visit to vacuum her house! The primary nurse refused, but worked with the woman to arrange a homemaker service.

4. "The considerate, wise physician-father and the tender, solicitous nurse-mother are ready-made love objects for suffering and frightened or unhappy and frustrated patients" (Schwartz & Schwartz, 1972, p. 13). In such instances,

dependence or genuine appreciation is converted by the patient into puppy love or sexual feelings and advances. It is important for primary nurses not to take these reactions too literally or personally. These feelings should be received with understanding but not reciprocated.

5. Intense anger from patients or families is often experienced by primary nurses. Sometimes patients or families are angry at someone else in the health care system, but feel that it is safer to be angry at a nurse. Usually, however, they are angry at their affliction and helplessness. Primary nurses must allow the anger to be expressed before other intervention will be useful. Patients and families should be helped to direct their anger at the right source without defensiveness from the primary nurse. If anger toward the nurse is justifiable, it should be addressed by the nurse. Sometimes explanations are in order. However, an honest apology usually goes a long way to getting the nurse-patient relationship back on a healthy track. The nurse-manager may have to help primary nurses acknowledge that they have made a mistake.

6. Devaluation of the nurse occurs when patients expect nurses to be waitresses or maids, call nurses honey, or do not listen to information. Usually, attempts to ignore the individuality of nurses or the importance of the nursing are not meant to be disrespectful. Nasty or chauvinistic comments often are the way that patients use to make nurses feel helpless and demeaned too. Nurses who are insecure personally or professionally are the most sensitive to the perceived disrespect. It is important that the nurses clarify the role of nursing to patients, because nurses cannot be professionally close if they do not feel professional or close to the patient. It helps greatly if nurses feel respected as professionals and supported in their approach by peers and the nurse-manager.

7. Even when offered an empathic link by their primary nurses, patients do not always respond with relief or appreciation. Because of their inherent preoccupation with their needs, patients sometimes continue to question—or test—the strength of the nurse's empathy and good intentions. Adults in particular are not used to being the center of another person's concerned attention. They may respond to their self-consciousness by changing the rules of the relationship, or they may seek the unselfish attention of the primary nurse through whatever means are available (often through physical complaints).

8. A very difficult reaction for a nursing staff to deal with is choosing favorites, when patients split the staff into good and bad nurses and inform the staff indirectly of these opinions, i.e. "Mary never takes care of me as well as you do—where did she go to school?" or "Can I have a different primary nurse? Mine never comes to see me." Once again, these actions are an indication of the patient's dependent position. Patients can respond to insecurity or fear by ingratiating the person they are with. If staff members hold the same opinion or need that kind of praise, patients continue to set themselves in judgment. The results can be disastrous to the cohesion of the nursing staff. Such patients should be encouraged to complain

directly to the nurse or to speak with the nurse-manager. If nurses look to each other for praise and constructive criticism of their work, they will be able to listen to patients' complaints without needing to take sides. Deep down the patient does not want to be deserted. In cases of malpractice, the nurse-manager will need to speak with the patient who has lodged the complaint.

9. Sometimes patients may idealize the primary nurse and say that the nurse is the most wonderful, skilled, caring person they have ever met. This can be rather sugary and embarrassing for nurses who know it cannot be true all the time, and it exerts the pressure of enormous expectations. Also, when patients idealize nurses, they feel inferior and are unable to view themselves as persons of equal worth and capabilities. Activities, such as patient teaching, become impossible because patients believe that only that nurse can do the cast care or change the colostomy bag. If nurses are confident, without needing to feel that they are God's gift to nursing, they can help patients interact on an equal basis.

These are some of the typical reactions that are difficult for nurses to handle in their relationships with patients. It is clear that these problems stem from an unrealistic view of the nurse and the situation. The reactions are distorted and are characterized by intense emotion and have little resemblance to the nurse's view of reality. They are the patient's view of reality which is a response to stress. The majority of these reactions are overblown defense mechanisms which are stimulated largely by unconscious needs. If these hidden needs are acknowledged, patients will not need to use such trying techniques in the nurse-patient relationship.

Becoming Professional

Being professional is always in the state of becoming. After a nurse learns pathophysiology and the necessary technical activities, the next area of emphasis requiring continuous, concerted effort is awareness of how the nurse can use the nurse-patient relationship. In primary nursing this awareness is mandatory. "The task of becoming a professional person means that the nurse should learn to deal with the conflictual distortions in her own life and attempt to resolve contradictions that interfere with her nursing behavior" (Schwartz & Schwartz, 1972, p. 15).

Individual nurses have their own patterns or characteristic styles of relating to patients which are sometimes based on unresolved conflicts. There are always patients whom nurses want to avoid or with whom it takes a great deal of effort to work. However, if nurses respond to all patients the same way, are unable to care for a majority of primary patients, or feel over- or underinvolved with most patients, this is evidence that nurses are not aware of or able to manage certain elements of the nurse-patient relationship. The female nurse who is not yet comfortable with her own sexuality may have difficulty interacting with male patients or may be seductive without realizing it, or she may show her discomfort by forgetting to inform a woman having a radium insertion when she can have intercourse. Similarly, female nurses may experience great anxiety about catheterizing a woman, often because of their own emotional discomfort and lack of knowledge about the perineal area.

Subconscious reactions to patient care can easily be overlooked or worked around by regular staff nurses because someone else can usually step in or take over every shift. However, for primary nurses, repeated discomforts in the nurse-patient relationship become apparent over time, if not to the nurse then hopefully to the nurse-manager.

The nurse-manager is in a position to recognize a primary nurse's difficulties. For instance, a primary nurse "may not recognize or accept her own dependent needs, and may thus react with hostility or avoidance to the very young, or the helpless of any age, who may wish to lean upon her emotionally for prolonged periods of time" (Schwartz & Schwartz, 1972, p. 14). The nurse's irritability may not be expressed verbally or may be directed at some other segment of work, such as the time sheet or the day's schedule, but the nurse-manager should have the perspective to see that the nurse is irritated with a patient, if, indeed, that is the case.

The nurse-manager should have a mental list of clues to help determine when an individual primary nurse or a group of primary nurses are unaware of distorted or personal need-fulfilling roles in their relationships with patients. Some clues are when a primary nurse:

- treats one patient very differently than most other patients
- forgets details, treatments, names of significant individuals, and other aspects of a patient's needs
- makes mistakes, such as in medications or in not monitoring a nurse's aide closely enough in the care of a patient
- reports having dreamed about a patient
- excludes the rest of the team in making important decisions or does not inform them about significant events
- develops unrealistic expectations for the patient
- shows signs of possessiveness about certain patients
- gets hurt or hypersensitive by what a patient says
- has not looked into pathophysiology and other specific information necessary to care knowledgeably for a certain patient

Once clues have been noticed, the nurse-manager can assist the nurse in gaining awareness and, thus, in growing professionally close. First, the nurse-manager must encourage all primary nurses to base their practice on knowledge of biological, behavioral, and nursing sciences.

Therefore, professional closeness requires continuing inquiry on the part of every nurse in order that the common elements (universal) in similar nursing situations can be continuously refined, and the relation between problem and nurse action can be formulated and explained. However, although the nurse is constantly looking for universals in cases or situations of like kind, she always starts by seeing the patient (or family unit) with whom she is working as if he were unique. Preconceptions derived from her theoretical knowledge or from other cases are constantly checked against new data; and the results of these checks may alter previous views to a considerable extent. Therefore, the nurse must be a sensitive observer with many techniques of inquiry at her fingertips so that she can get to know the patient fully, in as many dimensions as possible, from data obtained directly from him (Peplau, 1969, p. 351-2).

The nurse-manager can expand the awareness of primary nurses by asking about the similarities and differences between past and present patients. Relationships with former primary patients can be used to evaluate present relationships with questions. "How does this patient irritate you more than Mr. D, who has the same diagnosis?" "I think your approach to older childrens' parents needs revision since they don't seem to be learning from your teaching. What can you do differently?"

A systematic review of primary patients' current status will help primary nurses make associations with past experiences. Accurate formulation of the patients' health status and personalities will help primary nurses to judge whether reactions and approaches are appropriate. This kind of reality testing between peers and with the nurse-manager increases awareness and provides built-in checks and balances.

The nurse-manager can help increase awareness of roles with different patients by asking primary nurses to describe their interactions with patients and by listening when nurses blow off steam. Getting nurses to talk about their responses to patients before rushing to quick solutions can be a valuable expenditure of time.

When clues are picked up during times when the nurse-manager is absent, the nurse-manager may still want to talk with the primary nurse. The nurse-manager may ask a primary nurse about what happened with a family on the previous evening shift, even though the encounter is over.

Sometimes it takes a long time for primary nurses to become fully aware of their roles with certain patients. Often, complete awareness does not occur until after the relationship has ended. However, both satisfaction and bad memories can last indefinitely. It is never ancient history for a nurse to discuss previous relationships, as long as it increases awareness.

The nurse-manager can hope that most primary nurses will gain awareness on their own. However, people usually need help, especially when beginning careers, changing positions, or entering new clinical areas. Primary nursing requires added awareness and appropriate response to patients over periods of time. Preventing distorted relationships is better than working them out after they are recognized.

Autonomous primary nurses will recognize distortions and correct them, leading to

> constructive attitudes and changes within the nurse. One of the best methods of maintaining perspective in one's relationship with patients is a periodic review by a constructive critic. Thus, the nurse may wish to systematically share her professional experience with a reliable colleague, an understanding supervisor, or a professional psychotherapist. Sharing various experiences is vital to maintaining a realistic view of oneself (Schwartz & Schwartz, 1972, p. 15).

If the agency has mechanisms such as primary nursing conferences and constructive evaluations, autonomous primary nurses can use what is available. Autonomous primary nurses also know when to request assistance, such as a psychiatric nurse consultant, to gain awareness and perspective. "Members of the nursing staff request psychiatric nursing consultation in order to review the problem identified, add to their assessment, receive assistance in understanding the psychodynamics of the situation and plan appropriate nursing intervention" (Taylor & Abele 1977, p. 1). Autonomous primary nurses also know when problems with patients are more personal than professional and seek outside help.

Primary nurses who are not yet autonomous will need help to become aware. Sometimes the nurse-manager will have to address primary nurses' difficulties very directly. The nurse-manager in primary nursing has as much responsibility to teach nurses about relationships as to teach them other aspects of nursing. Technical and interpersonal learning should go hand-in-hand, because primary nursing will not be effective if either skill is excluded.

Base Three: Alternatives

The third principle in developing professional closeness with patients is to use professional knowledge and skill when offering patients an alternative to their actual physical condition or to their perceived condition. The professional relationship of primary nurses and their patients could be viewed as "an instrumentality through which a professional nurse aids a patient to recognize and formulate his needs, to cope with these needs more and more through his own efforts, and to take at least a tiny step toward self-development" (Peplau, 1969, p. 355).

The nurse-manager has an active part in helping primary nurses offer alternatives to their patients. Once primary nurses have achieved empathy and awareness, they can explore alternatives, options, and varieties of nursing interventions.

Because they are free from distorted nurse-patient relationships, their flexibility will be felt by their patients and families.

An alternative may decrease helplessness and anxiety and can lead patients to exercise their own "life-force" muscles. It is ultimately a growing experience—a journey in which the end is not always in sight.

Patients and their families may not have the slightest idea of what may be an alternative as they confront their expectations of the nurse-patient relationship. Even in primary nursing, patients are pleasantly surprised to receive such knowledgeable, thoughtful care. Unfortunately many patients and a surprisingly large number of nurses still do not expect nurses to be able to make much of a dent in a patient's health maintenance or outcomes.

The nurse-manager must believe that nursing care can make a difference in both the quantity and the quality of health outcomes because of its importance and potential effectiveness. This belief and enthusiasm can make a big difference in the energy that staff primary nurses are willing to exert. There will, of course, be times when both the nurse-manager and the staff will despair about their efforts and feel quite hopeless and often unappreciated! However, a general feeling of competence will carry a staff through brief periods of doubt.

It is also useful for primary nurses to be able to distinguish a patient's desires from a patient's needs. Often what patients want is not what they need. In fact, what they want may even be dangerous, such as the patient who wants a drink of water before surgery. "Demands and needs are not necessarily synonymous. Putting the patient in the position of being a 'customer'—a person who defines the services he wants and possibly gets—may even be detrimental" (Peplau, 1969, p. 355). So primary nurses need a clear idea of what is wanted, needed, and possible for each primary patient in order to propose ideas for alternatives to peers and the nurse-manager. A few examples will be used to illustrate this.

A patient, who was also a nurse, received results of moderate to severe cervical dysplasia from a Pap smear. She went to the clinic where she was seen by a nurse practitioner who quickly established an empathic link with a serious and concerned approach. Through an interview, the nurse found out the patient's gynecological history and fear that she had cancer. In the interview the nurse identified what the patient needed to know about upcoming treatments and appointments. The nurse became aware of personal reactions to the nurse-patient relationship which centered around some identification with the patient and some impatience that as a nurse this patient did not know more about gynecology. Once this was sorted out, the nurse was able to meet this patient's individual needs. The nurse drew a diagram of the layers of the cervix to show the extent of dysplasia. This relieved the patient greatly, and she was less frightened of the biopsy and more receptive to the cryosurgery that would follow. Although unable to change the Pap smear results or downplay the need for further treatment, the nurse offered the patient an alternative way to understanding the problem. The patient returned for all of the follow-up appointments.

In another example, the primary nurse of an adolescent named Paula who had taken an overdose, began dreaming about the girl. In the dreams the nurse was trying to pull Paula out of an iceberg. The primary nurse talked with colleagues about work with the patient and the dream. They helped the primary nurse to realize that empathy had definitely been established with Paula, although she was from a different socioeconomic background. The colleagues also noted how difficult this teenager had been for the primary nurse because she would often swear and refuse to talk. When the primary nurse began having iceberg dreams, Paula was getting ready to return to her family in the housing project.

Secondly, peers pointed out how invested the primary nurse was in Paula's improvement, suggested that the nurse was pushing Paula too much, and offered ideas of how to help Paula make the transition to home. They also agreed to become more involved with Paula to take some of the pressure off the primary nurse.

Through awareness of excessive expectations and frustration, which was evidenced in the dream, the primary nurse was able to modify the approach and help Paula get ready for discharge. When the primary nurse stopped viewing her role as that of some savior, the nurse was able to consider new alternatives. This freed Paula to accept other people's affection and help because she realized that she would not always have the primary nurse to confide in and to support her.

The primary nurse in a neonatal intensive care unit was assigned to a newborn with an immense facial hemangioma. The nurse was initially repulsed by the grotesque face, which tended to preoccupy all the staff who came in contact with the baby. The primary nurse and colleagues had to become aware of their strong dislike for the neonate's appearance while they were trying to help the parents adjust. As support from the primary nurse's peers increased and as the primary nurse began to establish clear lines of communication with everyone involved, the baby's functional level improved! The primary nurse became the hub of the patient's multidisciplinary care rather than waiting on the periphery to be told what to do. Eventually, the primary nurse involved the infant stimulation team to work with the parents.

Examples of how primary nurses can offer alternative adjustments to crises or acceptance of help are numerous. Because primary nurses must be relatively free of personal difficulties with patients, they must be willing to be empathetic and aware. Furthermore, primary nurses cannot let their own anxiety prevent them from being creative. If they can be creative, they can offer themselves and their patients good alternatives to seemingly impossible problems.

In short, professional closeness is not simply a matter of being generous, kind, affable, or obliging to sick people, but rather one of being knowledgeable about the practices and problems of nursing care. It is not so much a matter of being "closer" to the person who is ill, but rather one of being "closer to the truth" of that person's current dilemma and of having the know-how to use such understanding as the basis of effective help for the patient (Peplau, 1969, p. 352).

THE NURSE-MANAGER'S RESOURCES

The nurse-manager has the key role in the establishment of professional commitments to patients by primary nurses. But the nurse manager also needs reliable resources to maintain professional and psychological well-being. The role of nurse-manager of primary nursing is demanding, exciting, and cannot be accomplished without concrete supervisory and administrative support.

In primary nursing professional commitment is the first of five major areas requiring a nurse-manager's attention. The others are expertise in clinical practice, accountability, a professional milieu, and collaboration of energies. Each area of functioning in the nurse-manager's role involves specific activities and skills. Each of these five areas transcends the traditionally defined manager's role for patient care management, staff/personnel management, and unit management.

Whatever level the nurse-manager chooses to focus on, there are several managerial concepts that will help the nurse-manager stay committed to the nursing staff and their work without burning out. These concepts are: responsibility of command, anticipatory management through the nursing leadership team, and management by objectives. Ultimately, the nurse-manager is the clinical consultant to staff primary nurses.

To utilize these concepts to the fullest, the nurse-manager will need plentiful resources from people, supplies, and education. However, the most valuable resource is the support and validation that can be given only by management peers and supervisors. The ability to give and receive such support is enhanced by a responsive, competent nursing administration.

Management Concepts for the Nurse-Manager

Responsibility of Command

Every nurse-manager must settle the issue of responsibility of command before expectations for primary nurses are clear. Unfortunately, responsibility is often relative to the situation at hand, and thus the assignment or acceptance of responsibility is largely subjective.

To decrease subjectivity, all levels of the organization need to have clear role descriptions that are consistently carried out and enforced. Only with clear and clearly upheld operational guidelines can the nurse-manager know how much responsibility can be delegated to primary nurses. No nurse-manager wants to make a decision only to have it undermined or countermanded by someone at the same or a higher level of the organization. For example, the nurse-manager who schedules a primary nurse to attend a special conference does not want someone else to float that nurse to another clinic. Or the nurse-manager who is trying to keep clear distinctions between the roles of nurse aide and professional nurse does not want an evening supervisor to tell the aide to do something beyond the aide's role.

The same rule that applies to nurse-managers in regard to primary nurses also applies to nurse-managers in relation to nursing administration. Nurse-managers must be given enough formal authority to be able to fulfill their responsibilities. Just as the nurse-manager must give primary nurses the responsibility and authority to determine individual care management for primary patients, the nurse-manager must be given the responsibility and authority to run a clinic or unit. Just as primary nurses need help and encouragement to manage their patients' care, so do nurse-managers need what gives them confidence to be managers. Therefore, when considering responsibility of command, the art of delegation becomes crucial.

Finding the delicate balance of how much responsibility should be delegated to primary nurses is difficult, especially because primary nursing involves an expansion of the traditional staff nurse role. Many professional nurses feel very responsible and do not understand how they could be more responsible. In fact, the thought of more responsibility can be very frightening. Until the new role of primary nurses is clearly explained and until they believe that they have control and authority, the new responsibility will be confusing and induce pressure.

With inexperienced primary nurses, the nurse-manager will need to make definite suggestions about the directions to take in patient care. Many things cannot wait for a weekly care conference or even until the end of a shift. Therefore, the nurse-manager will need to specifically instruct, or delegate actions to, some primary nurses regarding interventions or decisions. New primary nurses need guidance about how to fulfill their responsibilities to patients.

Effective delegation of responsibility to primary nurses involves four steps as identified by Volante (1974):

1. "Define the task to be done." The nurse-manager needs to have a clear idea of what is expected of the primary nurse. "I want Amy to figure out why Mr. O is incontinent at night. He's making the night shift angry." The expectation may start as a desire ("I wish Mr. O wouldn't wet the bed") and turn into a direction.

2. "Relay your definition of the task." Giving directions to the primary nurse about the task must include answers to the questions who, what, where, when, perhaps how, and very definitely why. As primary nurses become more experienced in working with the nurse-manager and patients, the answers to the questions will become more obvious. The nurse-manager will merely have to pose the

concern to the primary nurse, who in turn will answer the questions. Until that time, the nurse-manager must individualize instructions for each primary nurse. For instance, one primary nurse will need to be told, "Talk to the night shift staff and find out what happens at 5:00 a.m. with Mr. O. They think he wants attention when they make their rounds. Maybe you could ask Mr. O what he thinks is going on—if he has control over his bladder, since he does during the day." Another primary nurse may already have researched the problem to a degree and merely need reinforcement from the nurse-manager that this is a priority.

3. "Establish controls and checkpoints." The nurse-manager needs to follow through on responsibilities delegated to primary nurses. Every piece of work does not need to be nor can it be inspected, but the nurse-manager can discriminately assess progress on the work which is delegated. The nurse-manager can ask the primary nurse to report or record the results of assessments and interventions. There are numerous ways that a nurse-manager can monitor a primary nurse's work, such as, shift report, care plans and charts, primary nurse conferences, and feedback from other professionals.

The most meaningful reinforcement for work which is delegated to primary nurses is personal attention from the nurse-manager. For example, the primary nurse who has been delegated the task of assessing Mr. O's incontinence may be told, "Let me know what you find," or "Come up with a new approach that the people on duty tonight can use." When the nurse-manager follows through, the staff primary nurses will learn the value of commitment to a project.

4. "Establish dialogue." When defining an assignment for a primary nurse, the nurse-manager should have a long enough conversation with the primary nurse so that both thoroughly understand the immediate issue. It is surprising how often two people think they are in agreement when they actually report two separate experiences. In the last example, the nurse-manager may think that the problem will soon be solved, while the primary nurse wants Mr. O catheterized! Even when both parties thoroughly understand the task, they may need to plan how it will be completed. In all cases the nurse-manager must be willing to help primary nurses succeed in their roles, and too much dialogue is preferable to too little.

Ultimately, the nurse-manager always aims toward complete delegation of responsibility for the decisions about nursing care to primary nurses. This is not as impossible a task as it may seem to the nurse-manager, because each nurse already functions within professional and institutional protocols. Thus, each registered nurse theoretically administers safe care and if given the right encouragement, education, and structure, will be able to go far beyond minimum functioning.

Primary nurses need not be frightened by responsibility if it is clearly defined and especially if they are allowed to grow in decision-making ability. Such growth requires that primary nurses be allowed to take calculated risks, particularly in experimenting with new nursing approaches. To foster independence and creativity in decision making, the nurse-manager must help primary nurses to "own" their decisions. Primary nurses must be able to claim their decisions and actions as their own and live with the consequences.

It cannot be overstated that for primary nurses to take on a high level of responsibility, the nurse-manager must take some risks in relinquishing control: "Risk-taking is of vital importance if primary nurses are to know the freedom of testing the 'rightness or wrongness' of their decisions. Staff must know that in some circumstances being wrong may be acceptable. It may not be ideal but it is human and sometimes the best a person can do in a given situation (Bartels, Good & Lampe, 1977, p. 27).

Along these lines, the nurse-manager has to find ways to control the quality of patient care so as to live with the challenge of responsibility invested in the nursing profession. The controls needed for primary nursing no longer lie in the realm of the doctor's order book or being switchboard operator for the nursing station. Responsibility for nursing care must be decentralized, while that for the smooth functioning of the clinic or unit round-the-clock must belong to the nurse-manager.

The nurse-manager's control in primary nursing must eventually be of the influential, consultative variety:

> As staff competence in decision-making develops, the head nurse's leadership emphasis shifts naturally from staff development to staff consultation. The strength of her consultation role is proportional to her excellence in clinical knowledge and nursing practice. Thus, her leadership power base evolves from personal expertise rather than merely ascribed power associated with the position (Bartels et al., 1977, p. 27).

In summary, the nurse-manager can only be as responsible as the persons on the staff. Responsibility is tenuous and grows or shrinks depending on the person or the situation. The nurse-manager needs to help primary nurses to learn responsible nursing and to stay responsible for their decisions and actions. The best role to facilitate responsible primary nursing is that of an interactive manager who is comfortable as a clinical consultant.

Anticipatory Management and the Leadership Team

Anticipatory management requires active participation by everyone on the leadership team (nurse-manager and assistants, clinical supervisors or coordinators, and the associated administrators). Ultimately, each staff member, especially primary nurses, should participate in planning and implementing changes in order to build a stronger unit.

For primary nurses to make and follow through with their professional commitments to patients, they need to feel that the stresses in their work are predictable and controllable. The leadership team's conscientious application of management principles can make the difference between a mediocre staff or one where each primary nurse functions exceptionally well. This is possible because anticipatory management decreases the crisis orientation that is present in most nursing staffs.

Anticipatory management entails planning ahead to minimize crises and, more importantly, preventing the frantic, vague feeling that things can fall apart at any minute. Decreasing the sense of impending disaster is essential to the smooth function of primary nursing. Whether primary nurses are working directly with their own or with other nurses' primary patients, the sense that everything is orderly and that their efforts lead to results is crucial to productivity and morale.

A dynamic leadership team identifies and attacks problems when they are still small and relatively simple. Through their frequent discussions, fact finding, problem solving, and energetic concern, they can make "solutions possible under the most advantageous circumstances, rather than at a time when procedures and attitudes are in disarray" (Frazier, 1966, p. 27). For instance, when someone on the leadership team notices that nurses are getting lax on medication administration procedures, the team can bring it to the attention of the nurses on all shifts. Medications are clearly an important aspect of nursing care, and proper administration affects all patients and nurses. If the problem is left uncorrected, chances are that a major medication error would be made in the future.

If the leadership team does not focus on prevention by involving all the staff in the process of planning ahead, the only alternative for the nurse-manager is crisis or corrective management. Not only is crisis management time and energy-consuming, it leaves the nursing manager feeling constantly behind. The old adage "a stitch in time saves nine" certainly applies to nursing leadership in primary nursing. If the nurse-manager is emotionally off-balance and disorganized by disruptions which could have been prevented, the primary nurses will also be disorganized.

One of the best ways to involve the leadership team in anticipatory management is to have regular meetings to discuss current issues facing each member of their respective shifts. At one hospital, these meetings are termed "vertical meetings" because they include nursing leaders from each rung of the supervisory ladder for a particular unit: senior staff nurse, nurse-manager, day clinical supervisor, evening and night clinical supervisors, and associate administrator (when requested). Normally, each leader meets with leaders in the same position. However, to manage an individual unit effectively, such meetings are not sufficient because the round-the-clock people never talk with or even see each other all together. After support for the concept and administrative planning, the evening and night leaders were scheduled to work on the same day once a month and to meet for one-hour sessions with their respective nurse-managers. Other evening and night supervisors covered their units and in turn had their shifts covered during their day-on days.

After a one-year trial, the results of vertical meetings have been outstanding. Everyone is satisfied with this concrete, administratively supported pathway for communication. The major improvements are:

- increased contact and familiarity with all the people who have direct responsibility for the policies, procedures, and professional development of the nursing staff on a given unit
- increased sense that the burden of unit management is shared but clearly delegated
- increased ability to discuss approaches and evaluations of nursing staff, especially those working on permanent off shifts
- increased objectivity in setting goals and evaluating unit progress toward objectives
- increased time—one hour a month together can save many hours spent alone in problem solving
- increased awareness of the administration about unit business because minutes of the vertical meetings are sent to the associate chairman of nursing

Primary nursing is one of the main subjects discussed at vertical meetings. Other subjects are related to primary nursing and the quality of care: staffing patterns, staff learning needs, orientation of new graduates, relationships between different units, and relationships with other disciplines and departments. Sometimes representatives from other areas are asked to join the discussion. Members of the primary nursing committee also attend when invited. In all cases, the meetings are results oriented and demonstrate to the nursing staff that the smooth functioning and good morale of a unit is high priority.

Evidence of anticipatory management must be demonstrated consistently at every level of a nursing department. In fact, one of the most useful categories of a staff nurse's evaluation is the one that measures the value of the nurse's responsibility for the effective functioning of an entire unit. Nurses can be evaluated by which statement below best describes their behavior in this area:

- a) Assumes responsibility for the effective functioning of the total unit at all times.
- b) Assumes responsibility for the effective functioning of the total unit when in charge of the unit.
- c) Fulfills responsibility for effective functioning of the areas of the unit to which she has been assigned.
- d) Others must assume responsibility for the effective functioning of the total unit, including those areas in which she has been assigned to work (Bower and Twyon, 1978).[1]

---

[1]This and other quotes in the text citing this source are reprinted with permission of Sandra Twyon, Chairman and Kathleen Bower, Associate Chairman, Dept. of Nursing, TNEMC, Boston, Massachusetts, 1979.

For a top rating, the nurse must consistently demonstrate full attention to the entire unit or clinic. The nurse must see beyond the immediate assignment to the complete needs of all the patients and to the position of the unit in relation to the whole institution. The nurse should be aware and responsive to the many pressures involved in decisions about the patients or staff of the unit, and must show evidence of participating in problem identification and solving at staff meetings and at other opportunities. Indeed, an emphasis on this high level of professional practice definitely sets an expectation that all nurses will participate in anticipatory management. Nurses need to focus on the health of a unit or clinic in much the same fashion as they are actively concerned with the prevention of complications in their patients.

Anticipatory management techniques must be built into the structure and expectations of the department. This commitment can be reflected in the role descriptions of each member of the nursing leadership team, in the manner in which a nurse-manager is supported, in attention to productive meetings, and ultimately in the work of every primary nurse.

Management by Objectives

Excellent primary nursing takes a long time to establish and can only be accomplished in manageable time periods with realistic goals to make progress. Because management by objectives (MBO) uses goal setting and organization of resources to meet them and because MBO is an employee-involving process that places high priority on change and progress, as opposed to ritual and crisis, its methodology is more conducive to primary nursing than any other management system.

What makes MBO so vital to primary nursing in the institution and to primary nurses professionally?

MBO can and should be adopted by all levels of the nursing department, thus giving credence and sanction to goal-focused productivity. In industry the goals usually involve money, whereas in nursing the goals are not always so obvious. Safe and therapeutic nursing care is a regular event that can become routine and tedious unless it can be defined and improved upon. MBO provides the nurse-manager and primary nurses with a vehicle to mark time. MBO turns infinity into interesting, often exciting, segments.

MBO asserts that line workers, in this case the primary nurses, are as important to the patients and to the organization as the nursing hierarchy. Nurses in upper-level positions enhance primary nursing, and primary nurses likewise enable the organization to achieve its standards and goals, such as cost containment, retrospective audits, clinical placements for nursing students, and good working relationships with other departments and the community at large.

When objectives become the framework and measuring stick by which people work, the impact of personality quirks and perceived status is greatly minimized.

The primary nurse with a master's degree works toward the same objectives as the primary nurse with a diploma.

> The concept of management by objectives helps in meeting many of the common problems arising in the management of professionals and other managers by allowing for measurement of the real contribution of these personnel and by giving definition to the shared goals of the organization and its people. Without giving up the aspect of personal risk-taking, defining goals stimulates coordination and teamwork (Palmer, 1971, pp. 17-8).

The MBO process requires more active efforts from administration and management to seek out and listen to advice from primary nurses regarding directions for the organization. If the administration wants all primary nurses to be certified in cardiopulmonary resuscitation but the primary nurses are complaining that the code (crash) cart equipment is outdated, both sides must listen to each other before a realistic goal can be determined. In MBO objectives should be set mutually, only after participation by everyone who would be influenced. In this way, "Managers are assured that their own organizational objectives will be met, since the combination of subordinate's objectives, when added up, should equal the manager's major objectives" (Labovitz, 1975, pp. 3-13).

The MBO process is analogous to the nursing process; the only difference is that MBO is the nurse-manager's nursing process applied to the whole staff rather than objective setting for the outcomes of an individual patient. Just as primary nurses determine realistic outcomes for primary patients through consultation, the nurse-manager develops and makes a commitment to accomplishment of unit objectives through consultation. Thus, the atmosphere of purposeful, meaningful activity is always present in a primary nursing unit.

The formal evaluation of primary nurses should also be made using the MBO process. What do the primary nurses want to accomplish professionally over the next months and how can the nurse-manager help them achieve it? Within an overall climate of MBO, primary nurses learn how to formulate their personal goals: "I want to learn more about chemotherapy." "I want to learn leadership skills by covering for the nurse-manager on vacation." "I want to force myself to speak up more in staff meetings." "I want to research the possibilities of joint mother-child admissions."

In primary nursing, MBO becomes more individualized—like a participative care plan for each nurse and each unit. MBO enhances autonomy. Each primary nurse becomes

> directly responsible for decisions in planning his job, and the plans provide a method of self-control. It is no longer necessary for his

supervisor to continually point out his problems; he is perfectly aware of how he is doing in relation to what he has said he will do. The subordinate becomes less dependent upon his supervisor and begins to view the relationship between them as supportive. This, in turn, leads to greater commitment of his efforts to meet organizational goals (Cain & Luchsinger, 1978, p. 37).

Setting new objectives and evaluating old ones on a three-month cycle is ideal for primary nursing management. Three months allows enough time for the necessary building activities, such as meetings, classes, and events, to take place. It is also long enough for common fluctuations, such as patient census and staff turnover, to occur, thus giving an accurate control when progress is being evaluated for feasibility and stability factors. It cannot be said too often that solid primary nursing can only be established over a long period of time. However, the time must be broken into workable segments, with a few specific goals stated for each time period.

Like any other aspect of primary nursing, setting and achieving objectives is most effective when the nurse-manager has administrative backing. The nurse-manager actually is the synthesizer of the goals that flow through that position:

Administration $\rightleftharpoons$ Nurse-manager $\rightleftharpoons$ Primary nurses
　　　　　Supervisor(s)

MBO is the easiest for everyone concerned, especially the nurse-manager, if the overall goal is the same, with portions of it delegated to the level that has the appropriate power and authority to deal with the task. To preserve sanity, the nurse-manager has to do a lot of talking with both sides of the nursing organization. The more that people are aware of and are in agreement with objectives, the easier it will be for the nurse-manager.

However, even if the whole department does not use MBO, a nurse-manager of primary nursing would still benefit from goal setting with the staff. This requires a great deal of formal and informal dialogue with primary nurses, followed by definite steps from the MBO process.

Step 1: The nurse-manager formulates a problem as precisely as possible. The problem does not have to relate directly to primary nursing because any improvement will also improve primary nursing. In fact any area of nursing service that the staff or the nurse-manager feels is not up to par should be considered.

Safety measures such as knowing CPR or familiarity with the side effects of medications, take priority over the more intellectual or interpersonal issues. However, the nurse-manager cannot underestimate how staff knowledge and attitudes can directly affect patient care negatively or positively. For instance, if primary nurses are preoccupied with anger at physicians, they may start making medication errors or avoiding the patients of those physicians. If a primary nurse does not understand adaptation to body loss, the nurse may omit important details about an amputee at the change of shift report.

In defining a problem, the nurse-manager must work with the staff to decipher the "chicken or egg" puzzle. The nurse-manager must also be free to seek consultation from the leadership team to determine the root of a problem. The nurse-manager must not be afraid to expose problems in an effort to do something about them.

Step 2: The nurse-manager then uses the objectivity and creativity of the individuals influenced by the problem to help determine a reasonable three-month goal which will indicate at least a partial resolution of the problem. For instance, the nurse-manager of a general surgical unit identifies that primary nurses feel guilty and frustrated when they cannot always give direct care to their primary patients and that the more senior nurses are talking of transferring to an ICU where they believe this frustration does not exist. The nurse-manager panics at the prospect of losing the senior staff and asks the clinical supervisor for some perspective. Together they narrow the issue to one that is typical of staffs with many new nurses and a core of senior nurses: the senior nurses were being assigned their own primary patients but were also helping the newer nurses with their critically ill primary patients. The staff agrees that this is the real problem and sets a three-month goal with the nurse-manager: "By March, Judy, Paula, and Nancy will be more competent with fresh post-op patients. Competency will be measured by their ability to take report from the recovery room nurse, to set up a schedule of treatments to be followed by all shifts, and to assess daily changes in condition. To do this Judy needs to spend a few days in the recovery room to follow patients through (nurse-manager will set this up with recovery room); Paula will take report on more primary patients who are just up from surgery and will be monitored by Fran (who would have less patients because she is working with Paula); and Nancy will work with the nurse-manager in assessing changes in her primary patients' conditions every day."

Step 3: Objectives must be written behaviorally with details about who, what, where, when, and how. Typical statements for managing primary nursing by objectives may include:

- For a pediatric unit where primary nurses do good assessments but need sophistication: "By April each primary nurse will have spent a few hours in a pediatric clinic to observe nurse practitioners doing assessments. In April we will meet to review our current assessment form for revisions based on our findings."

- For a VNA where nurses say they have more primary patients than they can handle: "In the next month, we will schedule a compulsory meeting to discuss the problem and detail a plan of action. Before the meeting, a committee of three will be selected to present the agenda. Results of the meeting will be reported by the nurse-manager at the regional meeting."
- For an inpatient psychiatric unit where primary nurses use terms in report and conferences that they do not understand or where there is no consistency of meaning: "Over the next three months: (A) Each primary nurse that presents at the primary nurse conference will include a term (discussed beforehand with the nurse-manager that applies to the patient to be presented: (B) The nurse-manager will ask for clarification of vague or misused terms as they come up in report: (C) the nurse-manager will put emphasis on behaviorally descriptive terms for patients rather than more abstract, psychological terms. The nurse-manager will read one different chart each day to assess progress.
- For the rehabilitation unit where new nurses are afraid they may hurt spinal cord injury patients by touching them: "By July each new nurse will be assigned and precepted on one spinal cord injury patient. The nurse-manager will ask a more senior nurse to give a presentation on the anatomy and physiology of spinal cord patients in the next month."

Consequently, MBO involves more than stating an objective in writing and crossing your fingers that it will be achieved. Writing an objective merely establishes a contract that necessitates further actions geared toward achievement. In other words, objectives are prescriptions for action.

Step 4: The nurse-manager should formulate two-tiered objectives that state where the staff should be and what the nurse-manager intends to do to help the staff meet that objective. For instance, the nurse-manager may say, "In the next month, each primary nurse must show evidence of short-term goals from one progress note to the next." In identifying any objective, the nurse-manager evolves the management role. This is true MBO because the manager's role hinges on the staff's achievements in a kind of interdependence. In the example, the nurse-manager has many options and can decide on one or more of the following:

- give a class or invite a speaker on short-term goals in patient care
- review one primary nurse's charting each day or week and discuss findings with the nurse
- ask one or more senior nurses to review charting by primary nurses
- get staff nurses involved in the concurrent auditing committees of the agency so that they can see their own clinic or unit strengths and weaknesses

- ask off-shift clinical supervisors to help check charts or to make suggestions that the staff document their interventions when they occur
- bring up the problem of primary nurses not reading each other's notes or not charting follow through on another nurse's primary patients
- suggest to the staff education department that there be more emphasis on short-term goal setting and charting in orientation classes
- suggest to the nursing department that it review present systems and formats for documentation because the current forms do not facilitate short-term goals
- xerox and post written material about short-term goals

The nurse-manager will need to determine carefully which approaches would be most effective. Even in a department where some objectives are assigned to a nurse-manager, the nurse-manager should have the freedom to select a means to the end:

> This allows administrative control without squelching initiative and independence. The manager's selection of means can be judged adequately by the results they produce. For example, if all head nurses are directed to give priority to reducing patient falls by fifty percent, each unit might be allowed to devise its own strategy, provided the objective is met. Clearly, where objectives can be quantified as in this sample (50%), it is easier to compare and evaluate strategies. In addition, successful strategies later can be combined and shared with others (Stevens, 1976, p. 61).

Step 5: Written objectives for a unit or clinic should be signed by all members of the leadership team and submitted to the associated nursing administrator. The nurse-manager should keep a copy and post a copy of the broad unit objectives for all primary nurses to use as a reference. In addition, the nurse-manager should add planned activities to a personal calendar—three months go by very quickly!

Step 6: If responsibility for achieving objectives is carefully delegated beforehand, evaluation of the objectives and those working toward them is simplified. The pressure of evaluation encourages nurse-managers to keep three-month objectives obtainable as well as progressive. Objectivity and kindness must be used in evaluating progress towards objectives. There are several rules of thumb that should be applied:

- Any approximation or improvement toward the objective should be acknowledged and commended. Sometimes maintaining the status quo during a period of severe organizational stress (financial cutbacks, community disaster, or labor union turmoil) is an achievement in itself!

- Any obvious achievement should be viewed as an accomplishment by all levels of nursing, but special recognition should be given to those who are involved in the activities listed with each objective.
- Falling short of an objective should be viewed as a shared responsibility, although individuals must be helped to identify their roles in the situation.
- If each person carried out the defined activity but the objective was not met, the objective itself must be analyzed. Perhaps the problem was not what it was thought to be, or maybe a crucial person was overlooked in the planning. A key person who is not part of the problem is definitely part of the solution.
- One unit or clinic can never be miles ahead of the whole agency because so much of nursing is interwoven, especially with centralized administration. Meeting objectives should be analyzed in the context of the entire organization.
- In measuring long-term projects (implementing primary nursing or developing triage in the emergency room), each three-month objective must be solidly met before moving into a new phase, although related objectives may be at various stages of completion; i.e. as shown in a PERT chart or other program performance plans. Each achievement is a building block for the next, and the blocks must be firmly established.
- All achievements contribute to the development of the staff group. Nothing is completely lost in the changes that a staff undergoes, and sometimes new ideas go underground until people are ready to work with them.

Objective setting and measuring can be an exciting process. The nurse-manager can enjoy planning strategies if there is openness and support from the leadership team, nursing administration, and the primary nurses. Continuous rapport and dialogue are essential in MBO. Nothing is as rewarding as meeting objectives and knowing that it could not have happened without committed, creative management. The nurse-manager's satisfaction is multiplied when shared with staff and supervisors, because they have some idea of the energy and efforts needed to manage by objectives.

Supervisory Support for the Nurse-Manager

In a majority of agencies, a first-line nurse-manager is only one member of a larger leadership team associated with a primary nursing unit. Because primary nursing involves round-the-clock activities and because the nurse-manager cannot always be present, the nurse-manager is dependent on colleagues to reinforce primary nursing. It is also imperative that the nurse-manager have an immediate supervisor who understands the elements of primary nursing and who actively supports the nurse-manager's role in primary nursing practice.

Supervisory support for the nurse-manager of primary nursing can be divided into two categories: support from the nurse-manager's immediate supervisor and support from off-shift supervisors who reinforce the policies, procedures, and objectives of the agency and the nurse-manager's unit. The immediate supervisor develops and evaluates the nurse-manager while the off-shift supervisor(s) assists the nurse-manager in promoting and evaluating the work of primary nurses and other staff members.

Although all the supervisory positions attached to a unit are complementary to the nurse-manager's role, each should have clear responsibilities in regard to primary nursing. Marram, Schlegel, & Bevis (1974) make a crucial point about the differences between the traditional supervisor's role and the requirements for primary nursing:

> No matter how the services of the hospital are arranged, one point is worth noting: if hospitals continue to use supervisors, they need to be readily accessible to nursing units as nursing care consultants for specific patient problems. Their accessibility is increased and their knowledge is better communicated if the number of units or specialties that they are assigned are kept to a minimum . . . (p. 105).

In other words, effective primary nursing requires more people in resource and staff support positions than have been used in most institutions. This may not increase budgeting allocations, but it definitely involves a rethinking of resources.

The director of nursing will have to examine closely administrative and clinical positions to determine which are most advantageous to primary nursing. For instance, if day and evening staffing is equalized, supervisory positions should also be equalized between the shifts. In other cases, the staff education instructor may be traded for a day-shift, acute care clinical supervisor, or a large unit with an assistant nurse-manager may need to be divided into two smaller units, each with a nurse-manager sharing the same immediate supervisor. The possibilities are endless.

The more authority and autonomy that is given to units and their supervisors, the fewer administrators are necessary. Therefore, for the best primary nursing, a department should be heavy in the middle with clinical supervisory and managerial positions filled by persons committed to primary nursing. These people will discover that when the other elements of primary nursing are in operation, their supervisory roles will be in a teacher/consultant mode rather than a "snoopervisor" position.

One of the main reasons nurses say that they have "primary" on weekdays but "team", or pot luck, on weekends and evenings stems from the myth that real nursing happens on the day shift. Staffing is done accordingly, and off-shift nurses and supervisors find themselves just getting by. Clearly, putting primary nurses and supervisors where and when they are needed most will create some upheaval as each agency defines what is meant by quality care given by professional nurses.

Role of the Nurse-Manager's Supervisor

Each agency defines the role of the person between the nurse-manager and nursing administration somewhat differently. In all cases, however, the person in that role must view development and evaluation of the nurse-manager as crucial to the maintenance and quality of primary nursing. In addition, the nurse-manager's immediate supervisor must have some influence in formulating the overall policies of the department so that interventions with top-level organization will enable the nurse-manager to reinforce primary nurses at the unit or clinic level.

The nurse-manager of primary nursing has an intensely dynamic responsibility that never ends but only shifts into new gears. Because the nurse-manager's engine is always running, refueling and a tune-up are needed occasionally. This support must come from a nursing supervisor, as opposed to the staff primary nurses, which would make the nurse-manager too dependent on them. Similarly, physicians should be colleagues of nurse-managers, and not used as their supervisors. Nursing as a profession must validate and refresh itself. The nurse-manager at the least needs a role model and at the most needs a mentor.

Although it would be ideal for the supervisor to be expert in the nurse-manager's clinical area and to have been a primary nurse or nurse-practitioner for an extended period of time, what matters most is willingness to be involved with issues that the nurse-manager needs to discuss and willingness to allow the nurse-manager to develop autonomy and skill.

There is a direct relationship between the way the supervisor works with the nurse-manager and the way the nurse-manager works with the staff. The supervisor sets the model for how problems should be dealt with, how staff should be confronted, how patients should be viewed, how administration should be perceived, and how the overwhelming emotions involved in health care delivery should be integrated.

Above all else, the nurse-manager's supervisor needs to be mature, secure, and responsive. The major responsibility of the supervisor as a representative of administration is to engage in dialogue designed to explore questions and find answers that are useful.

The extreme example of the nondialoguing supervisor is the highly defensive individual who seeks calm at all costs, even at the expense of a nurse-manager. This kind of person wears people out and outlives them all in their organizational lives. Such a supervisor

> tends to lead others to expectation, one she is unwilling to follow through on. She uses people and things to affirm herself. She deals with others in terms of their usefulness and function to her. For the monologi-

cal person, dialogue means an opportunity to convince others that she is right. She does not want to be disturbed; her mind is made up. She is a model of the dictum: "Don't confuse me with facts; my mind is already made up!"(McNally, 1975, p. 53).

This kind of person is dangerous to primary nursing, which tends to create new problems and needs of its own.

For a supervisor to be responsive to a nurse-manager, a supervisor needs the following qualities and needs a small enough span of control so they can put these qualities into action:

- daily face-to-face contact with the nurse-manager for as long as needed
- easy access to the supervisor by the nurse-manager
- provision of quick answers for high-priority decisions involving staffing or patient care emergencies
- familiarity and comfort with the clinical specialties covered by the nurse-manager
- objectivity about the unit or clinic and its personalities and special stresses
- experience and comfort with group dynamics
- belief in the advantages of primary nursing for patients and staff
- accurate evaluation of the nurse-manager's strengths and weaknesses, with emphasis on potential and confidence building
- honesty in issues between the supervisor and nurse-manager
- willingness to identify and accept differences in values
- attention to anticipatory management based on a mutual assessment of the nursing staff as a group and individually
- willingness to "go to bat" for the nurse-manager over issues involving nursing or hospital administration, interdisciplinary policies, or intrastaff conflicts
- skill in identifying staff learning needs and helping the nurse-manager develop, deliver, or locate appropriate programs

The nurse-manager of primary nursing should have a minimum of supervisors to report to—preferably only one. For this reason, it is probably most desirable for the supervisor to have administrative (line) responsibilities and to be clinically based. Indeed, this combination can be a very exciting, as well as streamlining organization. This arrangement minimizes red tape while providing the nurse-manager with a person who has advanced clinical knowledge. The supervisor can also offer objectivity on management problems that the nurse-manager may use in order to make difficult decisions. For this pairing to work well, each person must respect the other and must not be threatened by the other's competence or power.

The supervisor is both the translator of organizational policy to the nurse-manager and the translator of unit needs to nursing administration. The supervisor is both the buffer and the consultant. A good arrangement for primary nursing is "the supervisor who can supplement rather than replace the communication between the director and head nurse" (Marram et al., 1974, p. 103).

In addition, the supervisor must evaluate the nurse-manager on a regular basis. Evaluation is fair and accurate only if there is an objective evaluation tool which has heavy if not complete emphasis on primary nursing management and the nurse-manager and supervisor have honest, daily dialogue. If the nurse-manager uses MBO, the attainment of objectives will help to evaluate the nurse-manager's effectiveness and initiative. Without exception the nurse-manager's evaluation should be positive, aimed at personal and professional development.

Role descriptions for supervisors need to be consistent with the nursing department's organizational chart and with the goals of primary nursing. Activities specific to primary nursing should be incorporated into the formal evaluation of the supervisor's work. In this way, the supervisor will feel, and be, as accountable for the functioning and development of the nurse-managers who are supervised as the supervisor would like primary nurses to feel about their patient's care.

Off-Shift and On-Call Supervisors

If there are off-shift or on-call clinical supervisors involved in a primary nursing agency, they will need specific role descriptions for how to support primary nurses and their nurse-managers. If these supervisors do not understand or accept the concept of primary nursing, they can almost single-handedly impede implementation and development. If they understand and accept the concept but are not knowledgeable or skilled in their expanded roles, they can easily become the weak link in the nursing leadership chain.

It can never be assumed that supervisors will automatically know how to function, especially in relation to primary nursing. This is particularly true if a supervisor has never been a primary nurse. The predicament is compounded because off-shift or on-call supervisors are generally out of touch with the mainstream of meetings, classes, and activities regarding primary nursing due to their hours. This group of professionals has been the most neglected in primary nursing literature.

The truth is that all the responsibilities of the nurse-manager must be extended to off-shift or on-call supervisors in the nurse-manager's absence. In fact, the nurse-manager is often present on a unit less total time than other supervisors.

Off-shift and on-call supervisors must view their role in the light of primary nursing. Unfortunately, this new role is hard to imagine because these supervisors have been depicted as authoritarian administrators for decades. Finkelman (1976) describes the administrative aspects well:

Usually, she is called when there is a personnel problem, a staffing problem, or a question of policy or procedure. After solving the problem, she is expected to leave the unit. Frequently, she is also involved in getting equipment and supplies, and in housekeeping problems. In some hospitals on the evening and the night shifts, she becomes the pharmacist and the medical records librarian. Then there are the rituals of "getting report" and "rounds" which vary in purpose and quality. It is no wonder that with so many of these administrative functions, the supervisor must struggle with adaptation of the standards [1973 ANA Standards of Nursing Practice] which are clinically oriented while her administrative position is not (p. 31).

Primary nursing demands that off-shift and on-call supervisors, in concert with the director of nursing, require other departments to pick up nonnursing functions on a 24-hour basis. Otherwise the supervisors are not even administrators, they are the proverbial go-fors—go for this and go for that. As go-fers there is never time or energy to be involved in clinical assessments and staff development. Instead, each shift is spent maintaining the status quo.

Even when there are plenty of supervisors and other departments are consistently doing nonnursing tasks, off-shift and on-call supervisors need to get involved in the units which they cover. Anticipatory rather than crisis management is necessary. "The supervisor who is acutely alert to preventive action can stimulate and encourage her subordinate employees to be more sensitively attuned to significant situations that develop in their specialty areas" (Frazier, 1966, p. 24).

In revising the supervisor's role description to suit primary nursing, the Tufts-New England Medical Center Hospital developed the following criteria (Twyon, 1979):

1. Monitors primary nurse assignments to see that all patients are assigned within 24 hours of admission. If they are not, the Associate Nurse Leader [off-shift supervisor] will:
   a. Discuss the situation with the off-shift charge nurse who should relay it to the ANL.
   b. The night Associate Nurse Leader should tell the Nurse Leader [nurse-manager's supervisor] in AM report.
   c. Bring up persistent patterns in vertical meetings.
2. Help the staff evaluate whether the nursing care plan and treatments recommended by the primary nurse are appropriate and safe for the patient at that time. If deemed appropriate and safe, reinforces that the plan gets carried out.

3. Support nursing staff in changing the nursing care plan and treatments temporarily or permanently when necessary in the absence of the primary nurse.

4. Supports peer confrontation in resolving plans which are felt to be unsafe or inappropriate.

5. Participates in conferences and meetings about primary nursing and patient care on the assigned units and within the nursing department.

6. Actively brings up questions and findings about primary nursing in vertical meetings and to the primary nursing committee/consultant.

7. Works with senior staff nurses on permanent off shifts to develop them as leaders so that they can support primary nurses.

8. Contacts primary nurses directly through notes, messages, discussions and phone calls when necessary.

9. Refers questions about the care of specific primary patients to their primary nurses whenever possible.

10. When significant, identifies who the primary nurse is for a patient needing attention at intershift report between Nurse Leaders and Associate Nurse Leaders.

11. Assists primary nurses in identifying their individual learning needs.

12. Counsels primary nurses about their relationships with their primary patients.

Nurses who have been primary nurses and who can carry responsibility independently need to be recruited for the supervisory positions. However, they also must be comfortable with sharing territory with other supervisors. Above all they must be willing to be associates with the nurse-manager, collaborating at leadership team meetings, such as vertical meetings, and less formal occasions on matters of unit objectives and other facets of primary nursing.

Everyone in nursing leadership positions must believe that a primary nursing staff is only as good as the combined leadership behind it. ''Primary nursing care works for us because the values and structures underlying the practice are congruent with the values and goals of the medical center's leaders and clinicians'' (Smith, 1977, p. 2).

REFERENCES

Bartels, D., Good, V. & Lampe, S. The role of the head nurse in primary nursing. *Canadian Nurse,* March 1977, *73* (3), pp. 26-30.

Bower, K., and Twyon, S. *Performance appraisal of in-patient staff nurse.* Boston: Tufts-New England Medical Center, 1978.

Cain, C. & Luchsinger, V. Management by objectives: Applications to nursing. *Journal of Nursing Administration,* January 1978, *8* (1), pp. 35-38.

Frazier, L. Preventative management for supervisors. *Hospital Topics*, Nov/Dec 1966, pp. 21-9.

Finkelman, A.W. The standards of nursing practice and the supervisor. *Supervisor Nurse*, May 1976, 7 (5), pp. 31-4.

Labovitz, G. Importance of organizational objectives. *Motivational Dynamics*. Unit III. Minneapolis, Minn.: Control Data, 1975, pp. 3-5-3-15.

Marram, G., Schlegel, M. & Bevis, E. *Primary nursing – A model for individualized care*. St. Louis: C.V. Mosby, 1974.

McNally, M.J. The battered administrator syndrome. *Supervisor Nurse*, February 1975, 6(2), pp. 47-55.

Palmer, J. Management by objectives. *Journal of Nursing Administration*, January 1971, 1(1), pp. 17-23.

Peplau, H. Professional closeness. *Nursing Forum*, 1969, 8(4), pp. 342-360.

Schwartz, L. & Schwartz, J.L. *The psychodynamics of patient care*. Englewood Cliffs, N.J.: Prentice-Hall, 1972.

Smith, C. Primary nursing care—A substantive nursing care delivery system. *Nursing Administration Quarterly*, Winter 1977, 1(2), pp. 1-8.

Stevens, B. *First-line patient care management*. Wakefield, Mass.: Contemporary Publishing, 1976.

Taylor, M. & Abele, S. (Eds). Patient-focused psychiatric nurse consultant—New, expanding role developing at Tufts-New England Medical Center Hospital. *Nursing Pulse of New England*, January 10, 1977, 2(1), p. 1.

Twyon, S. *Role of the associate nurse leader in primary nursing*. Boston: Tufts-New England Medical Center, 1979.

Volante, E. Mastering the managerial skill of delegation. *Journal of Nursing Administration*, January-February 1974, 4(1), pp. 21-3.

Zander, K. Primary nursing won't work . . . unless the head nurse lets it. *Journal of Nursing Administration*, October 1977, 8(8), pp. 19-23.

Part II

"I Will Be Responsible for the Outcomes of the Nursing Care You Receive While Here"

Once primary nurses introduce themselves to their assigned patients and their families, they have begun a professional contract. As in any contractual agreement, primary nurses must know what they are expected to provide, and then be able to translate this information to their clients. This is an extremely difficult aspect of primary nursing because it implies liability.

Nurses generally view themselves as relatively free from liability (being sued), and indeed they are. So much of professional nursing is still done behind the scenes and out of the public eye. Even the laws that legitimize nursing are worded to make nursing activities hinge on physicians' dictums and licenses. The result is that nurses are still defining nursing, and until there is consensus about nursing, contracts with patients will be relatively nonspecific.

So, what should a primary nurse offer patients or their families? Answers like a good nursing care plan, safe treatments, or the nursing process have not sufficiently satisfied or impressed nurses or the public because they are too abstract. Even patient advocacy and patient education are relatively new services with which most people, and many nurses, are unfamiliar.

Nursing researchers have also had difficulty measuring actual results of primary nursing for patients. They have measured patient satisfaction levels, amount of documentation, and cost-effectiveness, but still scratch their heads in an attempt to grasp and quantify the essence of primary nursing (Primary Nursing Research Conference, Note 1).

The logical conclusion is that nurses are buried in the processes of patient care when they should also be attending to the outcomes of nursing care. When realistic outcomes of nursing care are delineated and consciously sought, nursing appropriately becomes results oriented. This is not to devalue the "hand on the fevered brow," but it is to assert that nurses have more to offer than a strong body and a big heart!

Defining what nurses mean by wellness and consciously working toward that goal through specific activities makes a primary nurse effective. Translating that work into the patient's framework makes the primary nurse an accountable professional.

Responsibility for the outcomes of nursing care involves several factors. First, primary nurses must be competent clinicians who have the skill to define outcomes and personally assist a patient toward them. Second, primary nurses are professionally accountable for those outcomes—successful or not. In other words, the primary nurse becomes known for results.

The results of primary nursing care are recorded and validated through audits of each nurse's documentation. Results are also recorded by the nurse-manager in preparation for the primary nurse's evaluation.

With these responsibilities, no primary nurse will feel confident in saying, "I will be responsible for the outcomes of the nursing care you receive while here," unless assured of supportive management and in-service education. Therefore, the nurse-manager must know about the systems and techniques for managing toward expertise in clinical practice and in the accountability of primary nurses.

REFERENCE NOTE

1. Primary Nursing Annual Resesarch Conference, North Central Regional Medical Education Center, Minneapolis Veterans' Administration Hospital Nursing Service, October 1978.

Chapter 3

Managing Toward Expertise in Clinical Practice

Expertise in the clinical practice of all staff primary nurses is a joy to see and to be part of as a peer or a nurse-manager. There is nothing in the world like primary nurses who are confident and competent. They are able to integrate many types of data, including their own feelings, and be responsive and effective with patients and colleagues. They are not threatened by the nurse-manager and are often comforting, complementary resources for the entire staff.

The nurse-manager who feels jealous of this description should not despair, because there are many things that can be done to recruit potential primary nurses and develop them to a high level of functioning. The nurse-manager actually has more power and influence than anyone else to develop clinically solid primary nurses.

Because not every RN is interested in or qualified for the role of primary nurse, the nurse-manager will need to use good interviewing techniques to attract and attain staff nurses. Their future expertise in clinical practice will be built upon the skills and attitudes they bring to the employment process.

Once the nurse is hired, the nurse-manager can advance the clinical capabilities of each primary nurse by establishing a "working alliance." The working alliance is a concept most familiar to psychiatric mental health nurses in their work with patients. It generally means that two people have agreed to work together using the potential of both persons to arrive at the goals of each person. In a nurse-patient alliance the relationship becomes an instrument of change; it is the prototype through which a patient can enact or verbalize concerns that are then evaluated together with the nurse. When either partner sways from active involvement, the other seeks a way to hold the partner accountable for the initial contract. The confrontation results in continued commitment to the alliance, a new contract, or termination of the relationship. Termination ideally occurs when both parties conclude that the goal of the working alliance is satisfactorily completed.

Similarly, a nurse-manager forms a working alliance with each primary nurse. Nursing management is almost completely an interpersonal phenomenon and should be approached with the principles of helpful, facilitative relationships in mind. This is not to say a nurse-manager should be the primary nurse's therapist! It does mean, however, that the nurse-manager must have a good working relationship with all staff members in order to secure optimal primary nursing.

Crucial to the nurse-manager's personality is "the ability to trust and be trusted. The staff must not only feel that the head nurse is competent but approachable, open and equitable. When the head nurse and staff work together in an atmosphere of open communication and mutual respect, the potential for excellent patient care and professional development is unlimited" (Bartels, Good, & Lampe, 1977, p. 28).

Managing toward expertise in clinical practice requires a working alliance at every phase of staff development. Three steps can ensure that primary nursing functions at its best in a unit or clinic: (1) nurse-manager control over interviewing and hiring of primary nurses; (2) a structured program for registered nurses new to a unit; and (3) flexibility and skill in clinical teaching aimed at development of competent thought and action. These steps are a three-pronged management approach to develop the clinical expertise of primary nurses.

INTERVIEWING AND HIRING PRIMARY NURSES

The nurse-manager must be given the authority and training to take an active role in interviewing and hiring primary nurses. This may involve several adjustments in traditional, centralized nursing departments. However, there are many benefits from giving the nurse-manager final accountability for the quantity and quality of nursing care:

- The nurse-manager knows best who can function well as a primary nurse in a particular unit and therefore makes a relatively low-risk choice.
- The nurse-manager has more of an investment in the new nurse.
- The nurse-manager is forced to define what is expected of a primary nurse.
- The nurse-manager owns the decision to hire, even if making the decision is stressful.
- The trust and respect shown by the administration increases the nurse-manager's authority with the staff.
- The staff can be included in interviewing and decision making.
- The candidate can see the unit or agency and sense its mood.
- The candidate gets an accurate picture of expectations and what the boss is like.

- Regardless of which department is recruiting, the nurse-manager makes the final decision.
- The nurse-manager knows from the beginning what the new nurse's strengths and weaknesses are.

Methods for Managing Prospective Primary Nurses

Health care organizations may need to change procedures for interviewing and hiring, but when coupled with some specific techniques and attitudes that may be used by the nurse-manager, these changes will greatly improve the chances for primary nurses to begin a working alliance.

Advertising

Attracting quality nurses to an interview is always a challenge and is often expensive. There does not seem to be any foolproof formula. Candidates may be motivated by salaries and benefits, nearby recreation areas, their family's needs, additional education, or a need for change.

Advertisements are usually placed in professional journals and should accurately describe the degree to which primary nursing has been implemented. An institution cannot honestly say it has primary nursing if only one unit has converted to it. False advertising is destructive to an institution's reputation as well as to the primary nursing movement.

In addition to journals, there are two other options. Regional seminars or conferences which are held for the purpose of continuing education can offer stimulating current topics or provide a new way to convey old material and thus put the institution in a good light. If they include theoretical or clinical material about the work of primary nurses, seminars and conferences will surely enhance an agency's reputation—no matter how good it is already.

The other option is to consider the future resources of student nurses. Undergraduate students are often eager to be part of a primary nursing system. When they have finished placement, the agency should know from student evaluation forms whether the student has an adeptness for certain kinds of nursing. Similarly, newly graduated master's degree students can be valuable employees, especially if they have done clinical nursing or research.

An agency may put some effort into arrangements with schools of nursing to place students in the clinical area. Of course, any level of nursing student is additional work for a nurse-manager. However, the time and energy that is invested in nursing students can bring excellent results, such as a waiting list of people who want to work on a certain unit with a certain nurse-manager! If time is devoted to building a working alliance with students, the nurse-manager can build up a good supply of potential candidates as well as a reputation among other students and their friends in nursing.

The agency's own nurses also act as recruiters through their personal contacts, who come to know whether the agency is a good place to work as a nurse. Because like attracts like, it is advantageous to have good primary nurses spreading the word. An institution must never underestimate the power of a good reputation.

Role of the Nurse Recruiter

The person responsible for initial contacts with candidates is designated the nurse recruiter, although not always a nurse. This individual must have good interpersonal skills, clear procedural guidelines, and a basic understanding of primary nursing.

The nurse recruiter sets the tone for future transactions with the applicant and therefore must be able to convey interest in the person. The nurse recruiter should also have the interviewing skill to screen candidates and know enough about primary nursing to answer basic questions.

Departmental guidelines must be clear so that the nurse recruiter will know how to process an applicant, especially in regard to arranging for an interview with the nurse-manager. The nurse recruiter should always be informed by a designated person if staff openings are expected in the coming weeks.

Each nurse-manager must have easy access to the nurse recruiter, because full staffing must be maintained to ensure effective primary nursing. The nurse-manager and recruiter should know about staff changes, and the nurse recruiter must know what qualities the nurse-manager looks for in primary nurses. The nurse-manager can be given a run down on the latest applicants and then share impressions of interviews with the nurse recruiter.

The role of the nurse recruiter is only that of a screener, and the nurse-manager should make all decisions about employment in consultation with the leadership team. A concerted, organized effort is necessary to keep a primary nursing staff at full force.

Preparation for the Employment Interview

Either the nurse-manager or the nurse recruiter should instruct the applicant to bring a sample of nursing documentation that shows the ability to organize thoughts into words. Sample care plans, progress notes, or nursing assessments are most indicative of logic and clarity of thought. New graduates as well as experienced nurses should have something they can use as samples. The nurse-manager should read the material ahead of time if possible with an eye for descriptive, problem-solving ability and with a focus on the nurse's attitude toward patients. The nurse-manager can tell a lot about an applicant by doing this.

The nurse-manager should read the application and any references before the interview in order to formulate questions and avoid wasting time on information already given. Gaps in the written application should be pinpointed for discussion at the interview. Thorough preparation will undoubtedly impress the prospective primary nurse with the forethought of the agency and the interest of the nurse-manager. "This place takes me seriously!"

The nurse-manager's interview should be a minimum of a half hour but not longer than an hour, although more time may be spent in a tour of the clinical area. The date of the interview should be arranged to ensure that the nurse-manager will be available.

Time spent in the unit should include:

- A private interview with the nurse-manager to begin a working alliance. It should take place in a fairly comfortable area, away from the hassle of daily nursing with all its interruptions.
- An opportunity for the applicant to observe primary nurses in action at report, rounds, or conferences and to speak with individual staff members. Allowing staff RNs to informally interview applicants alone or in a group gives them some input into the choice of candidate and fosters pride in the unit. The staff members are also able to offer the nurse-manager feedback on borderline applicants. Although this takes a little more time and planning, peer interviewing is fairer for the applicant and better for primary nursing.
- A chance to view the nurse-manager's skill and leadership style in action, since the applicant for a primary nursing position will be very interested in what a potential leader will be like.
- A chance to see some of the patients. The nurse who wants to work with burn patients but gets nauseated at the sight and smell of dead skin needs a chance to rethink choices. Potential primary nurses need an opportunity to reality test their notions about certain kinds of nursing. Likewise, the nurse applicant who offers to call the fire alarm code as the staff race to put out a fire stands a good chance of being hired!
- A chance to see nursing documentation in care plans and medical records.
- Time for the nurse-manager to get a summary of the applicant's experience and to ask and answer last minute questions. At this time, the nurse-manager can also clarify remaining steps in the hiring process and get a sense of whether the applicant should be seriously considered for a primary nursing position.

Attitudes That Affect Hiring

There are several questions that may cross the nurse-manager's mind during an interview. They are important questions to consider because they deal with the nurse-manager's expectations of future performance. These issues concern longevity, professional commitment, and qualifications of the primary nurse applicant.

What Can Be Fairly Expected from an Applicant?

Too much time can be spent convincing an applicant that the best benefits are offered at this institution. Primary nursing is a drawing card, but the recruiting emphasis is placed on salary, vacation time, and other benefits. Journal classifieds are full of promises or reminders of an area's cultural and recreational activities. Nursing is following the trend to meet everyone's needs, down to braces on teeth and tax-sheltered annuities. Thus, applicants tend to be preoccupied with what they will receive rather than what they have to offer the position.

Consequently, the nurse-manager should focus on what the applicant has to offer! Rather than sell the unit and the institution, the nurse-manager should expect to be convinced that the applicant is the right person for the position. Ideally, details on salary and benefits should be left to the nurse recruiter at the initial interview. The nurse-manager is then free to focus on the candidate's qualifications.

Even if staffing is low, the nurse-manager should not plead or be apologetic because that tone may pervade the working alliance with a future employee. The applicant should never be viewed as doing the nurse-manager a favor to come and work as a primary nurse. It is very important that the applicant knows that the nurse-manager is looking for a primary nurse, not a body to cover shifts. Respect and courtesy should be given all candidates, even the ones who will obviously not be hired. The experiences gained about primary nursing during the interview will give them valuable models for professional practice.

It is fair to expect that primary nurses will work hard for their salaries and benefits, or as the Ganongs state about a professional person, "to be known as a giver rather than a taker" (Ganong & Ganong, 1976, p. 29). Unfortunately, nurses traditionally have been exploited and abused by hospital administrations and other groups (Ashley, 1977). Nurses may even feel that they are more entitled than other groups of workers, and there has been abuse of the system, with false sick calls, strikes, and other strategies.

Fairness and honesty are needed in the relationship of the nurse-manager and primary nurses to avoid passive or immature reactions to unexpected work conditions. The boundaries of behavior should be made clear to candidates, such as whether compensatory time or overtime is used for special primary nursing situations, whether a time schedule can be arranged to allow for university courses, or what the limits to accountability and the legal protections for primary nurses are.

How Long Can a New Nurse Be Expected to Stay?

In nursing long-term employment often means a year at the same institution. However, high turnover rates are not conducive to primary nursing, which requires relative stability and rapid development of staff members. Although unable to reverse the trend of mobility and job-hopping alone, the nurse-manager can make a difference in a primary nurse's attachment to a unit and that difference starts with the employment interview.

The best way to cut down on turnover is to make it clear to applicants that the nurse is a person of worth in whom the institution is going to invest. A primary nurse's responsibility is unique in the profession, and a primary nurse cannot make work decisions as though that responsibility did not exist. Plans to take every summer off or to work only six months in an intensive care unit because it will look good on a resume are not acceptable in primary nursing.

Roughly, it is fair to expect a primary nurse to stay a time period equal to the time invested by the nurse-manager and institution in the primary nurse's professional development. Although the tallying of days and hours spent in orientation, preceptorship, continuing education, and evaluations seems absurd, the applicant must know that it takes a great deal of time and energy to become an effective primary nurse in each new clinical setting.

After a set period of time and good evaluations, the primary nurse may be allowed to transfer within the organization. Temporary transfer to broaden clinical expertise is a good way that the nurse-manager can conserve human resources. Some institutions have a formal rotation program between units and clinics for this purpose, while at other institutions the primary nurse may have to make a permanent transfer. Whether temporary or permanent, transfers should be thoughtfully undertaken in order to match individual and institutional needs as closely as possible.

In some ways, the situation in nursing education and employment has not changed much since the early part of the century: "To commit themselves to a profession was not expected of young women in nursing. The educational activities of hospitals benefited the public by preparing young women to be good wives and mothers, or so it was thought" (Ashley, 1977, p. 89). Primary nursing is the opposite of this view because to be an effective primary nurse entails remaining long enough in one place to gain solid expertise in complex skills. The nurse-manager's belief in the value of long-term employment will have a big influence on the whole primary nursing staff, beginning with their first contact.

Is It Fair to Expect a Commitment from a 22 Year Old?

Gail Sheehy (1976) in *Passages* refers to the time between ages 22 and 28 as the "trying twenties," when people pull up roots and try to learn what they do not want to do in order to master what they feel they are supposed to do:

> The tasks of this period are as enormous as they are exhilarating: To shape a dream, that vision of one's own possibilities in the world that will generate energy, aliveness, and hope. To prepare for a life work. To find a mentor if possible. And to form the capacity for intimacy without losing in the process whatever constancy of self we have thus far

assembled. The first test structure must be erected around the life we choose to try (p. 85).

Acknowledgment of the energies and conflicts of persons in this age group can make a great difference in the nurse-manager's ability to engage nurses in the challenge of primary nursing. The professional growth of nurses is facilitated when issues of inner growth are addressed. Although a nurse-manager cannot mold the work situation to individual needs, it is possible to channel the energies of young nurses and to offer them the challenge of mastery and commitment in primary nursing.

What Are Nurses Seeking from a Role?

Why do young nurses have difficulty staying committed to one place? Possibly they lack a mentor to help them resist the temptation to move on once they have mastered particular skills. Nurses seem to plunge themselves into situations where they feel insecure. As soon as they know basic medical-surgical skills, they want to work in an ICU. As soon as they have ten primary patients, they are ready to be nurse practitioners. Although some anxiety is necessary for learning and excitement, the high national turnover rate suggests that nurses either get bored very easily or are frightened by high degrees of competence.

In primary nursing the nurse-manager is the most readily available person to be a mentor.

Nurse-manager = Role model + Working alliance = Nurse-mentor

The nurse-mentor can help primary nurses balance the urge to be secure with the urge to be without security in their profession.

As a mentor the nurse-manager can offer advice and validation when primary nurses consider career options. Primary nurses often need a guide through the politics of nursing, ideally a concerned nurse-mentor who encourages self-examination. A mentor is a nurturer, a believer in abilities, and a validater of experiences.

An intelligent new graduate applying for a primary nurse position spoke excitedly about a professor from whom she had learned a great deal about nursing. The nurse-manager made a mental note that this nurse would have to shift mentors in order to stay involved in the new position. The primary nurse did well and eventually shifted the mentor role to the nurse-manager who enabled her to stay far beyond initial mastery of primary nursing skills. Otherwise, she may have joined the majority of persons who "skip through their twenties from one trial job and one limited personal encounter to another, [creating] a transient pattern" (Sheehy, 1976, p. 87).

When interviewing prospective primary nurses, the nurse-manager should consider the nature of a possible relationship: "Is this the kind of nurse I want to be a mentor for?" Nurses should be able to turn to other nurses for mentor support, as well as to the nurse-manager. However, the nurse-manager should keep this question in mind when considering the validity of managerial expectations of primary nurses: "Almost without exception, the women I studied who did gain recognition in their careers were at some point nurtured by a mentor" (Sheehy, 1976, p. 132).

Can a New Graduate Be a Primary Nurse?

Debates run high about whether a graduate fresh out of basic education is capable of being a primary nurse. Supporters contend that:

- primary nursing is an extension of the student nurse's case assignments
- new graduates have the most energy and idealism for the undertaking
- new graduates have had classes about primary nursing
- it is easier to form good attitudes and work habits with new graduates

The arguments against state that:

- a new graduate is not prepared or willing to do technical things as basic as counting IV drips
- new graduates are not ready to be in charge and manage an off shift, so how can they be in charge of several primary patients
- new graduates do not know the system
- new graduates do not know enough about specialties

The best way to resolve these arguments is to use the concept of structure. As defined previously, structure is a prearranged framework that sets the outside limits and expectations for behavior. If an institution's structure is firm and consistent with the mainstream of beliefs, it will be an effective guide for those within the structure.

It seems most practical for an institution to utilize new graduates as primary nurses as soon as possible. A new graduate is certainly capable of learning the primary nurse's role, if that role is reinforced at all levels.

What Is the Best Way to Approach an Interview?

During the interview two essential events must occur: information is shared and the working alliance is established. Both the nurse-manager and the applicant will have instinctive responses as information is exchanged. The nurse-manager will use both types of input as clues about the applicant and as a guide for the interview. Throughout the interview, both individuals will make judgments about the other, focusing on whether the working alliance will be more permanent than the duration of the interview.

It is difficult to define who might be a potential primary nurse. The applicant should show proficiency in application of the nursing process, potential to be assertive rather than aggressive or passive, evidence of trust and respect for former nursing colleagues, and a degree of perseverance and initiative.

Interviewing Techniques

John Drake (1972) suggests four areas of information that should be gained from the interview:

1. intellectual skills and attitudes
2. personality strengths and limitations
3. knowledge and experience
4. motivational characteristics (interests, aspirations, energy level)

The foremost question in the nurse-manager's mind should be, "Can this person be a primary nurse?" Combining the Drake method with the nurse-manager's needs, the following questions might be posed. They should be asked in a logical manner and the answers clarified along the way.

The questions should not be asked in a quizzing, interrogating manner, but rather as an honest attempt to get to know the applicant and establish even a temporary relationship. If the nurse is not hired or takes another position, the nurse-manager has given the applicant the interest and respect of a fellow nurse, something sorely lacking in the profession.

Motivational Characteristics

What makes you interested in this position?
What do you like about primary nursing?
What goals do you have that require a change in jobs?
What kinds of patients make you feel the most satisfied? The most frustrated?
Why are you looking for a staff position if you have a master's degree?
What are your plans if you don't get this position?
Would you want the job even if there are no leadership positions available in the near future?

Knowledge and Experience

Will you please tell me about your work with a primary patient (or patient you had as a student)?
Do you do any activities outside of nursing that have helped you be a better nurse?

Describe a patient or family for whom you felt particularly useful in teaching.
What do you know about patient advocacy?

Intellectual Skills and Attitudes

Review the writing sample, requesting the applicant to explain certain points.
How do you think the recovery room and ICU may be similar?
Please describe a crisis either in nursing or another experience that you think you've handled well.
What are the nursing skills you are proudest of?
How would you evaluate what you saw here today?
What helps you integrate theory with practice?

Personality Strengths and Limitations

What do you think would be your biggest adjustment in coming here?
A lot of our patients die or are readmitted. How would that be for you?
What kinds of supports have been most useful to you in the past?
"What would you say there is about yourself that could be improved or strengthened?" (Kowalski, 1975, p. 46).
How have you related to other RNs, nursing aides, your current manager?
Who has taught you the most about nursing?

Common Pitfalls to Avoid

- The interviewer talked too much, more than half of the time, and did not listen enough.
- The interviewer jumped to conclusions on the basis of inadequate data that were never validated.
- The interviewer consistently led the applicant into giving the desired responses to questions.
- The interviewer failed to apply the facts to possible on-the-job situations.
- The interviewer became emotionally involved in philosophical issues rather than remaining neutral or presenting a personal experience for the applicant to expand upon.
- The interviewer revealed management problems with current identified staff members.
- The interviewer unknowingly reversed the focus of the interview so that the applicant is giving the interviewer support.
- The interviewer began to oversell the position to a desired applicant. In this situation the interviewer may make promises that cannot be kept.
- The interviewer found out the other places the applicant is interviewing and tears them down rather than participating in an objective comparison.

- The interviewer offered false hope or prolonged saying no to someone not being seriously considered.
- The interviewer was overly impressed by a stellar resume and fails to ask the usual questions or go through the usual channels.
- The interviewer got into a one-upmanship competition by asking the applicant technical or theoretical questions that the applicant could not possibly answer.
- The interviewer refused to change preconceived notions about the applicant rather than listening to the data.
- The interviewer asked questions that do not pertain or are illegal to ask without the applicant's permission, such as are you in therapy or are you planning on getting pregnant in the next six months.
- The interviewer identified excessively with the applicant's situation ("I'm not appreciated enough," "the doctors keep me from doing the kind of nursing I believe in") and failed to compare the applicant objectively with other applicants.
- The interviewer was too pressured by low staffing or current staff problems and sought the applicant who was most moldable and compliant rather than a more challenging person.
- The interviewer, so disheartened by the loss of a valued staff nurse, sought someone who was exactly like the lost nurse.
- The interviewer forgot to give the applicant time to formulate new questions based on new information.

Hiring Primary Nurses

To hire a candidate as a primary nurse, the nurse-manager must know the proper channels for making the decision official. The nurse-manager may want to keep some people on hold until a first choice applicant decides between two agencies. Occasionally, the nurse-manager may want to recall someone for a second interview or negotiate certain aspects of employment.

In any event, the nurse-manager must juggle personnel so as to not leave gaps in the staffing quota. Sometimes, the risk of waiting for a particular applicant is necessary. However, the nurse-manager should decide when there are openings and how long to wait for an applicant's decision.

By making the final choice, the nurse-manager has a responsibility that few people would enjoy—having to select between qualified applicants. Hiring rarely becomes easier with time, for the dynamic nurse-manager becomes involved with each applicant. Therein lies the strength and the drawback of building a working alliance with staff, beginning with the initial interview! The benefits, however, are definitely felt with the nurses who are hired. And the nurse-manager is clearly established as a leader with the authority that goes with the responsibility of managing primary nursing.

ORIENTING PRIMARY NURSES

No matter how much education or experience a registered nurse has, beginning as a primary nurse in a new area requires an organizational structure that includes: (1) predetermined behavioral goals and (2) an individualized precepted way to obtain the goals. The roles of the nurse-manager and the clinical supervisors will have to be intertwined with the function of the staff education department and unit teachers according to these two components in orienting primary nurses.

Rather than propose massive changes in the way nursing departments have delegated responsibilities for incorporating new RNs, the focus here will be on the basic elements needed to orient a nurse to the primary nurse's role. As agencies convert to primary nursing, they will have to adjust their orientation mechanisms to the needs of new nurses and clinical units. Some of the traditional concepts about how to orient professionals need thoughtful revision.

Orienting primary nurses must be a shared responsibility between orienters and orientees. Orientation to the institution is both a socialization mechanism and a cognitive experience. Teaching and learning are active processes that require responsiveness from the instructors and the new nurses alike.

Orienting primary nurses should be a model or paradigm for the thoughtful, individualized approach the nurses will eventually take with primary patients and families. To this end, there must be a concerted effort on everyone's part to avoid the knots of teaching and learning so vividly described by Laing (1970):[1]

> There is something I don't know
>   that I am supposed to know.
> I don't know *what* it is I don't know,
>   and yet am supposed to know,
> And I feel I look stupid
>   if I seem both not to know it
>   and not know *what* it is I don't know.
> Therefore, I pretend I know it.
>   This is nerve-wracking
>   since I don't know what I must pretend to know.
> Therefore, I pretend to know everything.
> I feel you know what I am supposed to know
>   but you can't tell me what it is
>   because you don't know that I don't know what it is.
> You may know what I don't know, but not
>   that I don't know it,

---

[1]From KNOTS, by R.D. Laing. Copyright © 1970 by the R.D. Laing Trust. Reprinted by permission of Pantheon Books, a Division of Random House, Inc.

And I can't tell you. So you will have to
tell me everything (p. 56).

To avoid knots in an orientation program, there can be no face-saving maneuvers from anyone. Tendencies toward competition or one-upmanship should be avoided. Learning to be a primary nurse in a new environment is taxing enough without the added pressure of unduly needing to prove oneself. New people can be very easily traumatized in the early stages of professional development, acquiring scars that do not go away. An agency's efforts to avoid humiliation and mental injury will go a long way to bring about the confidence to develop clinical expertise.

On the other side, new nurses should not expect to be spoon-fed. An orientee's attitude about learning the ropes of an agency will be influenced by previous learning experiences, especially nursing school, as well as by basic personality style. Newly graduated nurses constantly, and often vociferously, challenge an institution to meet their ideals. Experienced nurses who have been angry or disappointed at former jobs often dare the new agency to be different. These phenomena are particularly true when orientees hope to be ideal primary nurses in ideal organizations.

The stresses of orientation often contribute to ridiculous mistakes by adequately educated nurses. Two errors made on an actual medication test point up an orientee's inability to problem solve and be practical during stress:

Quinidine 0.5 Gm IM is ordered. Each cc = 80 mg.
You give _____ cc. Orientee's answer: 625 cc!

Demerol 35 mg IM is ordered. Each cc = 50 mg.
You give _____ cc. Orientee's answer: 1750 cc!

How can such a person be expected to be a primary nurse? Legitimate question.

First, orientees should be encouraged to relax, because breaking in can be designed as a shared experience. Secondly, orientees have an obligation to help themselves by:

- being active, adult learners, energetically involved in the process of orientation
- demanding to learn what it takes to do the job well
- asking for clarification of expectations
- looking for positive qualities of the agency
- focusing on what can be contributed rather than constantly measuring what is received
- ceasing to pretend to be different than they really are

Orientation by Objectives (OBO)

Orienting primary nurses can be organized in the same fashion as management by objectives; that is, with predetermined behavioral objectives to be met by the new primary nurse within certain time periods. Optimally, there should be two sets of objectives: one for half-way through the probationary period as defined by the agency and one to mark the successful conclusion of the probation period. This practice necessitates a structure of orienters and orientees discussing progress before the person becomes a full-fledged primary nurse.

The major objectives should be consistent throughout the institution and should be formulated by key leadership personnel. Universal objectives may include areas such as medication administration, documentation, patient teaching, shift charge responsibilities, or professional attitude. In this way, standards of the nursing department become incorporated in each primary nurse's practice.

Similarly, each specialty area may develop secondary or contributory objectives. For instance, a new nurse in an ambulatory clinic may need to learn about the surrounding VNAs in the first few weeks in the clinical area, whereas a primary nurse in neurology would need to learn the principles of subarachnoid hemorrhage precautions. On the other hand, both neurological and psychiatric primary nurses may be expected to witness a CAT (computerized axial tomography) scan before their probationary period is finished.

Some objectives acknowledge that there are certain guideposts that mark events which all nurses must pass. Examples of this type of objective are (Bower & Twyon, 1979):

1. Develops a relationship with the patient that is professional (i.e. evaluates patient needs, provides for them to be met, and evaluates effectiveness of that interaction) and not based totally on a social nature.

2. Has done a CVP using correct technique, can give the normal range for CVP and what alterations might mean.

3. Can demonstrate the components of a good report:
   a) pre-organized systematic approach
   b) can paraphrase problems of previous eight hours
   c) summarizes present goals and guidelines for next shift
   d) communicates extra-departmental plans for the patient
   e) avoids socializing and interruptions.

4. Continues to develop and demonstrate skill in caring for the acutely ill surgical patient, concentrating on the area of particular difficulty which was encountered during the previous four weeks.

However, there is a definite need to phrase most objectives according to the concept of primary nursing and the timing required to meet the objectives. Objectives that specifically address primary nursing may read like:

- promptly introduces self to primary patients after receiving the assignment.
- sets appropriate long-term goals for each primary patient which are consistent with initial and on-going nursing assessments.
- willingly presents primary patients at conferences when requested to or when the need for advocacy demands it.
- by the end of six weeks, has admitted three primary patients.
- by the end of two months, has worked with the family of a dying primary patient.
- by the end of three months, has made one home visit to a primary patient.
- by the end of four months, has attended a class or seminar that would increase knowledge about the nursing care of the kinds of primary patients which are the most confusing to this orientee.
- by the end of three months, has completed discharge planning for two primary patients and written their nursing referrals.
- by the end of three months, audit reports are positive for documentation on one primary patient.
- by the end of three months, has formed good beginning working relationships with the physicians involved with each primary patient.

It should be obvious that efforts by both the orienters and orientees are needed to meet the objectives determined by the nursing department. A list cannot be handed to the new primary nurse without explaining what mechanisms and people will be available to help meet the objectives. The nurse will need to know whether the buck stops in staff education, with the nurse-manager, or with some as yet unfamiliar resource.

In orientation by objectives, nothing can be taken for granted. The primary nurse who knows that by the end of six weeks the objective of ''knowing when to send urine to the lab for culture and sensitivity readings'' must be met should know how to learn that function. Who is responsible for teaching?

Finally, who is responsible for evaluating the primary nurse's achievement of orientation objectives? The answer depends on how the program is structured. It is possible for some people to evaluate some aspects and other people to discuss particular objectives with the new nurses. Either way, primary nurses in orientation need to be encouraged to work actively on their objectives with leadership personnel. If the objectives are realistic and consistent with primary nursing, the new nurse will have a meaningful, goal-directed experience in orientation.

A Preceptorship Program

Without doubt, the difference between a mediocre and a dynamic orientation which addresses the many levels on which people learn, is intensive one-on-one interaction. Regardless of past experience, all new nurses benefit from a formal preceptorship program. The role of primary nurse cannot be learned alone or on a homework basis.

Because of the highly specialized role enactments of a primary nurse, primary nursing cannot be learned in a classroom. Furthermore, it cannot be learned in a specific length of time because of its interpersonal nature and the constant pressure to improve skills. Therefore, primary nursing must be learned in the unit where the nurse will be working, and the learning experience must be augmented by an assigned buddy or preceptor.

The preceptor must be a person who is available to the new nurse most of the time. The preceptor usually should not be the nurse-manager. The program works best if the preceptor is a senior staff nurse who can rotate to off shifts with the primary nurse. Precepting stimulates the nurse-preceptor and provides the novice with ready role models on a peer level. The nurse-manager will need to work with each staff preceptor to coordinate a new nurse's program.

Coordination

Exactly when a primary nurse should begin preceptorship is an individual decision for each agency. However, if primary nursing is the method for delivering nursing care, new nurses must be primary nurses from the beginning of orientation. Otherwise, primary nursing will be accurately perceived as something in addition to "real" nursing, rather than as the vehicle for professional nursing.

Therefore, internships, orientation units (Armstrong, 1974) or other programs must be carried out in the context of primary nursing. Not to do so would defeat the whole purpose of developing nurses within a role. Expecting new nurses to be primary nurses while they are learning about the agency, disease entities, and technical skills is the best way to teach. The primary patient becomes the anchor by which related tasks are learned. This creates a sensible, orderly, patient-focused medium for learning.

Assigning primary patients to new nurses is a slower orientation than having the orientee pass a checklist of tasks. However, the learning is more in-depth and helps the new nurse to integrate why things are done along with techniques for doing them. In the long run, patient-based orientation is more solid and organized than traditional methods of clinical orientation.

A solid primary nursing preceptorship within the first several weeks of orientation makes a difference in an individual's nursing as well as in the long-term quality of care on the unit. For this reason, the length of the probationary period must reflect the primary nursing preceptorship. In an agency where the probationary period is three months and the first six weeks marks the first set of objectives, the preceptorship program might be coordinated as follows:

- The nurse-manager assigns a preceptor and a primary patient to the new nurse based on the new nurse's previous experience and immediate learning needs.
- The orienting RN is assigned one primary patient sometime between weeks two and six.
- Accountability for patient care can be shared with the preceptor until a designated point when it is shifted to the primary nurse. (Recommendation: Orienting nurses should not be assigned a full case load of primary patients until weeks 7 through 12.)

Role of the Preceptor

The preceptor:

- makes a verbal contract with the orienting nurse, identifying mutual role expectations
- ensures that the orienting nurse meets the basic objectives of primary nursing
- explains the role of the primary nurse, nurse-manager, and other key personnel in relation to the new nurse's specific primary patients
- fosters autonomous practice by familiarizing the new nurse with skills at coordinating a multidisciplinary approach, introducing appropriate members of the multidisciplinary team, directing the nurse to resource literature and personnel
- reviews methods and evaluates each element of the nursing process as carried out by the orienting RN:
  assessment
  definition of problems and goals
  plan of care via nursing orders
  delivery of care
  communication of care via documentation, conferences, report, rounds
  evaluation of short- and long-term goal achievement
  revision of care plan
- communicates with the unit's leadership for input and feedback about the new nurse's practice of primary nursing, appropriate patient assignments, final evaluation, special needs (Recommended: Preceptor keeps anecdotal notes.)
- in conjunction with the nurse-manager, contributes to the evaluation of the new nurses' practice of primary nursing at the completion of the orientation program (adapted from Bower and Twyon, 1979)

It should be stated that the firmer an agency is with primary nursing, the clearer it will be what kind of orientation facilitates primary nursing. Even classes on the nursing process or the psychodynamics of patient care are only as useful as the degree to which they can be applied at the unit or clinic level. The stronger a unit is in regard to primary nursing, the easier and quicker it will be to orient new nurses to the role. The best way to help new primary nurses achieve success in the role and begin contributing to the agency is to invest in a total orientation program which includes objectives and preceptorship.

REDEFINING CLINICAL TEACHING

To manage toward expertise in the clinical practice of all primary nurses, the nurse-manager and others involved in staff development will need to redefine clinical teaching in relation to the new demands on primary nurses. Although primary nurses will be learning from many sources, the nurse-manager has greater influence than anyone else in creating an environment in which nurses can grow.

> The art of teaching is essentially the management of these two key variables in the learning process—environment and interaction— which together define the substance of the basic unit of learning, a "learning experience". The critical function of the teacher, therefore, is to create a rich environment from which students can extract learning and then to guide their interaction with it so as to maximize their learning from it (Knowles, 1970, p. 51).

In redefining the clinical teaching of primary nurses, the nurse-manager must follow two principles. (1) Primary nurses must be treated as adult learners, and therefore, traditional approaches used to teach children must be changed. Because primary nursing requires nurses to be committed to patients, teaching techniques must put them in control of when and what they need to learn. Malcolm Knowles' (1970) attention to the education of adults (andragogy) is directly applicable to the self-directed inquiry which is necessary for high level primary nursing:

> The important implication for adult-education practice of the fact that learning is an internal process is that those methods and techniques which involve the individual most deeply in self-directed inquiry will produce the greatest learning. This principle of ego-development lies at the heart of the adult educator's art. In fact, the main thrust of modern adult-educational technology is in the direction of inventing techniques for involving adults in ever-deeper processes of self-diagnosis of their own needs for continued learning, in formulating their own objectives for learning, in sharing responsibility for designing and carrying out their learning activities, and in evaluating their progress toward their

objectives. The truly artistic teacher of adults perceives the locus of responsibility for learning to be in the learner; he conscientiously suppresses his own compulsion to teach what he knows his students ought to learn in favor of helping his students learn for themselves what they want to learn. *This is not to suggest that the teacher has less responsibility in the learning-teaching transaction, but only that his responsibility lies less in giving ready-made answers to predetermined questions and more in being ingenious in finding better ways to help his students discover the important questions and the answers to them themselves* (p. 51).

(2) Nurses have valuable things to learn from other nurses, and they cannot rely on other professions to teach primary nurses what they need to know. Other disciplines can supplement primary nursing knowledge, but the nurse-manager and others must provide primary nursing know-how.

For example, the nurse-manager may love to send primary nurses to multidisciplinary conferences or seminars, but should not forget that primary nurses need teachers who are also nurses. A nurse-teacher can readily discuss the world the way nurses see it and put emphasis on the practical aspects of providing health care.

Opportunities for Teaching Primary Nursing

Primary nursing requires constant staff development at the unit or clinic level. The nurse-manager needs to be alert to the many opportunities for teaching primary nurses how to use the nursing process to the fullest. This entails teaching nurses how to integrate clinical data with nursing approaches.

Clinical expertise involves the ability to move easily and appropriately between a flood of disorganized information and a stream of organized action. Primary nurses need to learn how to function on several levels at the same time so that they can productively apply their ongoing assessments in constructive action.

The two main opportunities for teaching the complex science of primary nursing are spontaneous feedback during informal situations and primary nursing conferences (supervision), because they are clinically-based forums.

Informal Clinical Teaching

As every nurse-manager is aware, most teaching opportunities occur on the spot. A nurse-manager with a staff of primary nurses will find much of what used to be considered teaching was really telling staff what was expected. "Ms. S will probably need an enema today." "Don't let Mr. R out of bed until you check his neuro signs." With primary nursing, each nurse should have these particulars in mind and will be transferring them to other staff who may be caring for those primary patients. The nurse-manager's teaching role then becomes one of validating a primary nurse's plans and reports of patient care. Primary nurses will look to the nurse-manager for recommendations, reassurance, and praise, rather than messages and orders. Thus, the informal clinical teaching role of a nurse-manager in primary nursing resembles more that of a consultant from whom feedback is requested.

Feedback is the process of giving and receiving current data and opinions so they can be applied to future situations of a similar nature. A nurse-manager expends the most energy giving problem-solving feedback to primary nurses. The feedback can be a response to action already taken or action planned for the future. Unlike formal teaching, feedback is needed when it is requested. Besides being highly effective, immediate and informal feedback has certain advantages over more formal techniques:

> Problems are dealt with at the time they are happening; support can be given when it is most needed; subordinate anxiety can be alleviated by knowing that the job is being done according to design. Furthermore, employees often trust informal feedback more than formal communication because they feel that the communication is spontaneous and is given without the pressure of an organizational policy (Veninga, 1975, p. 41).

Constructive feedback gives the primary nurse information without detracting from a sometimes shaky sense of accountability for the primary patient's care. Ideally, all feedback from a nurse-manager should be of a consultative kind, reflecting the outlook that most people have inner resources with which to tackle new and confusing situations.

In situations that are life-threatening to patients, potentially dangerous to a nurse's life or career, or in violation of legal and/or institutional guidelines, the nurse-manager has to make unilateral decisions or give very definite orders. Otherwise, questions such as "What do you think is going on?" or, "I think you're missing a certain piece of data from the physical therapist," are more useful and often more accurate than telling a primary nurse what should be done.

The nurse-manager would do well to be aware that a primary nurse's request for feedback may be a mature way of asking for help in the clinical area. Help may require more knowledge or else confirmation that the primary nurse is capable of carrying out a certain plan with a patient or with another health care professional. Before responding to a request for feedback, the nurse-manager should think a moment about what kind of feedback is being requested. The immediacy of feedback should be tempered so that an appropriate response is given.

The subject of feedback always raises the related question of clinical responsibility. A primary nurse's request for feedback may be an unintentional maneuver to share or remove some responsibility for an action or decision. "What do you think," may be a way of saying "I'm afraid, so if I do what you want, then I am doing it on your say so, not my own." In these situations, the nurse-manager should avoid accepting any implied responsibility. Feedback should be given to increase the primary nurse's resources or confidence. To do this successfully, the nurse-manager has to accept the possibility that the primary nurse will not follow the nurse-manager's guidance.

A nurse-manager's natural inclination is to say "we did it" if things go well, and "you did it" if they go wrong. It is a fine line where individual action ends and group responsibility begins. However, when asked for feedback, the nurse-manager should give it with the attitude that the primary nurse may use it or not based on personal evaluation. Thus, the primary nurse is always individually accountable, no matter who gives feedback—solicited or otherwise.

Meanwhile, the nurse-manager should put energies into increasing each primary nurse's evaluative (data-processing) skills. This can be accomplished by offering feedback that expands the understanding of a clinical situation rather than giving advice on the solution to the problem. When primary nurses feel that the nurse-manager is an approachable, trustworthy consultant, their independence will grow as they continue to consult the nurse-manager for problem solving.

Primary Nursing Conferences

Primary nursing conferences or presentations provide group feedback. Recommendations for structuring the presentations are discussed in Chapter 1. Here, attention will be directed to the conference's uses as a forum for teaching toward clinical expertise.

Primary nursing conferences are directed, intensive learning experiences aimed at assisting primary nurses in work with their patients. They are an optimal way for both the nurse presenting and the nurses listening and responding to learn primary nursing. They are also an excellent way for the nurse-manager to learn about a primary nurse's work without being present when nurses are with their primary patients. Many levels of learning occur during a 20- or 30-minute session with a group of primary nurses and the nurse-manager. The nurse-manager must be in attendance to accentuate the conference's importance for the conduct of expert primary nursing.

For the primary nurse, frequent conferences are an opportunity to present professional work to others for review of the theoretical foundations and the actions taken in regard to patient care. The opportunity to review work must take place on a time-out, noncrisis, regular basis so that total attention can be given the primary nurse.

The role of the nurse-manager in primary nursing conferences is that of a tutor from the Greek classical period—someone who listens and asks questions that help people understand difficult ideas. This role is distinct from the duties and goals of the management role. As can be seen in the comparison in Table 3-1, both roles are a means of achievement and control, although the focus varies.

Table 3-1 Comparison of the Duties and Goals of Management and Teaching

Aspects of clinical nursing	Management duties and goals	Clinical teaching
Tasks	Assigning people and methods	Means of collecting observations and data to increase understanding of the patient and to stimulate new tasks
Time	A crisis orientation limited to shifts and usually viewed as an enemy	A flexible orientation determined by patient needs
Patients	People who need things done for or with them	People who are interesting and who present challenges that can be met through knowledge and inquiry
Staff tension	Relief via policies, benefits, personnel substitution, task completion, and sharing responsibility	Relief via group perspective and problem solving
Teacher role	Feedback on immediate problems—learning may be needed before learner is ready	Learning directed through identification of needs, discussion, peer collaboration, timing of suggesting—learner ready to learn
Dissemination of information	Meetings on one-to-one basis	Nurse-to-nurse in a concentric web as one nurse generally understands a concept. Increased internalization of the reasons for changes
Identification of learning needs	When a mistake is made	Staff expresses need before the skill must be used
Expertise	Teacher is the proven expert	Teacher is a co-learner but has been down similar roads before
Learning goal	Accomplishment of the organization's goals	Professional growth
Staff evaluation of learning	Minimal because of the crisis-orientation	Evident in clinical work over time, dialogues with nurse-manager for feedback and identification of ways to meet learning needs

The roles of manager and teacher are not mutually exclusive, although some institutions give them to separate people. However, in primary nursing the nurse-manager should be willing to move between the two roles. One role increases the nurse-manager's effectiveness in the other, because teaching and managing are both interpersonal processes.

When directing primary nursing conferences, the nurse-manager influences nurses' behavior. The best definition of clinical learning asserts that "learning is not soaking up information as a sponge absorbs water. It is an active process of transforming insights and understandings, attitudes, skills and values into one's own behavior. Changes in behavior persist or are dropped, dependent upon their usefulness to the individual" (Kaasch, 1968, p. 2).

Techniques for Teaching Primary Nursing

There are three areas of clinical practice that need particular attention and teaching skill from the nurse-manager

- Skills: technical; interpersonal; observational; expressive (writing, talking)
- Critical thinking: analytic, evaluative; cause-effect, consequential; priority-setting, logical; creative, questioning
- Assertiveness: advocacy; power politics

For each area there are some teaching techniques that work better than others. These techniques can be used by any nurse teacher and are especially effective when used persistently by the nurse-manager in the clinical area.

Skills

Teaching primary nurses technical skills such as the use of equipment or how to change sterile dressings is no different than teaching nursing skills in another setting. However, it should be remembered that the more competent primary nurses feel with technical demands, the more comfortable they will be in other aspects of primary nursing.

It is also essential that primary nurses have good observational skills. Primary nurses need to use all their senses in making observations. What a nurse smells is often more telling than what is seen! Similarly, touch and hearing are as useful to a primary nurse as eyesight.

To use every sense, the primary nurse cannot be anxious when with a patient. Allowing sensory input to register and to recall it afterwards requires heightened awareness to clinical situations. The nurse-manager can increase a primary nurse's sensory observations by:

- asking questions such as "What did he smell like?" or "Did you notice if the patient's skin felt dry or moist?"
- asking two or more nurses to compare observations of a patient and see how many senses have been used.
- playing an old, familiar party game at a staff meeting or class in which increasing numbers of dissimilar objects are placed on a tray and then removed. Each nurse must list as many objects as can be remembered. The person who remembers the most objects gets the award for Best Recaller that day.

Teaching primary nurses skills for responding to their patients is a complex, never-ending role for the nurse-manager. Interpersonal teaching can be best accomplished by learning experiences designed to expand some aspect or decrease some block to professional closeness:

- "He gives me the creeps the way he keeps staring at his stump. What should I do?"
- "I've had it! Everytime I cover him up he keeps exposing himself!"
- "I want to cry everytime I go in the room."
- "I really like feeding Tommy, but his mother keeps interfering."
- "I don't know how to bring up the subject of a nursing home."

Interpersonal learning requires honesty from the primary nurse as well as a willingness to explore with peers beyond the point where the primary nurse is stuck. For example, one patient with leukemia refused medications and verbally threatened nurses with violence. The primary nurse understood that the patient's anger was increased by strict bedrest and having to go for a venogram. The nurse, a woman, was seeking help for what to do next because she was frightened. With her peers she was able to imagine what the patient was experiencing and devise new approaches based on knowledge of the patient's stresses.

Interpersonal skills can be taught by:

- expressions of feelings related to the particular nurse-patient relationship always followed by discussion; pure emoting is not sufficient to stimulate new understanding which will be seen by future behavior changes
- role playing, especially when the primary nurse takes the part of the primary patient and other nurses tackle the role of the primary nurse
- classes in interviewing patients and families

Finally, the primary nurse needs to develop skill in conveying crucial information about primary patients to others. Writing and reporting skills are difficult to teach to a nurse lacking a strong background in language skills or to the primary nurse who is not convinced that there is information worth conveying. Basic learning needs such as these can best be approached through individual instruction, written examples, a structured format or checklist for change-of-shift report (Mezzanotte, 1976), feedback about documentation and reporting, and peer audit.

Encouraging Critical Thinking

"Critical thinking is the mental ability which undertakes to solve a problem, to define it, to limit it, to fence it in, and to see its relationship to things" (Kaasch, 1968, p. 9). Critical thinking is required to do a nursing care plan and to move independently through each step of the nursing process. The mental energy required is what makes problem-oriented charting difficult, sometimes to the point of frustration.

The natural inclination is to resist critical thinking, to be scientific and compulsive to a point and then to flee from thinking about the next logical step. Nurses have more opportunity to flee physically and mentally from a thought-task than other groups because there is always a patient who needs them or some other area to put their energies at the moment. The rationalizations to avoid time out for thinking can be heard everywhere. This can be seen by the way nurses organize themselves to be interruptable at all times. Thinking and doing seem to be mutually exclusive, and the tendency to flee into activity is stronger than that to apply analytic thought. Nurses often solve problems by activating a solution before the problem is clearly defined.

Because of the near-magnetic pull away from critical thinking, the nurse-manager needs to organize each day to include formal and informal times for critical thinking. Knowing that each primary nurse can think critically is a nurse-manager's only assurance that the staff is autonomous. Thinking is what keeps staff nurses functioning on a safe and therapeutic level, even in the nurse-manager's absence.

Critical thinking is not a subject that is learned, but rather a method of thinking that must be instilled as a style of nursing. The best way to teach the critical thinking method is to ask questions that will stimulate the processes of analytical and creative thought.

Through a series of preplanned and spontaneous questions, the teacher helps the students to understand a concept.

> The purpose of questioning is to bring about through reasoning an examination of the student's basic assumptions, influences or concepts. As this occurs, the student's concepts may be modified, as a result perception changes. It is possible through questioning to direct the attention of students to relationships by which diverse events in their world may be ordered and organized. As students acquire a concept, insight occurs. The teacher questions, but does not describe. Teaching is

primarily a process of helping another to structure and organize experience in such a way as to enable him to see (Connolly, 1974).

Identification of the area in which learning is sought is the first step in fostering critical thinking. This may require the nurse-manager to ask questions in order to refine a statement into a workable form. For instance, after a primary nurse says, "There wasn't enough time to do a complete nursing assessment," the nurse-manager must find out what that statement actually means. Never assume, but keep asking questions because the answers may lead to totally different responses:

- . . . so I don't know enough to present the case.
- . . . because the patient wouldn't stop talking about his symptoms.
- . . . because the doctor was doing the physical exam and I didn't want to interrupt.
- . . . because I have too many other primary patients.

It is very possible that the primary nurse had not thought about the reasons behind the reasons, so by asking questions the nurse-manager can encourage critical thinking. To this end, questions beginning with what and how are often better than why. Questions that ask for descriptions rather than reasons tend to free thinking rather than restrict thinking, which happens when people feel on the spot. The nurse-manager has to censor questions carefully so that they minimize resistance to new ideas by not threatening the learner's esteem. The more success a person experiences with a new attitude, the quicker it will replace the older one (Kaasch, 1968). The nurse-manager's questions must be geared toward helping primary nurses succeed.

Primary nursing conferences should be enabling experiences for the participants. However, because nurse-managers do not have the luxury of separating administrative from supervisory roles, they need to develop an active but non-penalizing style of teaching by asking questions during the presentation. The emphasis in primary nursing conferences should be on teaching, not evaluation. As different attitudes and patterns of primary nurses emerge during presentations, a nurse-manager can help individual nurses identify strengths and weaknesses in their practice, although this should be done directly in private meetings with the nurse-manager.

To be able to present their work openly and honestly in primary nursing conferences, primary nurses need to feel that the nurse-manager will not make hasty decisions about performance but will listen closely about the work and ask helpful questions that show interest and expand the ability to think critically. Any doubts about a primary nurse's work should be raised by that primary nurse. Negative comments from the nurse-manager and the others attending should be turned into positive suggestions. Other staff will follow the nurse-manager's example. A typical vignette may be as follows:

Primary nurse: Mr. P, recovering from a stroke, can't feed himself yet.
I've had to feed him each meal.
Staff nurse 1: He does okay when I watch him eat.
Nurse-manager: How do you explain the difference?

After discussion they both decide that they have set him up to eat identically except for the bib. The primary nurse does not like to see a grown man with a bib on, so leaves it off and helps him.

Nurse-manager: What is the goal you're working toward with him?
Primary nurse: To help him become able to carry out activities of daily living so he can become independent and go home. I also think he should gain back some of his lost self-esteem.
Nurse-manager: From your experience, which do you see a person gaining first, self-esteem or independence?
Primary nurse: They can both come together.
Nurse-manager: Yes, I think that's true. But I think stroke patients regain their self-esteem as they can do more things for themselves.
Staff nurse 2: Like Mrs. K.

Everyone nods in agreement.

Primary nurse: So I should let him spill food for a while? I guess I was expecting too much from him since he's made such a quick recovery.

If overprotection is an isolated problem, the primary nurse has overcome a roadblock to see the patient clearly. If the nurse-manager hears similar stories, help should be given for the immediate problem, and eventually the nurse-manager will need to discuss the pattern of overprotection with the primary nurse. However, primary nurses usually begin to see patterns in their own behavior through the nurse-manager's skilled questions.

Asking questions about any stage of the nursing process fosters critical thinking. It is most useful when right and wrong answers are not sought, but the focus is on tentative resolutions to complex situations.

Critical thinking is necessary to formulate a nursing diagnosis, which is the determination of a problem and its expected outcomes in terms that nurses can incorporate into action. The nurse-manager's questions can help primary nurses to clarify their understanding of symptoms, needs, and diagnoses. Primary nurses must be able to translate

- the patient's needs into nursing language and action
- the physician's language into nursing information

- the health care profession's language and understanding into the patient's and family's reality

The primary nurse's ability to put cause and effect together into a cohesive whole is a marvelous phenomenon. Combining theory, experience, and useful action is the most challenging part of primary nursing. Unfortunately, thinking analytically and creatively has been suppressed in nursing for the last century (Ashley, 1977).

Teaching nurses how to formulate nursing diagnoses involves encouraging them to think as far as they can on a problem. They need to be free of arbitrary, self-imposed limits to inquiry and curiosity which stem from fear that they are overstepping their bounds. Accentuating a person's normal curiosity and making learning fun and rewarding are two necessary attitudes for expanding nurses' thinking abilities.

Besides asking pertinent questions, the nurse-manager and other clinical teachers can foster critical thinking by using reinforcement techniques, which are used to reinforce or further elaborate on an idea or concept. They are creative ways to make a point without boring people with repetition, using:

- models—drawings, diagrams, plastic models, actual clinical equipment.
- examples—past case histories, articles from journals.
- analogies—describing something unfamiliar by comparing it to something that is familiar, as "the master problem list is similar to a grocery list in this way."
- paradoxes—using two ideas which seem opposite but are actually very similar, for example, "Good Grief!" conveys the idea that grieving is a necessary feeling after loss. It is even desirable in helping regain mental stability after the death of a family member or in helping a patient adjust to the loss of a body part. A paradox gets the learner's attention because it initially causes confusion and conflict. As the paradox is resolved, critical thinking takes place.

An optimal outcome of critical thinking is the primary nurse's ability to set priorities. This should be evidenced in work with primary patients as well as in the routine of the agency or unit. In fact, knowing when primary patients must wait until another unit need is attended to is an important decision which requires the ordering of priorities.

Teaching primary nurses to set priorities can be approached in several ways:

- protocols and guidelines which are either consistently reinforced or revised when necessary
- questions that are predictive, such as "what will you do if this patient gets a

pulmonary embolus" or "what can we use if we run out of IV poles"
- games that aim at problem solving, such as "if you were stranded on an island, what ten things would you need to stay alive and why would you choose them"
- value awareness exercises such as "if there were a fire and you only had time to save three patients, who would they be and why"

A nurse-manager's attention to the development of critical thinking among the primary nursing staff will be rewarded by improvement in the quality of care on the unit. The ability to think through a problem is a valuable tool for primary nurses in emergencies, when in charge, and when reviewing work with peers. Critical thinking cannot be learned in a vacuum because it takes a lot of effort. Therefore, the nurse-manager and other teachers need to be skilled critical thinkers and able to implement teaching approaches that help others to think through issues. Any patient-care setting has abundant opportunities to learn and utilize this skill.

Promoting Assertiveness

Assertive behavior is essential to primary nurses in fulfilling their responsibilities as advocates to patients and as colleagues to each other. Assertiveness can be learned through assertiveness training workshops, role modeling, and political consciousness raising. However, unless the nurse has clinical competence, there is nothing to be assertive about! If the nurse works in a climate in which assertiveness is not valued by others, there is no point in teaching assertive behavior to primary nurses.

Assertiveness is responsive, outward directed, self-assured, and self-owned behavior. "An assertive person demonstrates through words and actions that 'This is what I think. This is what I feel. This is what I want.' Assertive people set goals, act on achieved goals in a clear and consistent way, and take responsibility for the consequences of those actions" (Clark, 1977, p. 110).

Assertiveness stems from a strong belief in one's own worth as a person as well as a primary nurse. However, it does not mean putting that worth on the line. Assertive individuals know their worth but can separate it from their ideas and goals. Thus, they do not need to manipulate, depreciate, or disregard others to elevate themselves. Assertive individuals express themselves through self-disclosure, giving verbal and physical messages, but not to the point of self-exposure. Assertiveness may look risky, but it becomes second nature as new self-confidence and control is gained.

Because assertive behavior lies somewhere between passive and aggressive or impulsive behavior, the balance is not always possible to keep 100 percent of the time. In fact, the tendency toward one end or the other is very strong unless assertive behavior is learned by observing assertive people who are reinforced by a whole staff group.

The nurse-manager does not have to be an assertiveness training specialist to promote assertive behavior in the primary nursing staff. However, the nurse-manager would be wise to identify the ways that assertiveness can be learned and to conscientiously seek people and opportunities that will help nurses with approaches to familiar interpersonal problems.

Assertiveness training programs are sessions designed to help people define assertiveness and role play specific behavior, such as using "I" statements and avoiding "why" questions. The techniques are contrived, but the aim is to enable participants to incorporate new behaviors in actual situations. "Specific to nursing, the objective of such an increase in ability to express feelings would be to (1) improve nursing practice, (2) provide more nursing leaders, and (3) decrease role conflict, thus enhancing the ability of nurses to deal with bureaucratic and patient-centered goals simultaneously" (Grimm & Crawford, 1978, p. 61).

Unfortunately, there has been too much emphasis on assertiveness workshops and not enough attention to the daily situations that arise in a nursing organization. According to Belanger (1978) "many organizations have advocated workshops and seminars away from the work place. However, most of the good effects of these workshops are temporary because they do not deal directly with the organizational learning systems that created or permitted the problem to arise in the first place" (p. 38). This points to ways of learning assertiveness where it counts—at the unit level.

A second way that assertiveness can be learned is by studying role models and mentors. The nurse-manager will be carefully watched by primary nurses who are looking for a person they consider assertive and worthy of respect. They will be scrutinizing the nurse-manager's dealings with physicians, nursing supervisors, hospital administrators, and other key people to determine the level of assertiveness and the effectiveness of various behaviors. As the nurse-manager experiences administrative and supervisory support, the nurse-manager will grow in assertiveness.

More importantly, primary nurses will be very aware of how well the nurse-manager tolerates assertive behavior in the staff. Does the nurse-manager actually believe in assertiveness or merely give it lip service? Worse yet, does the nurse-manager allow the staff to be assertive, except when they need to be assertive with the nurse-manager? Is the rule do not contradict or otherwise upset the nurse-manager or you will suffer the consequences? The nurse-manager's feelings about assertiveness are quickly felt by each new member of the nursing staff because "under a stressful situation, the leader's old style surfaces because the assumptions beneath it have not been altered" (Belanger, 1978, p. 37).

It is very hard to be assertive and not defensive when managing the complex operations of a nursing unit or clinic. Just as the primary nurse needs a base of clinical expertise to be genuinely assertive, the nurse-manager needs a base of sound management skills to be able to promote assertiveness. Nurse-managers need to be patient with themselves as well as with primary nurses as they support each other in being assertive.

A third way to promote assertiveness is to teach primary nurses the art of influence, which is essentially increasing their skills in the area of collaboration. When nurses attempt to influence patients, it is called patient-teaching. When nurses hope to influence other health professionals, it's called politics! The process, however, is the same and calls for assertive behavior.

Primary nurses need to learn the ins and outs of working within a very formal and emotional health care institution. Because workers in an institution are in some way dependent on each other, something as simple as getting a blanket for a patient may be extremely complicated. Since nurses are usually the link between the patients' needs and the institution, nurses must receive materials or get action when they and the patients need it.

The nurse-manager can help by telling primary nurses useful channels of action and by actively discussing verbal approaches. Primary nurses who are condescending to secretaries will find that results come more slowly, if at all, when they need something. If that primary nurse was genuinely assertive, there would be no need to request something in a way which devalued the secretary.

There are many clues to problems with assertiveness. The nurse-manager may hear comments such as:

- I feel like the rest of the staff are neglecting my primary patients' intake and output sheets.
- I'd have to work overtime to get everything done for this patient.
- Why are the social workers always asking me who to call for a discharge disposition?
- I wasn't invited to grand rounds about my primary patient.
- No one listens to me when I say this patient isn't ready to go home.
- That family won't leave me alone!
- The evening shift leaves too many things undone.
- They said we'd have to wait until tomorrow.
- Ha Ha, I see you're changing my time schedule again.

The nurse-manager who is alert to early signs of surrender to pressures can help point out what is happening before it becomes another burden for the nurse. Together they can analyze the situation and decide on a more productive approach.

So the nurse-manager has several immediate alternatives in promoting the assertive behavior of primary nurses. Assertiveness will not cure all the ills of primary nursing, but it can help ease some of the frustrations of demanding, intense, clinical situations. As primary nurses learn to respect themselves, they will gain the respect of others and will be on the way to being experts in their clinical areas.

REFERENCES

Armstrong, M. Bridging the gap between graduation and employment. *Journal of Nursing Administration,* November-December 1974, *4* (6), 42-48.

Ashley, J. *Hospitals, paternalism, and the role of the nurse.* New York: Teachers College Press, 1977.

Bartels, D., Good, V. & Lampe, S. The role of the head nurse in primary nursing. *Canadian Nurse,* March 1977, *73* (3), 26-29.

Belanger, C. Do you confront the boss? *Supervisor Nurse,* December 1978, *9* (12), 36-40.

Bower, K. and Twyon, S. *Role of the preceptor.* Boston: Tufts-New England Medical Center, 1979.

Clark, C. *The nurse as group leader.* New York: Springer Publishing, 1977.

Connolly, A. *Concept attainment.* Boston: Boston University School of Nursing, 1974.

Drake, J. *Interviewing for managers.* New York: American Management Association, 1972.

Ganong, J. & Ganong W. *Nursing management.* Germantown, Md.: Aspen Systems, 1976.

Grimm, L. & Crawford, J. Viewpoint: Assertiveness training for nurses. *Nursing Administration Quarterly,* Spring 1979, 2 (3), 59-63.

Kaasch, B. Principles of learning and teaching. *Management of nursing care.* St. Louis: Catholic Hospital Association, 1968.

Knowles, M. *Modern practice of adult education.* New York: Association Press, 1970.

Kowalski, K. Job interviewing: An effective tool for hiring staff nurses. *Journal of Nursing Administration,* January 1975, *5* (1), 43-47.

Laing, R. D. *Knots.* New York: The R. D. Laing Trust, 1970.

Mezzanotte, J. Getting it together for end-of-shift reports. *Nursing 76,* April 1976, *6* (4), 21-22.

Sheehy, G. *Passages.* New York: E.P. Dutton, 1976.

Veninga, R. Interpersonal feedback: A cost-benefit analysis. *Journal of Nursing Administration,* February 1975, *6* (2), 40-43.

Chapter 4

Managing Toward Accountability for Nursing Practice

The central ideology in a primary nursing system is the dictum that a nurse has responsibility and accountability for the total care of a patient over a 24-hour period from a patient's admission to discharge. It is an extremely important concept in that it distinguishes primary nursing from other care-giving systems, especially the case method where nurses are responsible for total care but only for the eight hours that the nurse is present. If the philosophical construct of 24-hour accountability is not internalized and operationalized, a primary nursing system is not in effect! (Spoth, 1977, p. 224)

Accountability is the most elusive element in primary nursing, as it also is in general nursing practice. It "constitutes form without substance until nurses agree to whom and for what they are accountable, and until systems for monitoring and regulating nursing practice are developed" (Passos, 1973, p. 17).

Ironically, primary nursing provides the profession, the majority of whose members work in hospitals, with a mechanism by which to be accountable. However, there has been a great deal of confusion about the meaning of accountability in regard to primary nursing, and in particular, about holding primary nurses accountable for measurable practice.

How can primary nurses be responsible and accountable for the 24-hour care that primary patients receive when they are not actually present much of the time? The answer lies in the distinction between responsibility and accountability and in the use of operational systems to measure each function of primary nursing.

Twenty-four hour accountability is a catch phrase that needs to be clarified. It means that primary nurses are accountable for what happens to each primary patient regardless of shifts and length of stay. Primary nurses must account for the results of patient care given under their jurisdiction, from admission to discharge. Furthermore, they are evaluated on the degree to which clinical practice achieves patient care outcomes.

125

Responsibility differs from accountability because it is the means to an end, while accountability is answering for the results or outcomes of responsible actions. "Responsibility expresses the 'ought's' or expectations of performance, while accountability implies that our 'dids' or actual performance will be judged against expected performance" (Passos, 1973, p. 18). Responsibility refers to the activities of nursing care, while accountability refers to the outcomes of care.

An example will highlight the differences between responsibility and accountability in primary nursing. A primary nurse completes an excellent nursing assessment and care plan for a patient who has just had an ileostomy due to severe ulcerative colitis. An identified problem is lowered resistance to infection due to high doses of steroids used for immunosuppression. The primary nurse continues writing appropriate nursing interventions for the problem, such as, "Mr. J should not have contact with visitors or nursing staff who have colds or other infections," "check vital signs every four hours looking for increases in pulse, respiration, or temperature," and "watch WBCs for elevation and if elevated notify MD." The primary nurse carries out the responsibility of assessment and care planning and may even set a discharge goal for this problem, such as, "Mr. J will be infection free at discharge as indicated by normal TPR and WBC." However, if Mr. J contracts an upper respiratory infection while still in the hospital, the primary nurse will be asked to account to the patient, peers, and the nurse-manager for the occurrence of infection. Similarly, the primary nurse is accountable if Mr. J does not get an infection and is discharged according to plan.

Primary nursing involves both responsibility and accountability. The lack of clarity results from the traditional role in which nurses have responsibility without accountability. In primary nursing nurses have individual responsibility and therefore should also have individual accountability. For this to happen when nurses do not work 24 hours a day is a challenge to nurse-managers and administrators.

In order to manage effectively to gain accountability for nursing practice from all primary nurses, the nurse-manager must know the issues involved and must then review the systems which are used at the unit level to hold primary nurses accountable, such as documentation, audits, and evaluation of clinical expertise.

DOUBLE MESSAGES AND DOUBLE AGENTS

Accountability is difficult to deal with because it is the least defined concept in general nursing practice. Although the public and nurses themselves view nurses as highly responsible, the questions of responsible for what and accountable to whom remain. Two factors add to the problem of accountability: confusion about the role of the nurse and states' nurse practice acts which require nurses to work under the supervision of a doctor (Ashley, 1977). The lack of professional and legal clarity leaves the nurse-manager with the task of defining accountability within the bureaucratic structure of the health care agency. The nurse-manager synthesizes the double messages into a single message for the staff primary nurses by defining nursing practice in the context of the unit and department and specifying the tasks for which primary nurses are responsible and the outcomes for which they are accountable.

The Veil of Anonymity

Because nursing practice lacks consistent definition regarding process and outcomes, the profession and the nurse-manager have discredited themselves and the contributions of nurses. All the philosophical debates and theory building mean nothing unless nursing is defined and reinforced in all clinical areas by all nurse-managers. The power to struggle against anonymous nursing lies with the position of the nurse-manager.

Until primary nursing there was no way to hold nurses accountable for patient care, although they were certainly responsible for what they did on a shift or daily basis. They could be sued for gross malpractice; however, they could not be held accountable for the outcomes of nursing care because no one individual nurse could be cited as the person permanently assigned to a patient.

Nurses traditionally have exhibited a need to be anonymous, and the nursing staff has worked as "an unnamed conglomerate of interchangeable parts, who drops in and drops out of the patient's life experience" (Passos, 1973, p. 19). Upon close inspection many nursing routines seem to be mechanisms to help nurses remain anonymous by avoiding professional commitments to patients as well as patient care outcomes:

> Assignment lists are made and posted daily by the head nurse who may believe in "continuity of care" but cannot find a way to assign the same nurse to a patient more than three days in a row. Every day she intends to assign herself a patient or two, but usually ends up helping everyone else, taking off orders, or passing meds. From beginning to end of the shift, the staff, team leaders, and head nurse run from one crisis to the next, feeling isolated but dedicated. They feel overwhelmingly responsible as they rush to meet the needs of all the patients. No one but the head nurse checks the orders, goes on rounds, or gives report to the next shift or to the nursing supervisor. No one but the head nurse can answer a question from a family member because she is the only one with the information. Charts are left blank because no one can decide which of all the patients to write about. Citing lack of time as the eternal excuse, the staff does not document anything. They put in eight hours of frenzy but know it's over after report; the head nurse goes home later than everyone else, worrying about certain critical patients and wondering why nursing is so frustrating (Zander, 1977, p. 20).

Primary nursing will not solve the problem of anonymous nursing until primary nurses are sure of what they are accountable for and to whom they are accountable. The answer should be that primary nurses are accountable to the patient for the results of the nursing care delivered by the primary nurse and other staff members. The nurse-manager has the role of assuring that primary nurses fulfill their professional contracts with the public. As the patient advocacy philosophy stresses, primary nurses must first be accountable to the patient and carry through on professional commitments, even if the consequences displease other segments of the health care agency.

Nursing is complex because of its interdependency with other professions, and the boundaries of accountability can be fuzzy at times. Primary nurses may use this interdependency positively to facilitate patient outcomes or negatively to hide behind the complexities of health care teams where each group claims a piece of the patient-care pie as their jurisdiction. Of course, the most contention occurs at the boundary where nursing ends and medical practice begins.

How Nurse Practice Acts Create Double Agents

State nurse practice acts create confusion about accountability and in effect make nurses double agents—accountable to both patients and physicians. How frequently do you hear the refrain, "I was only following the doctor's orders" or "don't ask me, I'm only the nurse on the case"? When nurses try to please everyone, they tend to seek personal safety at all costs. Because of the diffuse way nursing is entwined in the bureaucratic, physician-oriented health care structure, nurses will always have an excuse for not defining or accepting accountability.

To add to the difficulty, nursing has a built-in disclaimer in the nurse practice acts: nurses must practice under the supervision of physicians. Few nurses consider the implications of these laws until they want recognition as independent practitioners. Until then nurses can practice comfortably under the liability insurance of the employing institution. Unfortunately, nurses may think that they function under the supervision of physicians, even when they are carrying out the nursing process with primary patients. The truth is that nurses are supervised by nurses in matters of nursing care. Physicians focus on cure, while nurses focus on health care. These two functions need to meet, but with equal legal sanction and public recognition. The nurse practice acts perpetuate dependence and subservience of nurses to physicians.

By incorporating the inequality of physicians and nurses into law, the nurse practice acts gave legal sanction to medical sexism: men were to supervise women, whether they were in the presence of these women or not. This supervision was then, and is still, literally an impossibility because physicians are not present in most of the settings where nurses are engaged in practice (Ashley, 1977, pp. 117-118).

For years nurses have believed that they need guidance from physicians in order to help patients. The suppression of medically related information and of attendance at intellectual seminars and rounds have also undermined the confidence of nurses in their thinking ability. Even collegiate nursing courses such as "physics for nurses" cannot help but make beginning primary nurses hesitant about their capabilities and certainly make them reluctant to set goals for outcomes of care.

Actually primary nurses work with physicians, not for them. If anything, nurses work for patients and therefore need to define their accountability in terms of patient outcomes. The authority of primary nurses comes from the nursing process which makes nursing systematic and scientific and from their personal accountability for the outcomes of care.

The clinical expertise of primary nurses comes from goal-oriented nursing which seeks many alternatives to reach goals. Consequently, primary nurses find pride and satisfaction in goal achievement from the recognition of the nurse-manager and nursing administration.

Minimizing Double Messages: Primary Nursing by Objectives

Primary nurses will only be secure in their responsibilities and effective in their activities if they view their role as that of a manager of nursing care. Nursing intervention must be regarded as a cyclical process through which preset patient care outcomes or objectives are attained.

Patient care outcomes must have certain characteristics in order to clarify the accountability of primary nurses.

- They must be patient-focused and therefore should be written behaviorally with the patient or family as the subject.
- They must be linked to a problem, need, or limitation of the patient or family that is identified at the initial or on-going assessments.
- They must result directly from nursing intervention, as opposed to the responsibilities of physicians or other providers. In many instances, a physician and primary nurse may work toward the same patient outcomes, but the responsibilities taken to reach the outcomes will differ.
- They must be limited to the period of time in which the primary nurse will have contact with the patient, i.e. "patient ambulates without assistance" may not be a realistic or fair outcome for which a primary nurse in an ICU should be held accountable.
- They must not exceed the limits of nursing responsibility as defined by the agency.

Consistent with these criteria, outcomes can include goals for health status, activity level, knowledge, and prevention of complications (Jacobs and Jacobs, 1975). The crucial factor for primary nursing accountability is that outcomes must be statements about the consequences of nursing responsibilities.

> In nursing, these goals must be operational so as to enable continuous evaluation and determination of the degree or extent of goal determination. It is begging the problem to state general goals such as "to restore to self-dependence" or "to optimize well-being". Such statements are more directional than operational and are not conducive to credible evaluation. Goals must of necessity be as quantitative as possible. Quantitative standards can then be factored to produce criteria as tests and indices of the more general qualitative goals. Goals should be as operational as possible and should not be confused with the methods determined to achieve the goals (Ryan, 1973, p. 51).

Patient care outcomes for a middle-aged woman who has undergone a modified radical mastectomy could look like this sample nursing index.

Problem, need, limitation	*Inpatient outcomes/goals*
1. Hesitant to use affected area for activities of daily living	1. Can brush hair and teeth, wash face, feed self, and wipe self in bathroom by discharge date
2. High-risk of depression as an after effect of breast loss	2. (A) Has been seen by Reach for Recovery at least once before discharge (B) Expresses feelings about self-image and discusses her support systems with the primary nurse
3. Hematoma	3. Absence of hematoma
4. Lack of knowledge about home care of incision line	4. States directions and plans for incision line care at home

Source: In Column 2, nos. 2 (B) and 4 from "Discharge Mastectomy," patient-teaching plans, by Pat Phillips (Boston: Tufts-New England Medical Center, 1978).

Any nurse observing the patient may define a need or problem, but only the primary nurse knows the patient well enough to determine realistic outcomes. All the staff share the care of this patient, but the primary nurse is solely accountable for the results. The primary nurse is responsible for determining and ordering nursing interventions that ensure achievement of the expected outcomes. Outcomes are stated so that they can be accomplished by the expected inpatient discharge date, barring premature discharge by the physician or the patient signing out against medical and nursing advice. The nursing staff is responsible for carrying out the orders of the primary nurse and physician, but only the primary nurse is accountable for the outcomes listed. Ideally, objectives should be determined by the patient, family, primary nurse, and physician together.

Primary nursing accountability typifies the concept of nursing by objectives:

> Managing patient care involves the concept of one nurse and one patient working together to carry out the medical care plan and the nursing care plan for that patient. While this concept can rarely be implemented without modification, application efforts to carry out the concept are being made by nurses with such titles as nurse practitioner, primary nurse, and clinical specialist.
>
> Nursing by objectives is a results-oriented technique using mutually-established patient care objectives, an implementation schedule, and evaluation of results and patient progress. It applies the management-by-objectives approach at the unit level with the focus on the one nurse/one patient relationship. The emphasis is not the performance of tasks for patients. It is upon helping the patient achieve his goals. This means establishing a helping relationship between nurse and patient, a relationship in which the patient is recognized as being in charge of himself (insofar as he is able) and the nurse is a facilitative manager of goal achievement in accordance with the medical care plan (Ganong & Ganong, 1976, p. 97).

It is essential that goals or outcomes be written in specific behavioral terms. Only in this way can a primary nurse's accountability be objectively evaluated. Many statements that are often considered goals, such as, maintain good hygiene and give emotional support, are only broad approaches. Results-oriented primary nursing entails thinking through each patient's problems, needs, or limitations to derive a description of outcomes for the current admission.

Some outcomes for actions of physicians and nurses may be stated in the same way, such as, patient oriented to time, place, and person upon discharge. However, nursing interventions will be quite different from the physician's responsibilities, and the primary nurse is only accountable for those which fall under the jurisdiction of nursing.

Problem	Outcome/goal	Nursing orders
Patient disoriented secondary to ICU psychosis	Oriented to time, place, person	a. Assess mental status every hour
		b. Primary nurse to talk to family about bringing familiar objects into hospital
		c. Limit visitors to one at a time for 5 minute stays
		d. Have same staff giving care every shift
		e. Notify MD of disorientation

Physician orders

a. Give Haldol

Here the primary nurse is accountable for the outcome to the extent that nursing interventions are carried out by the nurse and staff colleagues. The primary nurse should not be accountable for anything that is beyond nursing practice as defined by the agency. Although the physician and primary nurse are dependent on each other to accomplish the outcome of this case, the primary nurse uses very specific and creative approaches from the realm of nursing.

Some standardization of expected outcomes is probably necessary as primary nurses carve out the territory for which they will be accountable. However, this does not exclude individualism in need identification, outcome determination, and approaches used to achieve them.

Some routinizing of established patient-care goals, especially for new primary nurses who are learning their roles, can improve clinical expertise. Without sanctioned objectives, how can primary nurses have clarity of purpose, as well as the firm backing of the nurse-manager and administration? Standardized outcome goals can provide consistency for expectations from each primary nurse's work and also add weight to the patient advocate role. If the agency supports and expects predetermined outcomes, quality care can be more easily guaranteed.

DOCUMENTING AND AUDITING PATIENT CARE

In managing toward accountability primary nurses must be given blame or praise for the outcomes of their care by measuring it against predetermined standards and criteria. This information can be obtained by auditing the documentation which shows the steps of the nursing process that were taken and the progress made toward patient care outcomes or goals. Therefore, primary nurses and fellow staff members must have systems of documentation to facilitate their work during a patient's admission as well as to prove the worth of their work in retrospect, after a patient's discharge.

As whole agencies convert to primary nursing, they must make sure that their documentation and auditing mechanisms are consistent with the role of primary nursing and the measurement of accountability. This can be an institutional problem because nursing documentation must include all aspects of patient care, not only those ordered or provided by the primary nurse. However, there are documentation systems that record all interventions with a patient and specifically, identify those functions performed by the primary nurse.

The next two sections tackle the problem of documenting and auditing patient care. Because every agency wants its own forms, attention is given to the common elements that all agencies must include in their nursing records to promote accountability. Nursing has the right and the obligation to insist on documentation methods which reflect personal accountability.

Documenting Results-Oriented Primary Nursing

"What I do is *give up* autonomy by creating a high-demand situation, so that I must always jump from project to project, never really allowing time to think about what I'm doing it all for" (Sheehy, 1976, p. 333). This quote is a 40-year-old man describing how he avoids scrutinizing what his life is all about. How closely it describes the difficulty that many nurses have with taking time out to reflect and record what they are doing it all for! A nurse-manager needs to have an answer to this problem and a format to guide accurate and significant documentation.

Rationale

Phaneuf (1976) lists seven functions of professional nursing. If predetermined outcomes are included in the seventh, then every function listed, except the fourth, requires documentation by primary nurses and other nursing staff:

1. application and execution of physician's legal orders
2. observation of signs and symptoms and reactions
3. supervision of the patient
4. supervision of those participating in care (except the physician)

5. reporting and recording
6. application and execution of nursing procedures and techniques
7. promotion of physical and emotional health by direction and teaching

In addition, documentation by primary nurses is necessary because:

- The primary nurse has the total patient in mind, while others on the nursing staff have a task-completion focus.
- Only a primary nurse with the total picture can help a patient to set and understand realistic goals of care.
- Only a primary nurse can determine if changes in condition are significant for the patient and if they indicate movement toward or away from goals.
- The primary nurse is the identified patient advocate who pursues the patient's right to quality care by using the medical record.
- The primary nurse reviews what other health care providers have observed, assessed, and done in regard to a primary patient.
- The primary nurse prescribes nursing interventions for the primary patient that must be written to insure consistency during all shifts and over periods of time.
- The primary nurse is evaluated on the effectiveness of nursing interventions used to achieve identified outcomes and manage complications.
- Primary nurses must allow time to think about their work and to give themselves credit for assessments and interventions. They show accountability for the patient's clinical course and for future plans by committing themselves by name.
- Good documentation serves to clarify the professional nurse's role.

Primary nurses strengthen their position and professional identity when they use recording systems that reflect professional thinking and responsibilities. Good documentation shows areas of responsibility as graphically as medications transcribed on a medication sheet. Primary nursing-based charting tools, thus, reinforce a serious attitude toward responsibility and assigned accountability.

Documentation as Part of a Total Admission

Nursing documentation is only one facet of the patient's admission, yet it represents the core of the patient's total experience with the health care agency. Therefore, nurses must view documentation as an essential part of the patient's care rather than as an additional responsibility which is secondary to the real work.

Because the nurse-manager has the authority and influence to set priorities, expectations about documentation should be communicated to the nursing staff at every turn. Primary nurses must develop a set of responses that sends an alert, "this is something I should chart" or "I need to begin that care plan before I leave today."

Although integrated charting in which all health care professionals record their work in the same place in the medical record, is not essential to primary nursing, it is important for several reasons. Integrated notes are the baseline for evaluation of what nurses have to say about patients, and they are the only way to get a complete chronological story of a patient's care. Furthermore, integrated notes are the safest way to convey essential information so that it cannot be ignored by any discipline.

There should be no such thing as "nurse's notes." The use of a separate section for nurses' charting in the medical record is a remnant of discrimination against nurses. In some hospitals all other disciplines, including physicians, social workers, dieticians, consultants, and occupational therapists, chart in one section while nurses are relegated to a separate section. Separate but equal is not the case here. Nurses can only assume that their information is not to be contaminated by other disciplines or that it is not worthy to be included with that of other disciplines. Rather, nursing administration should support the use of "Patients' Progress Notes."

Documentation as an Integral Part of Primary Nursing

Although primary nursing is complex, the tools used to document patient care must be uncomplicated. Documentation must do three things:

1. Identify the work for which primary nurses are responsible and provide information and directives for the rest of the nursing staff
2. Identify the outcomes for which primary nurses are accountable
3. Allow for recording of routine or crisis interventions by nonprimary nurses

In addition, the documentation system must allow for changes based on regular nursing assessments. The system must be as dynamic and flexible as primary nurses and the clinical situations demand.

The essential elements of results-oriented documentation for primary nursing, which include the above criteria, are described in Table 4-1. The documentation system must distinguish the responsibilities of primary nurses from entries of other staff members. Although other staff members may need to document something in an emergency, the primary nurse has certain responsibilities that are central to primary nursing.

1. The primary nurse conducts and signs assessments when present at admission or cosigns those done by other nurses after reviewing them and adding new data. Assessments should be appropriate to the unit and the patient; for instance, a pediatric unit would want to know about a child's toys, and a psychiatric unit would need a space for assessing suicidal tendencies.

Table 4-1 Documenting the Primary Nursing Process

Objectives	Identify factors that influence patient care	Identify patient/ family concerns that need nursing intervention	Determine measurable outcomes or goals of nursing care
Steps of the primary nursing process	Assessment ⟶	Problem, need, ⟶ limitation— nursing diagnosis	Short-term and outcome ⟶ goals
Documentation tools	Admission: Assessment form Ongoing: Progress notes	Admission: Nursing index Care plan Ongoing: Nursing index care plan	Admission: Nursing index outcome goals Care plan short-term goals Ongoing: Nursing index outcome goals Care plan short-term goals Progress notes
Documentation components	Assessment: Form should show unit's priorities Used as a data base for development of individualized plans and outcomes Includes patient and family's perception of needs Progress notes: Assessment of progress or lack of progress, complications Assessment of new needs	Contains statements of patient or family's need as identified on assessment Contains needs or problems that arise during the extent of contact with the agency Phrase problems in workable units which lend direction to future action; define a problem so that you can do something about it	Written behaviorally with patient/family as subject Linked to problem Direct result of nursing action Short-term goals are the immediate progressive steps taken, increments of the outcome goals Outcome goals must be realistic for that admission and consistent with the agency's limits on nursing practice

NOTE: Read Table 4-1 across two pages.

Table 4-1 continued

Direct activities to correct or ameliorate patient health deficits in a progression toward optimum health	Record/give proof that prescribed or critical nursing care was given	Provide continual input on the nurse/patient relationship and activities
Decision to be ──► Meeting(s) ↘ advocate per need ◄── ↗ Resolution Plans to reach ↗ ──────► Actual interventions ──► goals—nursing orders		Evaluation
Admission: Care plan Nursing order/treatment sheet Ongoing: Care plan Nursing order/treatment sheet Teaching plans Progress notes	Nursing order/treatment sheet Progress notes Teaching plans	Progress notes Audit
Should be "fluid," pertaining to the immediate patient needs Revised so that outcome goals can be approximated and reached Reviewed and revised daily by primary nurse Include discharge planning steps	Should be specific for routine and individual- ized nursing care Should show who completed the task Responsibility shown by signature	Assessment of nursing care effectiveness Concurrent or retrospective audits done per primary nurse

Sources: The first and second objectives are courtesy of Robin Thomas, Childrens Hospital Medical Center, Boston, 1979. The fourth objective is from Ryan, 1973.

2. Any nurse can identify immediate needs and write them on a nursing index, but only the primary nurse can accurately set outcome goals. Because primary nurses are accountable for outcomes, they should be the ones to determine them within the agency's standards.

3. Short-term goals for nonacute problems may be set by the primary nurse or by anyone who is on duty when acute problems arise. The primary nurse is responsible for reviewing and writing short-term goals when on duty. They should appear in a care plan, whether or not the plan is a permanent part of the medical record. Short-term goals can also be identified and addressed in progress notes written by the primary nurse and others. In progress notes, the primary nurse is responsible for recording movement toward outcome goals through achievement of short-term goals. Because the primary nurse is in the best position to compare a patient's status over time, depth is provided for revision of present goals or determination of the next step.

4. The primary nurse is responsible for developing an overall plan of care and for administrating the implementation of it by staff peers. Because a plan is only as stable as the patient's condition, it is really a worksheet suggesting protocols for nursing action to achieve goals and, therefore, is largely, but not solely, the responsibility of the primary nurse. The primary nurse's name should be written on the plan along with dates when the plan was revised. The nursing care plan is a guide to good intentions. Primary nursing entails plans, but more importantly, requires that plans be put into action and the actions be recorded.

5. Recording interventions directed and delivered by primary nurses is equally as important as planning them. That a plan is actually executed by the staff must be documented on forms, such as treatment records, teaching plans, and clinical data sheets. Primary nurses, in a role similar to the head nurse of non-primary nursing units, are responsible for monitoring these documents to make sure that their patients receive the required care.

6. In primary nursing circles the primary nurse is considered responsible for "discharge planning." It has been one staff primary nurse's research-proven experience that primary nurses need some guidelines in planning for a patient's discharge. A checklist can be incorporated into a care plan for use by the primary nurse, and results of discharge planning should be reflected in progress notes written by the primary nurse. A study of discharge planning is presented in Chapter 12.

7. Nursing orders given by the primary nurse must be written on a permanent treatment record that is signed off by those who give the treatment (see Exhibit 4-1). For easy access the treatment record can include treatment ordered by both physician and primary nurses. Nursing orders should be reviewed and revised by the primary nurse on a regular basis. The treatment record indicates that theoretical approaches have been implemented.

Exhibit 4-1 Sample Patient Treatment Record

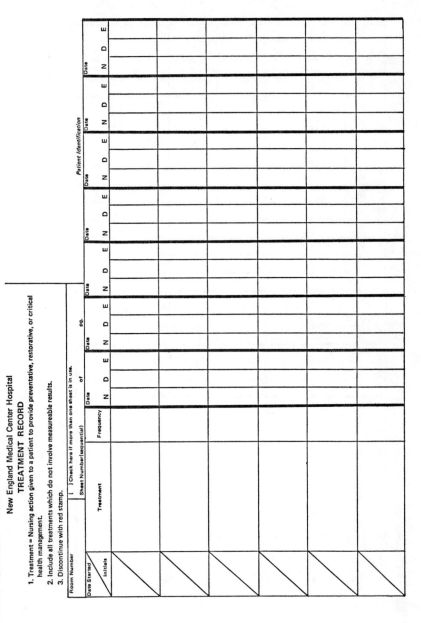

Exhibit 4-1 continued

Date Started / Initials	Treatment	Frequency	Date			Date			Date			Date			Date			Date			Date		
			N	D	E	N	D	E	N	D	E	N	D	E	N	D	E	N	D	E	N	D	E

Initials	Signature	Initials	Signature	Initials	Signature
	PN:				

Source: Tufts-New England Medical Center Hospital, 1979. Reprinted with permission.

8. Lack of patient knowledge regarding preventive or curative health measures is a legitimate category of need for nursing intervention. Standardized patient-teaching plans were developed by a retrospective audit committee and they proved a great asset to busy primary nurses who want to document patient education transactions (Zander et al, 1978).

9. Documentation of results from the patient advocacy loop of the primary nursing process is the responsibility of the primary nurse. Results of meetings, team evaluations, and consultations are necessary to show accountability for primary nursing practice. All patient advocacy actions should be recorded in progress notes, whether or not the desired resolutions are attained.

10. Formal evaluation of nursing care can be documented by the primary nurse in places such as progress notes, transfer notes, and discharge notes. In the absence of the primary nurse, writing these notes should be delegated to another nurse by the nurse-manager. If the primary nurse's documentation is comprehensive and up-to-date, other nurses will be able to take over with little difficulty. However, the primary nurse should be the person (1) to record when an outcome goal is met, thereby showing resolution to problems, and (2) to write nursing referrals for patients transferred to the care of other agencies. These notes not only provide a means for the primary nurse to record events, but also an opportunity for the primary nurse to evaluate the past days.

Adapting POMR Documentation to Results-Oriented Primary Nursing

If primary nurses are to be accountable for the outcomes of care personally directed and given by them, documentation must give priority to stating goals and evaluating progress towards them. Therefore, the current trend of POMR— problem-oriented medical record (Weed, 1972)—must be refocused on outcomes. The new focus might be called GOMR (goal-oriented medical record) or OOND (outcome-oriented nursing documentation). Whatever name is used, current systems must be adapted for charting the flow of nursing care from start to finish.

With minor revisions the problem-oriented nursing system of documentation, with its problem list and SOAP (Subjective, Objective, Assessment, Plan) format for progress notes, can be refocused on outcomes. This can be done by linking problems with outcome goals and by using the P (Plan) segment of progress notes to document the next goal increment and the steps to it.

For instance, the patient with a cerebral vascular accident may have the following problem list which when combined with outcome goals becomes the nursing index.

No.	Problem	Onset	Outcomes	Date Met
1.	Inability to ambulate secondary to left-sided weakness	3-1-79	1. (A) Can ambulate without assistance (B) Absence of contractures	
2.	Decreased ability to care for self	3-1-79	2. Can bathe and dress without assistance	
3.	Legally blind, secondary to cataracts	1960	3. Does not injure self	
4.	Immobility		4. (A) Absence of decubiti (B) Absence of pneumonia	
5.	Confused about what happened to him	3-2-79	5. Understands he had a stroke by: (A) Reviewing the day the stroke occurred (B) States why strokes occur (C) Asks questions about his concerns	
6.	Daughter overwhelmed by expected burden of father's care	3-5-79	6. Daughter makes decision about father's discharge plans after completing family teaching plans	

In this example, a progress note about the first problem could be written as:

3-6-79: No. 1. Inability to ambulate
  S "I want to go to the bathroom by myself."
  O Mr. L able to transfer to wheelchair today, although still very unsteady.
  A Is getting frustrated with his limitations and having trouble seeing that he is progressing.
  P 1. Should continue to use wheelchair for trips to bathroom.
     2. I will talk to physical therapy about Mr. L trying short walks with two people assisting in a few days. If they agree. I'll inform Mr. L of the plan.
              (Signature of nurse)

3-8-79: No. 1. Inability to ambulate
  S "So, you finally trust me."
  O Mr. L walked to bathroom today with two people.
  A Is strong enough now to be assisted by only one person.
  P Continue with one person assisting to bathroom until next week.
              (Signature of nurse)

As outcomes are achieved, the primary nurse records the dates they are reached. Those that state absence of complications should be dated on discharge. If the primary nurse uses the nursing index to guide the course of Mr. L's admission, the primary nurse will consciously be working toward outcomes.

In adapting a nursing care plan (Exhibit 4-2) to a goal-oriented charting system (Exhibit 4-3), the goals would have to be more specific, with patient as subject, and also divided into short-term goals entered in the care plan and outcome goals entered in the nursing index (Exhibit 4-4). The nature of the problem must be stated, but approaches must be entered in their own column and in the treatment record.

Exhibit 4-2 Original Nursing Care Plan: Patient with Abdominal Hysterectomy

Goal: Prepare patient to return home. Create and maintain therapeutic environment. Maintain good hygiene and physical comfort.

Date	Problems and needs	Approach
1	Requires medication for pain q 2-3 hrs.	Give medication as ordered. Turn, cough and deep breathe
2	Abd. incision draining slightly	Observe and report condition of wound
3	Indwelling cath.	Measure and record urinary drainage
4	Intake and output	Keep accurate intake and output
5	Requires assistance in getting O.O.B.	Assist out of bed
6	Observe for abdominal distention	Patient may need rectal tube or enema as ordered
7	Poor sleeping habits at home	Observe and report sleep pattern Offer back care and refreshments when awake
8	Crying at times	Facilitate awareness of self as an individual with varying physical, emotional and developmental needs

Age	Birth date	S(M)DW	Religion	Profession	Adm.	Date
44	05-04-30		pro	N/P		
Room	Name		Diagnosis		Doctor	
224			Abd. Hysterectomy			

Source: Ganong and Ganong, 1976. Reprinted with permission.

Exhibit 4-3 Adapted Nursing Care Plan: Patient with Abdominal Hysterectomy

(3 hours post-op)

	Problem, needs, limitations	Current short-term goals	Approach
2	Pain at operative site	1. Pain relieved by p.o. meds by 24° post-op	1. Observe for abdominal distention
3	Abd. incision draining slightly	2. Drainage should stop within 96 hours. Absence of infection	2. Check incision and record q shift
4	Indwelling catheter 2° inability to urinate voluntarily	3. Able to urinate without catheter	3. I&O until 24 hours post cath.
5	Difficulty getting out of bed	4. Able to get out of bed without assistance	4. Teach her how to support abdomen, how to raise head of bed to set up and swing legs
6	Crying at times	5. Regains emotional stability	5. Listen to her reasons for crying to determine whether she needs teaching and/or counselling. Facilitate awareness of self as an individual with varying physical, emotional, and developmental needs
7	History of poor sleeping habits at home	6. Gets adequate sleep to enhance healing	6. Observe and report sleep pattern. Offer back care and refreshments at HS

Exhibit 4-4 Nursing Index/Discharge Note: Patient with Abdominal
Hysterectomy

(On Discharge   Date 6-8-79)

No.	Problem, need, limitation	Onset	Outcome goals	Met
1.	Does not understand what will happen preoperatively	5-30-79	1. Completes pre-op teaching plan	5-30-79
2.	Pain at operative site	6-1-79	2. Absence of pain	6-8-79
3.	Abd. incision draining slightly	6-1-79	3. No drainage— incision clean and dry	6-5-79
4.	Indwelling catheter due to inability to void voluntarily	6-1-79	4. Able to urinate without catheter	6-2-79
5.	Difficulty getting out of bed	6-1-79	5. Able to move without assistance	6-2-79
6.	Crying at times	1 week PTA	6. Absence of crying	Not met
7.	Poor sleep habits	?	7. Define sleep habits as a problem	Not met
8.	Will need to take care of self at home		8. Completes patient teaching plan for abdominal hysterectomy	6-7-79

Additional Discharge Information:

6-8-79 Discharged at 10:00 a.m. to home with husband. Will be seen at surgical clinic next week, by C. Moore, RN on 6-15-79. Given appointment card.

Physical Status: V.S. stable, dsg clean and dry.

Emotional Status: States she is depressed but does not want further help. Thinks that husband will give her a lot of assistance when she gets home. Was told to contact her physician or her community mental health clinic if she continues to be depressed.

K. Zander, RN for
J. Gluck, RN

Because nurses will have difficulty transferring their thinking from problems to outcomes, they will need written and posted outcome criteria along with group and individual training sessions on how to determine goals based on agency standards and individual patient's strengths. A results-oriented documentation system will be useless unless primary nurses are taught to integrate outcomes.

The POMR-GOMR system also can be used alone or in conjunction with the medical staff. Although physicians may not be interested in setting outcomes or writing problem lists, they usually appreciate solid, scientific documentation.

Whether or not physicians approve of nurses using POMR, the system has benefits for primary nurses:

> Many nurses who have assisted in implementing PONS [Problem-Oriented Nursing System] have found that, for the first time, they have been able to develop a meaningful conceptual framework within which to view all their efforts, whether as clinical nurses, nurse-managers, or nurse educators. One of the reasons for this is that the PONS includes a number of components which once received lip service rather than committed application but which now have become . . . mandatory (Ganong & Ganong, 1976, p. 43).

With outcome goals added to the system, the cycle of the nursing process and primary nursing accountability is complete.

Results-Oriented Documentation from Scratch

Agencies that want to develop documentation systems for primary nursing have numerous options. Ideally, the system should reflect each step of the primary nursing process, as identified in Table 4-1, and must be useful during the admission as well as in retrospective auditing. Options include: (1) combining care plans with treatment sheets (Thomas, Note 1); (2) using WIG notes instead of SOAP notes—where the patient was (W), is (I), and should be going (G); and (3) using a statement of outcome as a heading for related progress notes.

The documentation of each primary nurse should be reviewed frequently by the nurse-manager aside from the regular search for specific patient information, because a results-oriented documentation format reflects how the nurses and their colleagues apply the nursing process. The nurse-manager can determine the level of commitment, empathy, problem-solving ability, and realistic goal setting and evaluation of individual nurses, because what they write is how they think, and how they think is what they do.

The documentation should be reviewed by the nurse-manager for the purpose of identifying learning needs of primary nurses in order to arrange seminars. There are several problems that nurses commonly have in thinking about and in documenting clinical work.

1. Nurses have difficulty discriminating between subjective and objective data and their assessment of the two. Learning need: To be able to step back from the clinical data to understand it, rather than be overwhelmed by it. Nurse-managers: Help primary nurses by discussing notes before they write them.

2. Nurses have difficulty discriminating which objective clinical data pertain to the problem being written about. For instance, in a nurse's note about a patient's severe postoperative hiccups, there was information about bowel movements that day. Unless there was a new medical connection between the two pieces of information that was not explained in the assessment section, the note completely lacked meaning and direction. Learning need: To understand the way signs and symptoms reflect underlying problems; to move from a task-completion to a theoretical nursing, diagnostic emphasis. Nurse-manager:

- reviewing body systems by distinguishing signs from symptoms by asking nurses to explain what their connection is
- reviewing treatment records because routine treatments are recorded in them, not in the progress notes
- reviewing change of shift report to watch how clinical data are put together to formulate a patient problem
- putting emphasis on sensory observation

3. Nurses often omit subjective comments of patients or their families. Learning need: More attention to and recall of the patient's/family's participation. Nurse-manager:

- routinely ask questions, such as, "what did the patient say he wanted?" or "did the mother ask you about the problem?"
- ensure patient participation in care plan
- have primary nurses do mini-process-recording to review together

4. Assessments are often too cautious, or as Kerr (1975) puts it:

> In the past when nurses were not supposed to have an opinion, we were all taught to write "appears" or "apparently" to avoid assuming the responsibility of making a forthright statement. I think that should be relegated to history. We are taught to observe and we should write down what we observe without apology or subterfuge (p. 36).

Learning need: To have the courage of the conclusions drawn from patient/family subjective and objective data. Nurse-manager: Help nurses put together clinical data with sensible judgments—the conclusions they draw and write should lead to plans.

5. Assessments are too general. In her warning to avoid basket terms Kerr (1975) states: "The only generalized term used to describe the patient's condition with a meaning that cannot be questioned is 'critical condition' " (p. 36). Learning need: To increase the vocabulary used to describe and assess. Nurse-manager:

- Strive for consensus of definition among your staff by asking questions such as, "what do you mean by 'regressed'?"
- Spend seminar time going through the alphabet and explaining meanings of commonly used words (McTiernan, Note 2).
- When nurses speak with the nurse-manager during a shift and at shift report, the nurse-manager should ask for descriptions beyond the general terms used.

6. Assessments can be biased or erroneous, sometimes placing the patient in a bad light and the nurse on precarious legal grounds. Learning need: To sort out intuition from fact. Nurse-manager: Provide a chance outside of the formal medical record for nurses to vent biases such as "I know that guy is a homosexual" or "she's probably a child beater." Although intuition is often accurate and can be useful clinically, it has no place in the medical record. The nurse-manager should help primary nurses to be curious enough to explore their intuition.

7. Historical information is most easily recorded under Objective. Learning need: To state the past concisely. Nurse-manager: Help nurses summarize patients' conditions concisely for report.

8. Plans are too often vague and lack specifics about who and what action is to take place. Learning need: To be able to think ahead. Nurse-manager: Put emphasis on preventive rather than crisis action. Primary nursing conferences should usually be focused on current goals of patient care as they relate to outcome goals.

The nurse-manager may elect to set up a staff review system for concurrently auditing records. The method and goals for this kind of peer review should be discussed and carefully implemented to make it a positive experience for everyone involved.

Developing Patient-Teaching Documentation

"One component of nursing that is universal to all clinical areas of practice is patient-teaching. Nurses have accepted and enjoyed this role and have increased the professional literature with knowledge on the rationale, content, and methodology for giving patients the information they need. However, with the growth of consumer pressure for informed consent and assurance of quality, and with the JCAH requirements for providing proof that the "patient knowledge" outcome criteria are met, nurses are faced with the tasks of evaluating and documenting what is taught to patients. Because patient-teaching involves a complex series of interactions between patient and nurse, documentation systems that reflect the teaching-learning process need to be developed.

"The Retrospective Audit Committee of the Department of Nursing, Tufts-New England Medical Center Hospital, began creating a system for documenting patient-teaching over two years ago. We assessed our concurrent audits and found that the POMR (Problem Oriented Medical Record) method of charting was too cumbersome for recording detailed content of every teaching session. We sensed that patients were receiving either "pot shots" of unorganized facts thrown their way from numerous well-meaning staff nurses or no information at all. Even with primary nursing it was unrealistic to expect one nurse to teach patients everything they may need to know in one session, despite the appropriate timing of the session. We also realized that nurses would not use a system that was too elaborate, time-consuming, or repetitive in addition to other forms already in use (Kardex, progress notes, flow sheets). We could find no prototypes that would meet both the needs of pediatric and adult in-patient and ambulatory settings as well as fulfill all our requirements for comprehensive patient-teaching. [Therefore], through trial and error, we have developed a format and protocol for a system of documentation that encompasses (1) the patients' rights to learn about their health care through individualized, organized communication with professional nurses, (2) the nurse's need for knowledge in a handy reference that exceeds policies and procedures, (3) the nurse's need for a useful documentation tool, and (4) the Retrospective Audit Committee's need for data that specific outcome criteria have been met.

"[The] teaching plans and guidelines are designed to be used by a registered nurse at any phase of a patient's education. They provide nurses with a means to organize the presentation of content and to evaluate, by way of learner objectives, the patient's response. The teaching plans are designed to be used either in conjunction with problem-oriented charting or as an adjunct to other charting methods. A nurse, optimally the primary nurse, places a specific plan in the patient's progress notes as soon as the need for teaching is identified. Since plans are usually printed on colored paper, they can be easily located among the vast array of other data in the medical record. The checklist nature of the teaching plans facilitates rapid, accurate, and complete documentation. Content and objectives are signed off with the date and the registered nurse's initials, giving their completion the same legality as the patient's medication record. Besides fostering accountability, the checklist format also encourages follow-through when teaching has begun in one unit and the patient is either transferred to another unit or discharged to an ambulatory clinic or VNA care. There is also space for the nurses to write an overall evaluation of the patient's movement toward meeting the objectives.

"Guidelines to enable the nurse to more effectively teach and evaluate the sessions are included with each plan. . . . They are correlated numerically with the plans to facilitate their use as a reference and have been a valuable asset for new or inexperienced nurses. In our setting we have found it useful to provide each nursing unit with a complete notebook of sample plans and guidelines. Each unit also has a stock of plans that are most frequently used, and a mechanism for ordering necessary plans is worked out through unit coordination.

"In addition to the plans and guidelines, handouts have been developed for patients' and their families' use on discharge or between clinic visits. Handouts can further enhance teaching that may already be completed. They ensure that regardless of how well patients and their "significant other" met the learner objectives, they have reliable information when they are away from the immediate hospital environment" (Zander et. al., 1978).

It is possible to formalize a system for documenting patient-teaching and for standardizing the content that is to be taught. Teaching plans and guidelines have to be consistent with standards of care but flexible enough to be used by any nurse in individualizing the content and methodology for a specific patient. The plans constitute a practical "no-frills" system of patient and family education. (See Exhibit 4-5.)

Auditing Primary Nurses

Measuring the outcomes of nursing care by auditing is the most effective way to hold primary nurses accountable for their clinical work. Outcomes transcend the eight-hour shift outlook common to nonprimary nursing systems, as described:

> Traditionally, the individual nurse has been held accountable within the nursing and medical hierarchy for performing nursing activities as prescribed by procedural manuals, physicians' orders, and hospital policies. Furthermore, accountability for patient care has been fragmented. Nursing tends to be a group activity, since many nurses participate in the care of each patient. Consequently, nurse performance has been measured largely in organizational, rather than patient terms, with criteria based on organizational goals and objectives. The "good nurse" came to work on time, carried out assignments promptly, adhered to hospital policies, never made mistakes, and always looked clean and neat. Such criteria have become increasingly irrelevant in today's complex health care system. Nurses can no longer rely exclusively on physicians' orders and hospital policy manuals. They are expected to exercise judgment and make decisions in new situations and in areas where there are few precedents to follow (Taylor, 1974, p. 377).

Thus, nurses need to individually account for the results of their work. Auditing outcomes crystallizes primary nursing as a patient-focused, quality assurance modality for delivering health care.

Exhibit 4-5 Patient-Teaching Plan: General Discharge Medication

	Content/re-inforcement delivered	Learner objectives met	
	Date and R.N.	Date and R.N.	Not applicable

Name of medication _____
Purpose
  • To facilitate a patient's compliance with his medication regimen on hospital discharge.
Content
  I. Medication
    A. Basic action
    B. Usual dosage and frequency
    C. Common side effects
  II. Medication management
    A. Administration schedule
    B. Special teaching needs
  III. Patient handout
  IV. Indications for notifying the physician
    A. Side effects
    B. Inability to comply with the medication regimen
    C. Indication for pharmacy refill
		(shaded)	

Learner objectives
  I. Patient describes the basic action, dosage, frequency, and common side effects of his medication.
  II. Patient describes the schedule for taking his medication.
  III. Patient identifies his medication by appearance and name.
  IV. Patient states indications for notifying the physician.
	(shaded)		

Evaluation			

If patient and/or significant others are unable to complete some or all of this teaching plan, document evaluation in progress notes.

Source: Reprinted with permission. Zander, K.; Bower, K.; Foster, S.; Towson, L.; Wermuth, M.; and Woldum, K. *Practical Manual for Patient-Teaching.* St. Louis: The C.V. Mosby Co., 1978, p. 25.

Nurse-managers and others can review the work of primary nurses by reading documentation and listening carefully during primary nursing conferences. However, an agency needs a formal means of assuring the quality of each primary nurse.

The retrospective audit which is required by the Joint Commission on Hospital Accreditation (JCAH) for quality assurance of patient outcomes is a useful tool for all nurses. In many ways, it is a useful research tool of clinical work which may settle the proverbial question of what is nursing. Answers are sought in the areas of desired patient outcomes, such as, health status, activity, and knowledge, and in the preventive and critical management nursing does to combat complications of diseases, conditions, and the side effects of curative drugs and treatments.

The results of these audits tabulated per unit, clinic, or service can be beneficial to the nurse-manager. They can indicate necessary changes in procedures, equipment, delegation of responsibilities, staff education, or staffing patterns. However, as long as audit results are tabulated for the institution, the individual nurse's accountability will not be fully accomplished.

An agency can use retrospective auditing to improve the level of primary nursing. The nurse-manager and the primary nursing staff may become involved in the auditing process in several ways:

- participating in establishing the criteria
- establishing criteria about subjects of interest to primary nurses and criteria that accurately state expected outcomes
- posting criteria and making them part of each primary nurse's practice
- tallying results for each primary nurse with follow-up as indicated
- sending reports to each primary nurse to give feedback
- re-auditing for improvements
- planning programs to improve deficits

Determining agencywide outcomes for a specific population of patients can be done by a committee, but it is best done in consultation with the primary nurses whose work will be measured. Primary nurses are the experts that Zimmer (1974) refers to:

> nurses who are experts in care of very specific patient populations *know* the patient health wellness results for which they are aiming and the observable evidence of patients' progress toward these outcomes. They either know or they have the communication skills and the trust needed to learn patients' expectations (p. 320).

Steps in Retrospective Auditing

1. Define the audit task utilizing current forms (see Exhibit 4-6, Study Objectives).

2. Instruct retrievers to code for each nurse throughout the audit. Have the auditor keep a key of which code number stands for which nurse. Note that this implies a redefinition of the aim of retrospective auditing (see Exhibit 4-6, Special Consideration).

3. Discuss overall results and individual findings with all clinical leadership personnel, including the nurse-manager, to determine justifications, deficits, patterns for each criterion and across criteria, and final recommendations (see Exhibits 4-7 through 4-13).

4. Send individual audit report to each nurse and ask for plans for improvement and signatures. Reports must be returned to the audit committee and individual personnel files (see Exhibit 4-14).

5. Incorporate audit report in each primary nurse's evaluation.

6. Use caution in determining group versus individual learning needs or deficits.

Exhibit 4-6 Audit Study Specifications

A AUDIT STUDY SPECIFICATIONS

TOPIC: YOUNG ADULT IN-PATIENT ADMISSIONS   DATE: 1978

STUDY OBJECTIVES
1. To study primary nursing care of a specific age group with multiple problems

2. To determine effectiveness of in-patient versus day hospitalization.

DESCRIPTION OF AUDIT TOPIC:

		INDEX CODES

PATIENT RECORDS

INCLUDE: All records with diagnosis: adolescent adjustment reaction, psychotic reaction, depression, borderline personality, schizophrenia

- ☐ Discharge Diagnosis
- ☒ Problem or Condition
- ☐ Surgical Procedure
- ☐ Special Procedure
- ☐ Other

EXCLUDE

AUDIT IDENTIFICATION DATA

- ☐ Original audit
- ☐ Repeat audit   Date(s) of prior audit(s) _____
- ☐ Medical audit only
- ☒ Nursing audit only   (Per Primary Nurse)
- ☐ Combined patient care audit
- ☐ Report to (PSRO, other agency) _____
- ☐ Other
- Committee: Retrospective Audit Committee
  - COMMITTEE CHAIRMAN: _____
  - AUDIT LIAISON: _____
  - COMMITTEE ASSISTANT(S): _____

PATIENT IDENTIFICATION DATA

AGE
- ☐ All ages
- ☐ Exclude pediatric, under age _____
- ☐ Exclude geriatric, over age _____
- ☒ Only between 15 and 22 years

SEX
- ☒ Both sexes
- ☐ Males only
- ☐ Females only

AUDIT STUDY SIZE AND TIME PERIOD

No. records available for audit topic in last
- 6 mos. _____
- 12 mos. _____
- 18 mos. _____
- 24 mos. X
- _____ mos. _____

No. of physicians with privileges for audit topic (optional) _____

No. records requested for audit _____

Method of selection:
- All, in period, from _____ to _____
- Sample, as follows: _____

SPECIAL CONSIDERATIONS, OTHER INFORMATION TO BE REPORTED

1) Please code primary nurses and do audit per nurse

2) Please record length of stay as in-patient and also length of stay as a day hospital pt or name of institution that pt was discharged to.

3) If transferred, check for presence of nursing referral

SIGN-OFF ON AUDIT SPECIFICATIONS, CRITERIA AND INSTRUCTIONS

_____ , Chairman

_____ , Audit Liaison

_____ , Consultant

_____ , Consultant

DATE

Source: InterQual, 1978

Exhibit 4-7 Audit Identification Data Display

AA AUDIT IDENTIFICATION DATA DISPLAY TOPIC: YOUNG ADULT IN-PATIENT ADMISSIONS DATE:

AUDIT STUDY TOTALS: NO. RECORDS ___ NO. PHYSICIANS ___ NO. NURSING UNITS ___

PATIENT DATA

AGE RANGE	TOTAL NO. PATIENTS	MALE	FEMALE	AVE. LOS DAYS	OTHER
15 yrs	4	1	3		
16 yrs	4	2	2		
17 yrs	4	4	0		
18 yrs	5	3	2		
19 yrs	3	0	3		
20 yrs	7	0	7		
21 yrs	7	1	6		
22 yrs	4	3	1		

ACTUAL LENGTH OF STAY — NO. OF PATIENTS

NO. OF DAYS	TOTAL	No. Days	Total	SPEC. CARE
1	1	34	1	
4	1	36	2	
5	1	41	1	
6	3	43	1	
7	2	46	1	
9	1	50	1	
12	2	54	1	
14	2	66	1	
15	2*	69	1	
20	3			
21	1			
22	1			
23	2			
25	1			
26	2			
28	1			
29	2			
33	1			

PHYSICIAN DISTRIBUTION

PHYS. NO.	NO. PTS.	PHYS. NO.	NO. PTS.	PHYS. NO.	NO. PTS.

NURSING UNIT DIST.

N.U. NO.	NO. PTS.	DISCH.
N1	5	
N2	4	
N3	4	
N4	4	
N5	3	
N6	3	
N7	2	
N8	2	
N9	2	
N10	2	
N11	2	
N12	1	
N13	1	
N14	1	
N15	1	
N16	1	

Source: InterQual, 1978

Exhibit 4-8 Audit Criteria

B AUDIT CRITERIA   TOPIC: YOUNG ADULT IN-PATIENT ADMISSIONS   DATE: _____

ELEMENTS	STANDARD 100's or 0's*	EXCEPTIONS	INSTRUCTIONS FOR DATA RETRIEVAL
ADMISSION	NO	NO	NO
Patient exhibits problems in 2 or more of the following categories:			
A) Evidence of thought disorder/psychosis			
B) Suicidal/Homicidal Attempt			
C) Drug/Alcohol abuse			
D) Withdrawal from family/friends			
E) Sleeping/eating/sexual disturbances			
F) Hx of School/work interference			
OUTCOMES			
1. Maintains personal hygiene	X	1. Pt had physical disability, ie: paraplegia. AMA. Physician notified of non-compliance	1. NPN or Nursing referral for evidence that patient can dress, feed, bathe self without assistance from nurse
2. Treatment plan includes structured daily activities as a day Hospital patient	X	2. Pt discharged to combination program of work/day hospital or school/day hospital. AMA. Physician notified of non-compliance	2. NPN or nursing referral, Discharge teaching plan for evidence that pt will continue in community day hospital program every day.
3. Returns to safe, supportive living situation	X	3. Pt not living at home before admission. Discharged to Half-Way house or Residential treatment facility. AMA. Physician notified of non-compliance	3. NPN for evidence that pts home 1) provides food and heat and 2) includes a person who is both associated with a family worker and who the pt feels he can depend on.
4. Demonstrates working alliance with staff	X	4. Physician notified of non-compliance	4. NPN for working alliance – Pt is involved in the group program and patient keeps appointments with primary nurse and evaluator

*Criteria Should Be Set For   Diagnosis: Surgery/Special Procedures/Admission Justification; Discharge Status (Patient Health and Knowledge Outcome), Mortality, Length of Stay (Pre-Op and Post-Op if Surgical), and for Other Indicators of Quality Such As Select Process Items, Complications and Injuries.

Source: InterQual, 1978

Exhibit 4-8 continued

B AUDIT CRITERIA

TOPIC: YOUNG ADULT IN-PATIENT ADMISSIONS   DATE:

ELEMENTS	STANDARD 100 - 1=0	EXCEPTIONS	INSTRUCTIONS FOR DATA RETRIEVAL
8. continued		8. continued	8. convinced that someone is after him, etc. b) Change in mental status - indication that patient is beginning to hallucinate, get increasingly agitated and uncontrollable patient states he is having thoughts or making plans for self-destruction. c) Room Program - Plan to limit patients activities on unit to his room, bathroom and dining room; ie no groups, or passes to go out of hospital.
9. Other	X 9.		9. NPN or nursing referral for evidence of homocide attempt, return to drug abuse, prostitution, etc.

*Criteria Should Be Set For Diagnosis/Surgery/Special Procedures/Admission Justification; Discharge Status (Patient Health and Knowledge Outcome), Mortality, Length of Stay (Pre-Op and Post-Op if Surgical), and for Other Indicators of Quality Such As Select Process Items, Complications and Charges

© InterQual 1976

Exhibit 4-8 continued

B AUDIT CRITERIA

TOPIC: YOUNG **ADULT IN-PATIENT ADMISSIONS**   DATE: _____

ELEMENTS	STANDARD 100 or 0	EXCEPTIONS	INSTRUCTIONS FOR DATA RETRIEVAL
4. continued		4. continued	4. and patient contacts hospital when crisis situation out of the unit on passes
5. Completes discharge medication teaching plan	X	5. Not discharged on any of listed medications: Thorazine (Chlorpromazine) Stelazine (Trifluoperazine) Mellaril (Thioridazine) Prolixin (Fluphenazine) Haldol (Haloperidol) Navane (Thiothixene) AMA Physician notified of non-compliance	
6. Death	X	6.	
COMPLICATIONS			
7. Suicide Gesture/Attempt	X	7. Preventative: RN assesses pt before and after passes from in-pt unit RN assesses pt every shift who is on 15 minute checks Critical: RN notifies MD	7. Master Problem List or NPN for documentation of suicide gesture/attempt – pt tries to do harm to self by actual physical injury or by placing himself in a situation that would potentially lead to his death. Look in order sheets for indication of 15-minute checks.
8. Reoccurrence of Acute Psychosis	X	8. Preventative: Milieu meeting held if pt refuses to take meds and/or is having trouble taking part in daily hospital program. Critical: RN notifies MD for acute changes in mental status Pt placed on room program	8. NPN for: Milieu meeting – meeting of at least one RN and an MD with the pt to discuss serious matters ACUTE PSYCHOSIS – Pt experiences return of scary illogical thoughts that brought him into hospital Pt may state he is seeing or hearing things that don't exist, that he feels unreal, that is

*Criteria Should Be Set For: Diagnosis; Surgery; Special Procedures; Admission Justification; Discharge Status (Patient Health and Knowledge Outcome); Mortality; Length of Stay (Pre-Op and Post-Op if Surgical); and for Other Indicators of Quality Such As Select Process Items; Complications and Charges

₂ InterQual 1976

Exhibit 4-9 Data Retrieval For Each Patient Record

DATA RETRIEVAL FOR EACH PATIENT RECORD   pep
                                                           JCAH

IDENTIFICATION DATA		
AUDIT	PATIENT	PHYSICIAN/UNIT
Topic: YOUNG ADULT IN-PATIENT ADMISSIONS Committee: Nursing Retrospective Audit Committee Asst: Date: 6/78	Record No.: Age: 16 Sex: F Other:	MRNo. XXXXXX Primary Nurse: N1 Dept./Serv: Psychiatry Units/Wards: Psychiatry

AUDIT CRITERIA DATA									
NOTES	CRIT. NO.	ELEMENTS EXCEPTIONS OR CRITICAL MANAGEMENT	STD. %. 100/0	MEETS EL	EX	CM	VAR	NO CM
Pt noted family and friends "different than her", superficially cut wrists, began experimenting with LSD, THC, pot. 12/76 picked up by police after ran away from home. Taken to City Hosp. for withdrawal behavior. Not attended school since 12/76. 1. No documentation 2. Primary nurse actively involved in plans for school and conjoint day program. 3. No documentation 4. Doc. that pt was initially withdrawn but gradually attended groups and worked with staff. 5. Discharged on Stelazine and Cogentin but no documentation of teaching. 7. 3/7 pt. cut wrists slightly: put on checks and MD notified. P.N. continues to assess. 8. Evaluated as chronically psychotic. Preoccupied with feelings of self-abuse. 9. No drug abuse. **Nsg. referral states pt. responds well to structured and caring limits (written by primary nurse)		Pt exhibits problems in 2 or more of the following categories: A) Evidence of thought disorder/psychosis B) Suicidal/Homocidal Attempt C) Drug/Alcohol Abuse D) Withdrawal from family/friends E) Sleeping/eating/sexual disturbances F) Hx of school/work interferences.	100	✓				
	1.	Maintains personal hygiene	100				✓	
	2.	Rx plan includes structured daily activities as a Day Hospital patient	100	✓				
	3.	Returns to safe, supportive living situation	100				✓	
	4.	Demonstrates working alliance with staff	100	✓				
	5.	Completes discharge medication teaching plan	100				✓	
	6.	Death	0	✓				
	7.	Suicide gesture/attempt	0			✓		
	8.	Reoccurence of Acute Psychosis Episodes of staring and voices put there by devil	0				✓	
	9.	Other	0	✓				
		Length of Stay as in-patient 43 days Length of Stay as a day hospital pt 64 days Name of institution patient discharged to Day Hospital nearer her home If patient transferred, was nursing referral in chart? X yes ____ no ____ n/a						

1 The committee can use reverse side for variation analysis notes
2 In a nursing audit note the unit number on which a complication was first documented in the patient record

Copyright 1974. Joint Commission on Accreditation of Hospitals.

Source: InterQual, 1978

Exhibit 4-10 Deficiency Analysis

Key
H - Pt Status or Noncompliance
I - Community Factors
J - Needs Further Investigation

1 - Environmental/community Barrier
3 - Feedback inadequacy
4 - ...

M - Minor
S - Serious

DEFICIENCY ANALYSIS

TOPIC: YOUNG ADULT INPATIENT ADMISSIONS   DATE:

CRITERIA		DEFICIENCIES			ATTRIB PER VAR ANAL
#	SUBJECT	PROV/CODE #	RECORD #	#DEF/PREC	

ANALYSIS: PROBLEMS AND CAUSES

SINGLE, ISOLATED DEFICIENCIES BY RECORD	CAUSE	SEVERITY
99-02-94 Parents would not turn in guns, so pt was discharged	H, 1	S

#	PATTERNS PER CRITERION ONLY	CAUSE#	SEVERITY
1	lack of documentation	1	M
2	pts who had no written plan were also the patients who left in an emergency	1	M
3	Either no doc. or discharged to difficult home situations	4	S
4	Patients too psychotic to make alliance	3	S
5	No documentation - no form	1	S

PATTERNS OCCURRING ACROSS CRITERIA AND RECORDS	CAUSE	SEVERITY
A) Poor documentation of mental status and other criteria when pt discharged in an emergency	1	M
B) Lack of xeroxed nursing referral to long-term hospitals	1	M

INCIDENTAL PROBLEMS DISCLOSED BY AUDIT	ATTRIB	CAUSE	SEVERITY
Emergency transfers occur at transition time to day hosp.	H, I, J	4	S
B) Alliance between staff and parents of teenagers found to be weak in some cases	G, I, J	3	S

UNJUSTIFIED EXCEPTION/VARIATION/COMPLICATION RATES	ATTRIB	CAUSE	SEVERITY

#	CRITERIA DEFICIENCIES, FORGOTTEN EXCEPTIONS
8	102-90-68 Patient was on sitters & room program but eloped from unit
8	96-77-35 Psychotic pt treated as an acting-out patient
	97-81-39 Had contracts not to drink but did drink and were discharged
	92-68-62

*, InterQual, 1976.

Source: InterQual, 1978

Exhibit 4-11 Selected Variation Exception/Complication Rates

Selected VARIATION/EXCEPTION/COMPLICATION RATES   TOPIC: __YOUNG ADULT IN-PATIENT ADMISSIONS__

PROVIDER		VARIATION RATES [✓/#] Variations [#/#] Deficiencies						EXCEPTION RATES [✓/#] Met Element [#/#] Met Exception					COMPLICATION RATES [✓/#] Complications [#/#] Not Meeting CM								
		CRITERION NUMBER						EXCEPTION NUMBER					COMPLICATION NUMBER					TOTAL # COMP. IN STUDY	# PTS. WITH COMP.
PROV. #	TOTAL # RECORDS IN STUDY	1	2	3	4	5		1	2	3	4	5	7	8	9				
N1	5	5/4	2/2	2/2	1/1	4/4		0/1	0/1	0/1	1/2	0/1	1/2	2/2				3	2
N2	4	3/2	2/1	2/2	1/1	2/2		1/1	1/1	1/2	2/2	0/2	0/2	1/2	0/1			3	3
N3	4	4/1	1/0	3/3	1/1	1/1		3/3	0/1	1/1	0/4	0/3		1/1	0/1			1	1
N4	4	3/2	1/0	3/3	1/1	2/2		0/2	1/1	0/2	0/2	0/2							
N5	3	3/3	2/0	1/1	1/1	2/2		0/1	1/1	0/3	0/3	0/1	1/2	0/2				3	3
N6	3	1/1	1/0	3/1	1/1	2/2		0/2	2/3	2/3	0/3	1/3	0/0	1/0				1	1
N7	2	2/1	2/1	1/1	2/1	1/1		0/1	0/1	0/1	0/1	1/1	2/1	0/1				3	2
N8	2	2/1	2/0	1/1	2/2	1/1		1/1	1/1	0/1	1/6	0/1	1/0	1/0				2	2
N9	2	2/1	1/0	1/0	1/0	1/1		1/1	1/1	1/1	1/1	0/1		1/0				1	1
N10	2	2/2	2/0	2/1	1/0	1/0		1/1	1/1	1/1	1/1	0/2							
N11	2	2/1	2/1	1/0	1/0	1/1		1/1	1/1	1/1	2/2	0/0	1/0					1	1
N12	1	1/0	1/0	1/0	1/0	1/1		1/1	1/0	1/1	1/6								
N13	1	1/0	1/0			1/1			0/1	0/1	1/0		1/1	1/1				1	1
N14	1	1/0	1/0	1/0		1/0			0/1										
N15	1	1/1	1/0	1/0	1/1	1/1		0/1	0/1	0/1			1/0	1/0				1	1
N16	1	1/1	1/0	1/1	1/1	1/1			0/1	1/1			1/0	1/0					
# OR % PER CRIT.		24%	4%	10%	10%	19%		52%	92%	80%	80%	80%	0	4	0				
PROBLEM (✓):																			

Source: InterQual, 1978

Exhibit 4-12 Actions and Follow-up

EE ACTIONS AND FOLLOW-UP   TOPIC: YOUNG ADULT IN-PATIENT   DATE:

		CORRECTIVE ACTION PLAN			FOLLOW-UP PLAN			
CRIT.#	WHAT	CONCURRENT MONITORS ✓	BY WHOM	WHEN HOW OFTEN HOW LONG	HOW	WHEN	BY WHOM	✓
1	Include category in:	X	K. Zander					
	Initial nursing assessment				Initial assessments	Mar. 79	K. Zander	X
	Nursing referral If Unresolved				Nursing Referrals	Mar. 79	K. Zander	X
	Discharge Note If Unresolved				Discharge Note	Oct. 79	K. Zander	X
	Nursing Index If Unresolved				Nursing Index	Oct. 79	K. Zander	X
2	Post criteria in each chart of young adult admission so it can be incorporated in care plans		Unit Secret.,	Every Adult	Post on Unit.	Mar. 79	K. Zander	
					Post in Chart.	April 79	K. Zander	
3	Include awareness of home living situation in primary nursing supervision		K. Zander					
4	Add "active psychosis" as exception Discuss criteria with Chief MSW and implications for more family contact. Discuss need for young adult group in the program with Chief of Service	X			Young Adult Therapy Group	Sept. 79	To be determined	
5	Use Medication Teaching Plan	X	K. Zander Concurrent Monitor	Every 3 months	Use Med. Teaching Plans	Jan 79	Staff	X
8	Improve documentation of critical management							
9	Increase awareness among staff of young adults as a group of patients with special needs	X	K. Zander		Present audit results to nursing staff	Mar 7,79	K. Zander	X
					Chief of Service	Mar 6,79		X
					Chief Social Worker Chart Rounds	Mar 6,79		X
	Copies of Nursing Referrals in chart on day of discharge	X	K. Zander		Unit Secretary to make copy	Mar 79	K. Zander	X
	Letter to each primary nurse describing their results and requesting plans for improvement	X	K. Zander		To be returned by	May 79	K. Zander	

CRITERIA REVISIONS NOTED ON CRITERIA NOS.:
WORKSHEET FOR CRITERIA   RE-AUDIT DATE

Source: InterQual, 1976

Exhibit 4-13 Audit Summary

F AUDIT SUMMARY   TOPIC: YOUNG ADULT IN-PATIENT ADMISSIONS   DATE:

| Original Audit [X] | No. records in study 50 | Physician data: | Nursing Audit Data: No. nursing units in study |
| Repeat Audit [ ] | No. adjusted records | No. in study / No. with privileges for topic | No. discharge units |

DESCRIPTION OF STUDY (SUMMARY OF CRITERIA, MAJOR FINDINGS AND PROBLEMS DISCLOSED, INCIDENTAL FINDINGS, PLANNED AND EFFECTED ACTION AND FOLLOW-UP)

CRIT. NO.	AUDIT CRITERIA	% MET	NO. VAR.	VAR. NO.	JUST. %	TOT. EXC.	NO. DEF.	PROBLEMS AND ACTIONS RECOMMENDED
1.	Maintains personal hygiene	34	33	9	27	52	24	Include category in initial nursing assessment, and discharge note (if an identified problem) and nursing referral.
2.	Treatment plan includes structured daily activities as a day hospital patient	58	21	17	81	92	4	Standardized care plan for young adults individualized to include special family work, core evaluations (#766) psychosis, alcohol and drug abuse, etc.
3.	Returns to safe, supportive living situation	64	18	8	43	80	10	Increase primary nurses' attention to the patient's home situation by increased discussions with MSW's more home visits.
4.	Demonstrates working alliance with staff	60	20	10	50	80	10	Include "active psychosis" in exception
5.	Completes discharge medication teaching plan	62	19	0	0	62	19	Primary nurses to begin using formal teaching plans, spot-checked
6.	Death	100	0	0	0	100	0	
7.	Suicide Gesture/attempt	88	6	6	100	100	0	
8.	Reoccurence of Acute Psychosis	76	12	8	67	92	4	Improve documentation of critical management
9.	Other	96	2	2	100	100	0	Transferred patients should have copy of nursing referral in their charts. Letter to each indiv. P. N.

REVIEWED BY:	AUDIT SUMMARY			FOLLOW-UP		
	DATE SENT	DATE SIGNED	SIGNATURE	DATE SENT	DATE SIGNED	SIGNATURE
AUDIT COMMITTEE CHAIRMAN						
DEPARTMENT CHAIRMAN						
PRESIDENT/CHIEF MEDICAL STAFF						
CHAIRMAN, MEDICAL STAFF EXECUTIVE COMMITTEE						

REVIEWED BY:	AUDIT SUMMARY			FOLLOW-UP		
	DATE SENT	DATE SIGNED	SIGNATURE	DATE SENT	DATE SIGNED	SIGNATURE
NURSING SERVICE DIRECTOR (NURSING/COMBINED AUDIT)						
CHIEF EXECUTIVE OFFICER						
HOSPITAL BOARD OR COMMITTEE						
OTHER						

Source: InterQual, 1976

Exhibit 4-14 Audit Report to Primary Nurse

To: Karen Zander RN
From: Retrospective Audit Committee, Department of Nursing

Dear Ms. Zander,
 A retrospective audit of the last 50 young adult psychiatric inpatient admissions was done in 1978. A copy of the criteria is enclosed. Of these you had 4 as primary patients. We would like to congratulate you on the fact that two of these young adults met all the criteria without complications. One of the other two did have a reoccurrence of acute psychosis, but the preventive management measures had been carried out and appropriate critical management was instituted.

 In the fourth patient, several outcome criteria were not met, largely due to lack of documentation in criteria nos. 1, 3, 4, and 5. Please outline your plans for improving future audits of young adult admissions in the space below, sign, and return to Box 38 by March 30. This report of your successes and plans for improvement will become part of your personnel file. A copy will be sent to you for your own records. Once again, congratulations.

Outcomes Based on Levels of Care

 Gluck (Note 3) has proposed that graduated outcome criteria be used to evaluate the effectiveness of clinical specialists. Exhibits 4-15 through 4-17 show her proposal for outcomes for patients with chronic obstructive pulmonary disease. If primary nurses can be considered clinical specialists for acute and/or institutional care, the spectrum of outcomes takes on interesting significance.

 A primary nurse on an inpatient unit would be accountable for the outcomes of patient care up to a certain level of wellness, while a primary nurse in an outpatient clinic would be accountable for different outcomes with the same patient. Graduated outcome criteria may be useful to agencies serving more than one level of acuteness in patients. Most important, such criteria would guide primary nurses in understanding the goals of their plans and interventions.

Other Benefits of Auditing

 The purpose of chart review in the nursing audit is to identify the degree to which actual performance meets the criteria applicable to a particular patient population. The gaps that occur represent potential for improvement and must lead directly to appropriate action to close the gaps or the audit becomes a hollow experience (Berg, 1974, p. 334).

Exhibit 4-15 Maintenance of Maximum Physical Status: Chronic Obstructive Pulmonary Disease (COPD)

1	2	3	4
Short of breath at rest, unable to perform even light work	Able to perform light work with minimal distress	Able to walk on level ground and/or climb one flight stairs with minimal distress	Able to climb two or more flights of stairs with minimal distress
Achieve 85% of maximum heart rate at 100 kpm during exercise testing	Achieve 85% of maximum heart rate at 400 kpm during exercise testing	Achieve 85% of maximum heart rate at 800 kpm during exercise testing	Achieve 85% of maximum heart rate at 1000 kpm during exercise testing
Flow-volume loop < 40% predicted	Flow-volume loop 40-60% predicted	Flow-volume loop 60-80% predicted	Flow-volume loop > 80% predicted
Rhonchi, wheezes and/or rales present during inspiration and expiration	Rhonchi, wheezes and/or rales absent	Rhonchi, wheezes and/or rales absent	Rhonchi, wheezes and rales absent
Unable to lie flat without distress	Able to lie flat without distress	Able to lie flat without distress	Able to lie flat without distress
At least one wheezing episode per week (requiring prn medication)	At least one wheezing episode per month (requiring prn medication)	Wheezing episodes intermittent, less than one per month (requiring prn medication)	Wheezing episodes absent and not requiring prn medication

Code:
1. Status on admission to inpatient
2. Minimum discharge criteria from inpatient
3. Status typical of outpatients
4. Optimum outcome of outpatient nursing care

Source: Exhibits 4-15 through 4-17 are from Gluck, J. *Clinical nurse specialist in pulmonary medicine: A prospectus.* Unpublished manuscript, Boston University School of Nursing, 1975.

Exhibit 4-16 Understanding of Disease Process and Treatment Regime: COPD

1	2	3
Cannot name or briefly describe lung disease	Can name and briefly describe lung disease with assistance	Can name and briefly describe lung disease independently
Cannot identify regularly scheduled medications, dose, or times	Can identify regularly scheduled medications, dose, and times with assistance	Can identify regularly scheduled medications, dose, and times independently
Cannot identify prn medications, dose, or indications for use	Can identify prn medications, dose, and indications for use with assistance	Can identify prn medications, dose, and indications for use independently
Cannot identify therapeutic or toxic effects of medications	Can identify therapeutic and toxic effects of medications with assistance	Can identify therapeutic and toxic effects of medications independently
Cannot describe purpose of equipment, method, or indications for use	Can describe purpose of equipment, method, and indications for use with assistance	Can describe purpose of equipment, method, and indications for use independently
Cannot set up or correctly use equipment	Can correctly use equipment after it is set up by someone else	Can set up and correctly use equipment independently
Cannot describe breathing exercises, purpose, or indications for use	Can describe breathing exercises, purpose, and indications for use with assistance	Can describe breathing exercises, purpose, and indications for use independently
Cannot describe chest PT (including postural drainage), purpose, or indications for use	Can describe chest PT (including postural drainage), purpose, and indications for use with assistance	Can describe chest PT (including postural drainage), purpose, and indications for use independently
Cannot describe relationship of exercise or heavy exertion to effects on illness state	Can describe relationship of exercise and heavy exertion to effects on illness state with assistance	Can describe relationship of exercise and heavy exertion to effects on illness state independently
Cannot describe short or long term goals of therapy	Can describe short and long term goals of therapy with assistance	Can describe short and long term goals of therapy independently

Code:
1 Status on admission to inpatient
2 Outcome criteria from inpatient admission
3 Optimum outcome from outpatient nursing care

Exhibit 4-17 Compliance with Treatment Regime: COPD

1	2	3
Rejects planning alterations in life style	Participates in planning alterations in life style only with encouragement	Participates freely in planning alterations in life style
Does not participate in devising treatment schedule	Participates in devising treatment schedule only with prodding	Participates freely in devising treatment schedule
Unnecessarily limits self in many or all aspects of previous social role	Unnecessarily limits self in some aspects of previous social role	Returns to previous social role as appropriate within physical limitations
Unnecessarily limits self in many or all aspects of previous or newly devised work role	Unnecessarily limits self in some aspects of previous or newly devised work role	Returns to previous or newly devised work role as appropriate within physical limitations
Sees health/illness state as uncontrollable	Identifies significant others as primarily responsible for controlling health/illness state	Identifies self as person primarily responsible for controlling health/illness state
Does not use regularly scheduled medications	Uses regularly scheduled medications inappropriately	Uses regularly scheduled medications appropriately
Does not use prn medications	Uses prn medications inappropriately	Uses prn medications appropriately
Does not use equipment	Uses equipment inappropriately	Uses equipment appropriately
Does not do physical therapy (chest PT, postural drainage, breathing exercises)	Does physical therapy inappropriately	Does physical therapy appropriately
Disregards all activity limitations; continues to perform activities until he finds them intolerable	Attempts many activities known to cause distress and ceases activities only when he encounters distress	Utilizes activity simplification methods to adjust to activity limitations and avoids activities known to cause distress
Avoids periodic professional assessment	Seeks periodic professional assessment with encouragement	Seeks periodic professional assessment independently

Code:
1 Status on admission to inpatient
2 Outcome criteria from inpatient
3 Optimum outcome criteria from outpatient nursing care

Knowledge and skill gaps can lead to new programs for primary nursing focused on improving particular aspects of patient care. When the subject is audited again, improvement in scores indicates the effectiveness of staff development programs as well as the quality of primary nursing care.

Gaps can also show areas requiring managerial emphasis. Because the gaps often result from lack of documentation, audit results also reflect the nurse-manager's ability to provide complete nursing care, both routine tasks and individualized approaches, through the whole nursing staff. As audits show, a primary nurse is only as good as the nursing staff that supports plans, orders, and suggestions.

Another benefit of auditing is that primary nurses feel more professional.

> As registered nurses develop and use sets of criteria, they may be stimulated to use the criteria as a basis for systematic recording of the patient's progress toward realistic outcomes. The intrinsic reward for the nurse of seeing goal-directed nursing activities assisting the patient to achieve realistic outcomes is a very powerful one (Berg, 1974, p. 334-335).

Lastly, using the auditing process provides a tool to research aspects of primary nursing care on a national level. As long as auditing is required of all major hospitals, nurses should use the process to their advantage.

EVALUATING PRIMARY NURSES

For primary nurses to be held accountable for their work with primary patients, they must be evaluated on the way they carry out each of their responsibilities. Evaluating primary nurses is a management function that is a process that helps primary nurses determine ways to excel in their areas of responsibility. Evaluations should stimulate personal introspection which allows them to grow in their abilities and actions. Only with feedback can primary nurses be fairly held accountable for the outcomes of those actions. This relationship is shown schematically in Figure 4-1.

Thus, accountability alone is necessary but not sufficient for primary nursing practice. To elaborate the relationship between clinical expertise and accountability further, a story reported by Passos (1973) makes the point: "A young boy was going into the boxing ring for his first fight. When the bell rang and the boy stood up, he made the sign of the cross. A young man watching the fight asked a priest sitting near him, 'Father, will that help him?' The priest answered, 'Yes, *if* he can fight'!" (p. 21).

Figure 4-1 Relationship of Evaluation to Outcomes for Which the Primary Nurse is Accountable

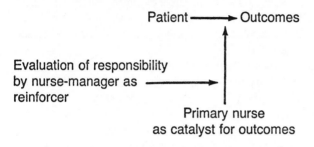

Therefore, the nurse-manager needs to treat evaluations of primary nurses as an important aspect of managing toward accountability. Evaluations are not simply paperwork, but can be used as tools for discussion about a primary nurse's career.

There are two kinds of evaluations used for primary nurses, daily refueling and formal. The nurse-manager will need to know how to make the most of each type of evaluation regardless of the particular system and forms used in each agency. For both types of evaluations a nurse-manager's responsibilities can be accomplished more easily with primary nursing than with other patterns of nursing care delivery, because the primary nurse's area of accountability and responsibility is directly defined and measurable. All of the principles of performance appraisals are applicable to the evaluation of primary nurses. However, the timing and manner in which the principles are applied differs in a primary nursing setting, as does formal evaluation itself.

Evaluating primary nurses differs because primary nursing involves application of the nursing process over time, rather than task completion per shift. The elongated time element benefits both the primary nurse and the nurse-manager because the nurse-manager has more opportunity to observe primary nurses' thoughts as well as actions. Does the primary nurse consistently identify subtle changes in condition? Where does this break down? Does the primary nurse collaborate with nursing peers? Does the primary nurse treat nonprimary patients with respect and interest?

Evaluations of either type should be done within the context of the working alliance that was begun at the first interview. Nurse-manager and staff nurse should never forget the tone of that initial meeting and the space traveled in between. Even if the nurse-manager forgets the particulars of the working contract, chances are that the primary nurse has not, because it is the nurse's career. More than subsequent interactions, the staff nurse remembers the tone or attitude of the nurse-manager's working alliance. In fact, much of the primary nurse's subconscious attention is riveted on the relationship with the nurse-manager, no matter how autonomously the nurse functions. There is no way to avoid it—trust is as important in a primary nurse/nurse-manager relationship as it is in early childhood development. If primary nurses believe that the nurse-manager has their interests as much in mind as the interests of the patient, trust will override the occasional inconveniences of assignments, overtime, and days when the nurse-manager is not functioning at top form.

The way a nurse-manager uses formal or refueling evaluation sessions is a hallmark of leadership style. When and how the nurse-manager holds the sessions may determine whether the staff views the nurse-manager as working as energetically for their development as for the care of patients. Personal attention from the nurse-manager is a productive experience designed to enable the primary nurse to fulfull the responsibilities that lead to accountable practice.

Refueling Evaluation Sessions

Refueling evaluations may be requested at any time by either the primary nurse or nurse-manager, and preparation time for them is not necessarily needed. They are off the record and may have many purposes. The nurse-manager may request a session when a primary nurse is doing exceptionally well or starting to slip. The nurse-manager may also need to discuss the primary nurse's role in future staffing needs or in upcoming educational opportunities. The primary nurse may request a refueling meeting for the same reasons as the nurse-manager or to discuss something else. The urgency of the "can I talk to you" from a primary nurse will give some clues about the content and need for the refueling session.

When the Nurse-Manager Requests Sessions

- The primary nurse is doing excellent work with a primary patient.
- The primary nurse needs a push to prepare patient and family for discharge or to talk to the physician.
- The primary nurse is withdrawing from patients and the rest of the nursing staff by not communicating essential information for continuity of care.
- The nurse-manager needs the primary nurse to be a preceptor for a new staff nurse and wants to discuss details.
- The nurse-manager wants the primary nurse to present a seminar on an unusual diagnosis at a primary patient conference.
- The primary nurse's documentation needs to be more concise because people are not reading the notes.
- The primary nurse has made two medication errors in a week and with one more will be put on formal probation. The nurse-manager wants to acknowledge the crisis and discuss ways to help avoid another error.

The nurse-manager should review the following guidelines when conducting a refueling session.

1. Speak with the primary nurse as soon as an issue or behavior is identified—never postpone because it will not go away, or if it is a positive behavior, it will be lost in the shuffle and not reinforced.

2. State the purpose of the session when it is requested. Do not leave the primary nurse in suspense because it may cause needless anxiety and difficulty responding to any positive or critical feedback.

3. Focus on the business at hand during the session. If the purpose is to change unwanted behavior, do not sugar-coat or sidetrack attention by first mentioning positive aspects of the nurse's performance: "you do this well, but . . ." A "but" always qualifies the positive statement, which can leave the nurse feeling anxious and confused about the evaluator's intent or, worse, believing that nothing is good about the nurse's work.

4. Request the primary nurse's evaluation of the issue or problem to make it two-way.

5. If undesired behavior is identified, the nurse-manager and primary nurse must explore how to change the behavior together, although each with a definite role. Never accept "I'll try harder."

6. Make the refueling session productive ending with a mutual decision, plan, or agreement.

7. Hold the session during the primary nurse's shift to reinforce that evaluations are part of each person's regular professional work.

When the Primary Nurse Requests Sessions

- The primary nurse needs the nurse-manager's approval for a plan about a primary patient.
- The primary nurse has complaints about the way other staff are treating a primary patient or other patients in general.
- The primary nurse needs to inform the nurse-manager about special needs, such as career and personal plans.
- The primary nurse wants to talk privately with the nurse-manager about their relationship.
- The primary nurse needs suggestions or borrowed power for patient advocacy interventions.
- The primary nurse may want consensual validation.

The nurse-manager should review the following guidelines when interacting in a refueling session requested by a primary nurse:

1. Talk to the primary nurse as soon as you can.
2. Wait to hear all of what the primary nurse has to say before jumping in with ideas, decisions, or judgments.

3. Listen to the primary nurse's evaluation of a situation, especially in regard to other staff nurses. Do not take sides for or against the nurse, but make the nurse tell you a way to improve situations.
4. Encourage the nurse to bring up general issues in staff meetings.

Use of Formal Evaluation Sessions

Formal evaluations are those required by the institution at specific intervals for multiple purposes including:

- maintaining or upgrading the general level of staff performance
- salary adjustment/promotion
- data for permanent employee record
- documentation of behavior that necessitates possible or actual dismissal

Formal evaluations traditionally are based on the traits and behaviors expected of all nurses in an institution. Although there may be standardized criteria, the nurse-manager can use the formal evaluation for the advantage of all concerned.

Adjustments to Primary Nursing

As primary nursing develops, tools which have traditionally been used for formal evaluations will need to be revised with attention to: quality assurance and standards of practice; autonomy and motivation of individual nurses through goal setting, goal attainment, and self-evaluation; and changes in management styles that emphasize the enabling process between a nurse-manager and each primary nurse. Therefore, formal appraisals should take the form of a performance evaluation, which puts priority on demonstrated performance rather than personality traits and nonpurposeful behaviors. Ganong and Ganong (1974) have clarified performance evaluation as "the measurement (the determination of degree of conformity with criteria of quality and quantity) of the results (consequences, outcomes) of a person's work effort (on-the-job activities and exertion) compared with (examined in order to note the similarities or differences) previously agreed upon (jointly developed in advance with accord by the manager and the employee) standards (acknowledged measures of comparison for qualitative or quantitative value; criteria; norms)" (p. 11).

The performance evaluation method is part of a program called results-oriented performance evaluation program (ROPEP), which connects organizational standards and objectives with the performance goals of individuals (Ganong and Ganong, 1974). In essence ROPEP extends the management-by-objectives (MBO) framework to the individual staff member by expecting everyone to achieve agreed upon objectives which contribute to the maintenance and growth of the organization.

By using ROPEP, primary nurses can manage and evaluate their own perform-ance in much the same way that nurse-managers coordinate unit activities. This method of evaluation increases the staff nurse's knowledge about and control over expected performance. ROPEP enhances ownership of behavior and active in-volvement of staff members with their manager.

The six steps in the ROPEP-MBO procedure are:

1. Identify purpose and performance responsibilities (to whom).
2. List the major job segments (details of performance responsibilities).
3. Develop measures of satisfactory performance.
4. Set goals, objectives, and target dates.
5. Work toward achievement of objectives.
6. Review performance results; plan new objectives and target dates.

"The hoped-for outcomes of this process are results that contribute to achievement of the purposes of the individual employee, the department, and the organization. In hospitals and other health care agencies, the expected beneficiaries are the consumers themselves" (Ganong and Ganong, 1974, p. 49).

Some primary nurse performance responsibilities that should be included in the evaluation process are:

- interactions with families
- effectiveness as a patient educator
- evidence of making realistic plans for patients
- interaction with peers
- willingness to cover other patients and carry a fair share of the total work load
- successful supervision of ancillary personnel
- ability to organize and verbally report on patient status and plans
- effectiveness as a patient advocate
- independent actions to define learning needs and attend educational pro-grams

In addition, audit results should be tabulated and included as a major part of a primary nurse's evaluation. In this way, the accountability loop is completed through documentation of individual performance results in accordance with standards.

Guidelines for Formal Evaluations

1. Schedule sessions well in advance to give the nurse-manager and primary nurse time to prepare.

2. Preparation includes review of old care plans, review of the last evaluation, especially goals, and review of anecdotal notes. Anecdotal notes can be kept on index cards for each member of the nursing staff throughout their employment. They are notations of both positive and undesired behaviors, recorded soon after the behavior is exhibited. They function as the nurse-manager's memory and can be used as data for formal evaluations. They are best utilized to record informal refueling evaluations, so that the primary nurse gets personal attention at the time and so that the nurse-manager does not forget the content of the refueling meetings. They are especially useful when there are long intervals between required formal evaluations.

3. The primary nurse should come to the session with a self-evaluation which may include objectives set at the last evaluation, a list of strengths and weaknesses, new objectives, or a form to be used as the primary nurse's worksheet.

4. Evaluation should accurately describe the entire period of time covered, not just the latest mistakes or the success of the first month in the position.

5. Evaluation should, as much as possible, be in the control of the primary nurse with the nurse-manager providing objectivity to the primary nurse's perceptions of performance. This process works best with employees who have internalized accepted standards of behavior, but it is possible to encourage others to participate actively in their own evaluations too.

6. Formal evaluations should not contain any surprises because any deviations from expected performance should have been addressed in refueling sessions. A formal evaluation is merely a summary of behavior and outcomes of which the primary nurse is already aware.

7. Do not expect the primary nurse to like or agree with every point.

8. Do not interpret a staff nurse's behavior by using armchair psychology. Keep any personal information you know about the nurse outside the evaluation.

9. Keep communication flowing during the evaluation interview by avoiding the common traps identified by Stevens (1976):

- conducting a one-way conversation
- interrupting the employee's thoughts, explanations, questions
- criticizing the employee rather than the performance
- smoothing over real deficiencies and problems too fast
- failing to investigate facts before expressing opinions
- passing the buck by claiming that one's corrective measures originate higher up
- allowing the interview to fall into charge-countercharge cycles
- allowing the interview to fall into charge-excuse cycles
- allowing the interview to deteriorate into a social visit (p. 161)

10. Write the permanent evaluation after the session, incorporating the significant points that were discussed. This insures a mutual discussion about the criteria because the nurse-manager is willing to adjust isolated evaluations about the nurse.

11. Give the primary nurse a copy of the official evaluation.

Evaluating the Nurse-Manager

The nurse-manager can use the individual refueling and formal evaluations to evaluate the staff collectively, and subsequently, the nurse-manager's own role with them. This can be done because the staff is a group with norms and values that is aware of each member's actions. Thus, the nurse-manager should never expect one nurse to be far removed from the others in behavior.

For instance, if one primary nurse is taking a back seat on the multidisciplinary team of a particular patient, other primary nurses are more than likely having difficulties being assertive—otherwise the other nurses would have influenced the unassertive nurse. The nurse-manager needs to point out at which points the primary nurse retreated into passivity and then, together with the primary nurse, to find out why and what can be done to change the situation. The nurse-manager may realize that the leadership style is sabotaging a primary nurse's position on certain multidisciplinary teams. Also evaluation sessions may show that the majority of the staff, including the nurse-manager, feel insecure about a certain type of patient.

The nurse-manager needs to risk learning reactions to leadership style. The nurse-manager should not be self-deprecating or defensive during an evaluation interview, but should listen quietly to the between-the-lines evaluation of the nurse-manager being given by the primary nurse.

The nurse-manager can invite an evaluation by asking, "what can I do to assist you?" or "where do you feel I didn't understand you?" This can be done during refueling sessions which are off the record so as not to allow a nurse to turn the formal evaluation into an evaluation of the nurse-manager. The manager's evaluation traditionally is discussed with the nurse-manager's own immediate supervisor.

The benefits of staff evaluation of the nurse-manager are identified by Marram, Schlegel, and Bevis (1974) in the areas below:

- Attitudes and strength
- Leadership
- Resource person
- Role model
- Staff development
- Areas needing improvement
- Help to individuals
- Unit suggestions

An evaluation conference can be more meaningful when a dialogue occurs. This dialogue implies that the staff nurse and head nurse evaluate each other. The staff nurse also evaluates the assistant head nurse and the unit service coordinator on a six-month basis. If the responsibility of unit leaders is to provide quality patient care standards and staff development, it is essential that they get feedback from the staff regarding their attitudes and performance. . . . (pp. 118-119)

Using individual evaluations, the nurse-manager should reinforce consensus of the primary nurse's role definition, but should not try to have all the primary nurses fit a mold. Having everyone fit a mold is not only an unrealistic goal, but the nurse-manager's dream may obscure what each individual has to offer the whole staff group. A nurse's personal style cannot be changed too much. Attempts at this can backfire by making the nurse feel stifled and pushing the anger about the evaluation underground, which may cause the nurse to work against some of the nurse-manager's expectations.

If attention is on individual professional development rather than personality change, the nurse-manager and the staff will have an enjoyable, thriving relationship. Both refueling and formal evaluations should be accurate appraisals, mutually determined. A nurse-manager needs to be free enough from impatience to be creative with all the primary nurses on the staff. Through evaluations the nurse-manager can give primary nurses the information, assistance, and security they require to be truly accountable professionals.

REFERENCE NOTES

1. Thomas, R. Unpublished manuscript, Childrens Hospital Medical Center, Boston, 1979.
2. McTiernan, E. *Assistant nurse leader.* Unpublished manuscript, Tufts-New England Medical Center, Boston, 1979.
3. Gluck, J. *Clinical nurse specialist in pulmonary medicine: a prospectus.* Unpublished manuscript, Boston University School of Nursing, Boston, 1975.

REFERENCES

Ashley, J. *Hospitals, paternalism, and the role of the nurse.* New York: Teachers College Press, 1977.

Berg, H. Nursing audit and outcome criteria. *Nursing Clinics of North America,* June 1974, *9*(2), 331-335.

Ganong, J. & Ganong, W. *HELP with results-oriented performance evaluation.* Chapel Hill, N.C.: W.L. Ganong Co., 1974.

Ganong, J. & Ganong W. *Nursing management.* Germantown, Md.: Aspen Systems, 1976.

Jacobs, C. & Jacobs, N. *The PEP primer.* Chicago: Joint Commission on Accreditation of Hospitals, 1975.

Kerr, A. Nurses' notes, that's where the goodies are! *Nursing 75,* February 1975, *5*(2), 35-41.

Marram, G., Schlegel, M. & Bevis, E. *Primary nursing: A model for individualized care*. St. Louis: C.V. Mosby, 1974.

Passos, J. Accountability: Myth or mandate? *Journal of Nursing Administration*, May-June 1973, *3*(3), 17-21.

Phaneuf, M. *The nursing audit, self-regulation in nursing practice* (2nd ed.). New York: Appleton-Century Crofts, 1976.

Ryan, B.J. Nursing care plans: A systems approach to developing criteria for planning and evaluation. *Journal of Nursing Administration*, May-June 1973, *3*(3), 50-58.

Sheehy, G. *Passages*. New York: E.P. Dutton, 1976.

Spoth, J. Primary nursing: The agony and the ecstasy. *Nursing Clinics of North America*, June 1977, *12*(2), 221-233.

Stevens, B. *First-line patient care management*. Wakefield, Mass.: Contemporary Publishing, 1976.

Taylor, J.W. Measuring the outcomes of nursing care. *Nursing Clinics of North America*, June 1974, *9*(2), 337-348.

Weed, L. *Medical records, medical education, and patient care*. New York: Appleton-Century-Crofts, 1972.

Zander, K. Primary nursing won't work . . . unless the head nurse lets it. *Journal of Nursing Administration*, October 1977, 7(8), 19-23.

Zander, K., Bower, K., Foster, S., Towson, L., Wermuth, M. & Woldum, K. *Practical manual for patient-teaching*. St. Louis: The C.V. Mosby Co., 1978.

Zimmer, M. Guidelines for development of outcome criteria. *Nursing Clinics of North America*, June 1974, *9*(2).

Part III

"I Will Work with the Staff on Your Behalf"

The professional commitment to patients is not complete until the primary nurse can say, "I will work with the staff on your behalf." To patients and their families the staff is a mass of faces and names on whom they are forced to depend. To the primary nurse the staff is composed of specific nurses, aides, physicians, and other health care providers who share responsibility for this patient's care.

The personality and skill of the nurse-manager in working with the nursing staff are crucial aspects of primary nursing. In fact a nurse-manager who can interest the staff and help them to motivate themselves for the challenge of working with patients can be more valuable than a nurse-manager who is solely a clinical expert.

In making it possible and desirable for primary nurses to work well with all health care providers, the nurse-manager has two goals: to establish a professional setting, or milieu, where peer support and consultation are daily realities; and to create an environment in which everyone's energies are well spent in the service of patients. This requires pride in one's own work and respect for the work of others.

Despite the autonomy and self-directedness of primary nursing, patient care in every area, except private practice, is a group activity. Because professional nurses must depend on each other, the interpersonal dynamics of the staff strongly influence group morale and productivity. Experienced leadership can make the difference between an exciting work setting where people are proud of their own competency and each other's work or a situation in which people lack motivation and respect for each other.

179

Chapter 5

Managing Toward a Professional Milieu

A professional milieu is an environment in which professional behavior is valued and reinforced by the majority of the people in the environment. The professional behavior of a nursing staff which is conducive to primary nursing may be delineated as follows.

- The patient is the primary focus.
- Professional closeness with patients is a constant goal.
- Individual, personal, and professional development is a strong motivating force.
- Competition is healthy rather than destructive.
- Destructive reactions are sublimated.
- There are internal and external checks and balances on decisions.
- Although each professional discipline views experiences through different conceptual frameworks, all strive towards unanimity and joint resolution of cognitive dissonance.
- The easiest solution is not necessarily the best.
- There is a demonstrated belief in the value of planning ahead.
- Quality of care is documented and intrinsic to patient care.
- Confidentiality about a patient's problems is maintained within the confines of the task at hand.
- Staff work is carried out on a task or project basis rather than on an hourly time clock.
- Attention is paid to cost-effective policies and procedures.

The most powerful force on a nursing staff is the effect of the staff as a whole on individual staff members. The group is composed of all staff members, whether on or off duty. The staff group differs from staff groupings, which are composed of the daily contacts staff have with each other both formally and informally.

The nurse-manager's interactions with the staff group can make the difference between optimal primary nursing or primary nursing in name only. Because the staff should be considered as a group at all times, knowledge of group dynamics is valuable for the nurse-manager to have. Unfortunately, it ranks among the least used.

Those chosen for the nurse-manager position usually have good clinical skills, are established as role models, and have done well in charge positions. Their management skills lie in dealing intuitively with individual staff members. At best, their background is in team leadership and functioning on a one-to-one basis with patients. Even for nursing education in psychiatry, group experience is limited and not focused. Thus, new nurse-managers lack both theoretical and applied knowledge about role theory, group dynamics, and creative problem solving.

A nurse-manager walks a fine line between being part of the staff group and being isolated from it by virtue of rank. The best nurse-manager is someone who can support and influence the group, but not rely on it for personal support. This is a bitter lesson that new nurse-managers usually learn when the group is disappointing in some way. To combat multiple frustrations that may cripple an effective leadership role, the nurse-manager must incorporate group concepts into everyday functioning.

In managing toward a professional milieu, the nurse-manager benefits by integrating theories of group dynamics into the daily operations of the unit or clinic. Conscious application of group leader techniques will encourage motivation and peer collaboration.

MOTIVATING THE PRIMARY NURSING GROUP

Studies of task-oriented groups indicate that both motivation and successful task accomplishment are strongly influenced by the way group members respond to each others' work and ideas. These interactions determine the extent to which the available resources are applied to the task objective or to some other, personal objective. . . . Especially important is the way the manager or other person with the most authority behaves toward the others in the group (Chopra, 1973, p. 55).

The Dynamics of Staff Groups

"Good group relations is more than the absence of conflict; it is a positive condition of mutual reliance which the manager must build. . . . The violation of accepted common law principles of justice in handling group relations is a manager's most fatal error" (Ganong & Ganong, 1976, p. 212). The Ganongs list the common aims of every group as:

- an economic order favorable to the attainment of its objectives
- cooperation, natural or imposed, of other groups in the attainment of its objectives
- the right to utilize its skills to the greatest advantage
- the maximum amount of freedom in the exercise of its skills
- a maximum return for the skills of its members

The nurse-manager's understanding of the general characteristics of groups will provide a solid background for working with the primary nursing group. Converting group theory into positive action is then the next challenge for the nurse-manager.

The Nursing Staff as a Task Group

A task group is a collection of people organized to complete work either once or repetitiously. Common task groups include the garden club, a community orchestra, or Equal Rights Amendment supporters.

The task or cause serves to unify a diversity of members, no matter how the task is valued. The more valued the task, the more dedicated the members are to the group.

People can easily belong to several task groups at any one time, such as work, PTA, and church committee. Membership in a task group is usually, if not always, motivated by individual needs. Some of the rewards of task group membership are socialization, status, and remuneration in the form of salary and benefits or by self-actualization through task achievement.

It is advantageous for the nurse-manager to consider the staff as a never-ending task group, rather than a periodic task group during planning meetings or care conferences, in order to:

- emphasize the continual high priority on performance, problem solving, and decision making
- emphasize cohesion and collaboration and a sense of belonging during all hours of the day, giving staff a sense of continuity
- force conflicts to be resolved rather than ignored, denied, or postponed

These qualities are necessary for the smooth functioning and development of primary nursing.

Membership in a nursing staff task group is voluntary to the point that the nurse or aide has freedom to quit and go elsewhere. This is an interesting dynamic because the possibility of staff leaving can be used either by the staff or by the leader—somewhat similar to a married couple's perception of the likelihood of ever getting a divorce.

It is best to operate as if the staff is not voluntary, because then the nurse-manager is in a position of power to set standards and expect productivity. Even in voluntary organizations, the task is formulated as a given and the expectation is that all who belong to the group will work toward it. The group's collective power is in achieving its goals.

Of course, the nurse-manager knows there may be mutiny—the modern form being ostracism, backstabbing, or mass resignation. For this reason the style of working with the staff group must take into consideration that the staff is for the most part voluntary and prepared to disassemble. The nurse-manager must pay full attention to the degree of cohesion or "interpersonal glue" present among the staff. The nurse-manager must also develop a leadership style that creates cohesion around the task and among the people working toward the task:

> Some measures of cohesiveness are arrival on time, full attendance at group meetings, a high trust and support level within the group, the ability to tolerate individuality and have fun, the ability to work coopera- tively with other group members to enforce agreed-upon norms, and ease in making statements of liking for the group or for group members (Clark, 1977, p. 31).

The membership of the staff group is composed of individuals who by virtue of personal and educational background view and value the task of patient care differently. The nurse-manager must be aware of the individual motivations of each staff member in relation to the delegated workload and the overall task of dealing with the particular kinds of patients that the staff serves. Although surveys and research may give the nurse-manager a general idea of why people want to be nurses or nurse aides, the best sources of information are the staff members themselves. If the nurse-manager listens and watches, answers to the following questions will reveal the personal motivations of staff members.

- How does the staff member talk about patients?
- Where does the staff member spend a majority of time, assigned and nonstruc- tured? Where are the priorities?
- How does the staff member view health and sickness?
- How important does the staff member feel in relation to other staff, to patients, to the decision-making process?
- What does the staff member do when various changes are discussed or implemented?

The members of a nursing staff are forced to deal with degrees of intimacy unlike those of any other task group. Lawyers and clergy are exposed to the facts and emotions of intimacy, doctors are exposed to brief periods of physical and emotional intimacy, but only a nursing staff is exposed to prolonged periods of touching, smelling, hearing, and participating in intimate reactions with patients. The pressures and conflicts that such intimate contact arouses are processed by the staff members in various ways.

Theoretically, staff groups have an idiosyncratic processing system, and therefore, nursing staffs unintentionally strive to form a shared understanding of the nature and meaning of their collective work. They evolve and share a general opinion about the larger organization in which they work as well as some opinion about the kinds of patients they serve. A nurse-manager can have a tremendous influence on a staff group's perceptions of the presssures and conflicts that are constantly at hand.

The members of a nursing staff are particularly sensitive to time. The way time is perceived by each member is related to the way the nurse-manager, as pacesetter of the group, organizes the tasks in relation to time. Time in a hospital is unlike time in any other setting. On one hand, it goes on forever, 24 hours a day, every day. It is amazing to think that in a nursing unit, there has been a nurse present around-the-clock since the day the unit was opened. Such infinite time must have an impact on each person in the setting. On the other hand, time in a health care setting can be reduced to seconds in a crisis, such as a cardiac arrest, a woman going into labor, or a call to a poison prevention center. The job of primary nurses is shortening infinity and extending crisis time. In order to do this, primary nurses must feel that they control time.

The role of a nurse-manager is to help make time manageable. Do the nurse-manager and the staff view time as something to be harnessed or as something that has a harness on them? Is time to be used or to be used up? What constitutes a crisis? What are the patients' perceptions of time?

Group time perception can be illustrated by the staff that staunchly contends that charts cannot be done until the end of a shift because, "what if something changes with a patient between the time a condition is charted and the time the shift ends?" The assumption seems to be that the condition of patients works on eight-hour shifts, just as the staff does in a conventional nursing department. The sense that a patient's experience supersedes an eight-hour shift is lost.

Similarly, when discharge teaching is not considered until the last minute, nurses have lost sensitivity to the fact that except for wanting the relief of pain, discharge is probably foremost on the patient's mind at admission. Experience shows that nurses try to impose their own time frame on patients and also that nurses often function on a last-minute, crisis basis, even when they do not have to.

The nurse-manager needs to help the staff group believe that they can control time. This attitude can be developed from: (1) a sense of group cohesion; (2) an ability to set priorities; (3) attention to mutually set group goals; (4) reality testing about what it is possible to accomplish; (5) attention to people putting reasonable limits on their work time so they can get needs met outside of work; and (6) the kind of perspective that humor and positive feedback can create.

Group Behaviors Are Learned

Group participation is a natural way of life, and beginning with the family, each person learns group behavior. This learned behavior is repeated somewhat in the nursing staff group. Often the characteristic roles taken within the family are enacted again in the staff group; such as, the nurse who becomes the spokesman for everyone's complaints; the female aide who as earth-mother has the role of nurturing everyone with her humor and sage advice; the person who says I told you so; the constant devil's advocate; and the proverbial rotten apple who seems to spoil everything. It should be pointed out that, for the most part, these roles are not played consciously, but are nonetheless very strong and consistent. The nurse-manager has the power to enhance, reinforce, or play down various aspects of staff members' roles. When and how this is done has a profound impact on the norms and values of the present group. The nurse-manager cannot change people's psychological lives, but can manage the environmental factors in which the staff live for hours at a time.

Informal Groups

Each formal nursing staff group has within it a complex mixture of informal groupings called the "informal organization" by Davis. These subgroups arise "spontaneously as people associate with one another" (Davis, 1975, p. 2-22), and they have a strong influence on productivity and job satisfaction.

In any formal staff group, there are individuals who unite people around them for specific reasons, such as complaints about the leader, planning social events for singles, or convincing others that medication procedure is getting sloppy. Informal groups arise voluntarily and persist because they meet certain needs of the members, such as perpetuating cultural values or providing social status functions.

Thus some purposes of informal groups may detract from the formal group's delegated task, while other purposes may improve the quality or quantity of the task attainment. Although the informal group is usually smaller and more unstable than the larger, institutionally sanctioned formal group, it is an important influence and at least must be acknowledged by the nurse-manager. Due to the subjective nature of the causes around which informal groups form, there may be as many leaders as groups. People usually are unaware that they have attached themselves emotionally to various informal groups, and awareness peaks only when circumstances cause sides to be drawn.

However, one staff member usually emerges as predominant. Depending on the environment, one person could just as easily advocate primary nursing as another could suggest that people call in sick if they do not like their time schedules. If this person leads an informal group which questions current policy and standards, conflict in the staff group will result.

At this point, the nurse-manager's interventions are the key to the tone of the work environment. One good reason for frequent group events in a unit is that they provide the nurse-manager with firsthand information about group sentiments on certain issues. Using the group modality as a management tool, the nurse-manager can learn to identify the informal group themes and leaders and to actively participate in the ideas they express. The nurse-manager can even learn to predict new trends and help the staff mobilize their intense, informal bonds toward positive change.

Unless active during the activities of informal organization, the nurse-manager will be a passive onlooker and will then be in an untenable defensive position. The staff, however justified and adamant, will always feel somewhat guilty for emotionally deserting the nurse-manager.

A nursing staff wants a leader strong enough to interact with them in a meaningful discourse, to incorporate staff's ideas, and yet to keep at the task. The nurse-manager must be responsive within a defined structure. It should be remembered that before taking a formal, power-based position, the nurse-manager was most likely an informal leader who gave some people the impression of possessing leadership potential.

The Group Legacy

Each nursing staff has a legacy, or history, which is quickly learned by new members and often repeated until a major event changes the historic course. The presence of the legacy can be seen in the variety of ways that staffs carry out the same functions. It can also be felt in meetings of various staff groups or even in the nursing stations of different units. Although a group's history is influenced by the type of patients it serves as well as the physical environment, the main history maker is the nurse-manager. Examples of group legacies may be subtle or obvious, positive or negative in regard to the task:

- The staff on X unit are all doctor-haters.
- The staff on Y unit are good technically.
- Every summer half this staff leaves.
- Z staff pays more attention to who's dating whom than to the order book.
- If you leave on time, you must not have done all your work.
- No one puts in just an eight-hour shift here, but the rewards outweigh the time.
- Beware, or you'll be easily abused by the system. We need a union.

The nurse-manager must tap the past of the unit as well as the present ideas about it. The need for this can be seen in the way people drag up staff ghosts or interview and indoctrinate new staff. Another good indication of group legacy is what people say during times of extreme stress. Stress brings out the basic assumptions that staff members hold about the nature and purpose of their work and their supervisors.

Also, the nurse-manager should be attuned to the reputation the unit has within the larger group of the institution: "that unit is like the Jefferson Institute," "they're the most progressive unit," "their unit has 'Big Nurse' for a nurse-manager," or to an orientee on the first day, "if you don't like it there, you can always transfer in six months." These statements should convince any nurse-manager that the staff group is more than a collection of people, it is a composite of people who hold an opinion about the abstract idea of the group as well as about each member.

Developmental Stages of Groups

Any staff group can be identified as being at a stage of development because groups, like other living things, have the capacity to grow. A staff group is always at some point of the "working phase," as opposed to the orientation or termination phases which are more typical of time-limited or therapy groups. The working phase is "the middle phase in a group, when members know how to work together cooperatively, thoughts and feelings are shared more openly, and the leader needs to intervene less frequently to move the group along" (Clark, 1977, p. 174).

Getting and keeping a staff group in the working phase is the legitimate and necessary role of the nurse-manager. Because morale and productivity are so entwined with a group's life, the nurse-manager needs to intervene based on accurate assessments of the staff's working phase.

The cogs ladder model of group development attempts to delineate specific stages of the working phase of a group (Labovitz, 1975). It is outlined here as a guide for the nurse-manager to determine where the staff is located on the continuum. Examples related to primary nursing are added to show that primary nursing is possible at any phase of group development. However, it works best when the staff group is in the constructive or esprit stage.

Polite Stage. Members need to be liked at any cost. Primary nurses talk about their patients' situations, not involving themselves with issues or with each other. Conversations are of the please and thank you variety. Slip-ups in treatment are not investigated for fear of retaliation. All complaints go through the nurse-manager, who is expected to single-handedly solve the problems. Cliques are formed as nurses make judgments about which staff members share their views of patient care or opinions about aspects of personal life.

To help a group move from the polite stage to the "why we're here" stage, the nurse-manager has to be ready for uneasiness arising from more honesty among group members. The nurse-manager should use as many opportunities for group interaction as a day will allow, always being attentive to posing issues in a general, nonpunitive way. The willingness of the nurse-manager to nurture and be depended upon for attention, to be consistent with policies, and to be fair, is the most important indicator in group growth at this level.

Why We're Here Stage. Staff members begin to question the purpose and value of the work. There are many complaints about primary nursing during this stage, because primary nurses cover up their insecurities by attacking the system or the agency. They also have trouble feeling useful to particular types of patients and speak of being ineffective or defeated at every attempt to be good primary nurses. Nurse aides begin to act or feel separate from the professionals, because identification with the staff group's work is low. Disagreements and questions are voiced again, even though they were addressed previously. The senior nurses feel frustrated by the newer nurses and begin to redefine their career paths. The newer nurses feel confused and lack complete commitment to the job because the group bonds are not firm.

To help a group move from the why we're here stage to the "bid for power" stage, the nurse-manager needs to maintain the sense of worthwhile work and adhere to any previously made commitments to new projects. Ideas and encouragement of professional growth should not be dropped during this stage. A charismatic leader can often superficially avoid this stage, but most nurse-managers will need to patiently clarify the goals and objectives of the task. The nurse-manager's willingness to be a primary nurse during this stage can make a positive difference in the staff's commitment to patient care. The newer nurses need to get a stronger working alliance with the nurse-manager who symbolically represents the group. The senior nurses may need to discuss their frustrations with the nurse-manager individually and revise the reasons that they feel needed by the group.

Bid for Power Stage. During this stage individual primary nurses will test their strengths, and competition emerges. The staff begins deciding which primary nurses are good and which are not so good. Sides are overtly drawn around nursing care issues: can Mr. B really help himself or does he need a nurse to do a complete bath; is Ms. V's regression manipulative or unconscious; is it the role of the VNA nurse or the social worker to help the patient get food stamps; who gave the student nurse the authority to write in the care plan when the primary nurse wasn't there; or why was the utility room left so dirty last night?

In this stage suggestions for districting of primary nursing are heard. In group development terminology, districting is a way of dealing with the nurse-manager's power by dividing a unit into smaller parts. Although this method is initially quite satisfying, it does not solve the problems of staff group development or individual autonomy of primary nurses.

Another indication of this stage is the suggestion that the nurse-manager role be dissolved. This is an attempt to deny the need for, and interdependency with, a person who reinforces the structure and standards of patient care.

Primary nurses will either monopolize primary nursing conferences or be too shy to present their work. The bid for power stage is best characterized by extremes in emotions and work performance, as well as exotic or impulsive suggestions for changes.

To help the staff group move to the "constructive" stage, the nurse-manager should firmly maintain basic policies and procedures. Assignments and praise should be evenly distributed.

The competitive energies can be redirected to constructive projects and learning opportunities. Primary nurses need to be encouraged to be the best nurses they can in relation to themselves, not to each other.

Constructive Stage. Staff members settle into roles for which they feel adequately prepared and committed. There is an increased sense that the work is valued and valuable, and that the unit or agency will survive through the idiosyncracies of individual staff members and patients.

This stage is probably the least preoccupying for the nurse-manager because things go smoothly and people's talents are consistently utilized. Ideas for changes which have sound, long-term benefits are expressed, but unless the ideas are seriously considered, the staff will become bored and create small crises.

The constructive stage is the best for primary nursing because all energies can be focused on patients. The nurse-manager can use this opportunity to move the staff group to higher levels of professional closeness and clinical expertise. Twenty-four hour responsibility and accountability for outcomes of nursing care become a reality during the constructive stage. Primary nursing conferences actually take place, documentation and advocacy really happen, and peer support is the fuel that runs the group's engine.

The nurse-manager's role is that of consultant for the clinical work of primary nurses. A primary nurse's need for the nurse-manager's input is always present, but it is easiest to meet during the constructive phase.

- Provide a climate where I can achieve!
- Give me a goal.
- Stretch me.
- Be honest with me.
- Reward me accordingly.
- Build my pride in our organization.
- Don't manipulate me.
- Make the best of what I have to offer.
- Know when to turn me loose.
- Help me to broaden.
- Recognize that I am a human being.
- Raise my sights (Davey, 1978, p. 93).

There will be brief periods when a staff group reaches a level of high morale and productivity. This is called the "esprit" stage and is probably the dream of all nurse-managers.

Esprit Stage. This stage is the group equivalent of Maslow's (1954) self-actualization stage of personality development. Like self-actualization, the esprit stage is relatively brief and intense. It usually occurs during "wartime" situations, such as a blizzard, the last days of a political campaign, or a party for a beloved staff member.

During the esprit stage, individual differences are secondary to the cause at hand. There is a euphoric sense that the task outweighs any inconvenience, effort, or expense. Group members feel very loyal, creative, unselfish, and productive.

The nurse-manager should enjoy esprit when it occurs, but not make major decisions or demands because the stage is short-lived. If a special patient's progress seems to be creating esprit in the staff group, the staff will suffer when the patient is discharged. The nurse-manager must help the group to keep their work in perspective so that they can feel good but not omnipotent. Otherwise, the staff will grow bitter that all needs cannot be met at work.

A staff group constantly goes up and down the stages of development. However, some staff groups tend to get stuck at one stage unless the nurse-manager, with the help of the leadership team, can counteract the tendency of a group to move backward rather than forward toward the constructive stage. Constructive group behavior is the goal of the nurse-manager of primary nursing and can be reached by actions that enhance group growth.

Enhancing Group Growth

Group growth refers to the positive abilities of individuals in a group to advance collectively to the constructive stage of group development. There are techniques that the nurse-manager can use to stimulate group growth.

Use of Meetings

The wise nurse-manager will have as many group meetings as possible with as many staff members as can be brought together at one time. Group growth takes place over time as a result of multiple interactions between the staff and the nurse-manager. Some guidelines for the nurse-manager's interactions with the group follow:

- Be present at all formal staff groupings such as, shift report, staff meetings, and primary nursing conferences.
- Have clear goals for each type of staff grouping and make them clear to the members.
- Have the same kind of meetings the same time each week in the same place whenever possible. Consistency enhances group cohesiveness and saves time. Members come to depend upon certain groupings and count on that forum to raise issues. People will plan their time in order to attend.

- Set up meetings with as few interruptions as possible. Rotate staff to cover the unit.
- Cancel groupings only in the most dire emergencies. Even if there is only the nurse-manager and one other staff member, carry on business.
- When a crisis emerges, call a crisis meeting. When the permanent night nurse gets the flu, get all scheduled staff together to help solve the staffing problem. Or when someone's primary patient dies unexpectedly, ask the primary nurse's permission to call a group together to discuss the facts and feelings about the death.
- Hold staff meetings at a minimum of once a week to provide a frequent forum for information sharing and discussion of staff concerns.

Once the basic structure is set, the nurse-manager can concentrate on refining group leadership functions. Although the best way to learn new styles is to watch other leaders in action, few nurse-managers have the opportunity to observe role models. To help fill this gap, some ideas on how to understand and facilitate staff group growth will be discussed next.

Recognizing Group Process

At any given moment in a group, there are two levels of experience for each participant—content and process. The nurse-manager is responsible for equal awareness of both levels and must make interventions accordingly.

Content refers to the subject being discussed. It is the overt, manifest data at hand. Content is that which can be recorded directly on paper or machine; it is the concrete reality; it is fact.

Process is the "constant movement as group members seek to reduce the tension that arises when people attempt to have their individual needs met yet work to help meet group goals" (Clark, 1977, p. 172). Process includes latent, or covert, content—that which has meaning ascribed to the concrete subject. Process differs from content as the theme of a novel differs from the action, such as the theme of will versus fate told through the actions of several generations of a family. Just as in literature, a staff group is rich with stories and themes. A typical story may be anger because promised pay raises were not seen in paychecks, while the theme may be that you cannot trust people in power.

In primary nursing, discussion at staff meetings may center around the appropriate role of primary nurses in a given situation while the underlying process may be complaints that all primary nurses are not pulling their weight. In this example, the words of conversation are used to convey an underlying staff group concern. It is important for the nurse-manager to separate the content messages from the process messages that are heard every day from the staff.

Because group process extends indefinitely over time, a staff group has multiple interactions each day, and the sum total of the atmosphere and results of these interactions indicates the direction in which the group is growing. The process is carried out by individuals, but it outlasts each individual's stay with the group. The process becomes the group's history or legacy.

Clark (1977) offers useful questions to help determine a group's process over time:

- What seems to lead to increased tension levels?
- What indicates conflict?
- When does the group seem to be apathetic?
- How are decisions arrived at?
- What types of leadership occur?
- What rules for behavior are in operation?
- What factors lead to effective movement toward and away from group goals?
- What signs of aggression and assertiveness are evident?
- What phase of group process does the group seem to be in?
- What themes recur? (pp. 20-21)

Managing Process Not People

The ideal role for the nurse-manager of primary nursing is to manage the process of the staff group rather than the people. This approach is most easily applied during meetings or what was referred to earlier as staff groupings. Because time is so valuable in health care settings, staff groupings must be managed so that they are participatory, productive experiences rather than wasteful or even destructive. "In a world of complex, interdependent systems, we can no longer afford win/lose solutions; we must find solutions in which everyone wins and the whole system improves. Win/win solutions do not need to be compromises" (Wong, Doyle, & Straus, 1975, p. 37).

The irony of using a group process approach in nursing management is the same in primary nursing: for better results that last over time, the nurse-manager must give up more traditional controls and adopt a more interactive, facilitative style. The nurse-manager must be more "laid back" so the group can move ahead! The rewards for the nurse-manager become helping each staff member take on responsibility for the group's actions and solutions to problems. However, laid back does not mean being apathetic or silent in group meetings. Rather, it requires the nurse-manager's thoughtful and intuitive involvement in the process of discussions rather than the content. Clark (1977) describes task functions and maintenance functions as areas "that must be fulfilled by the leader in order for the group to work at its highest possible level of performance" (pp. 28-29).

Task functions are directly related to accomplishment of group goals.

- getting the group going
- keeping the group moving toward its goal
- clarifying unclear statements or behaviors
- suggesting ways to move toward the goal
- pointing out movement toward or away from the goal
- restating more clearly what others have said (paraphrasing)
- refocusing discussion on the task or on a small step toward the goal
- giving information

Maintenance functions are directly related to improving interpersonal relationships within the group.

- giving support to group members who are unsure or anxious
- relieving extreme tension levels
- encouraging direct communication
- voicing group feeling
- agreeing or accepting
- helping the group to evaluate itself

Managing group process involves listening to both the process and the content of group discussions. The group leadership functions that have been delineated are inappropriate unless they are actions in response to attentive listening. That involves concentrating on the key points the speaker is making and the tone in which things are said. VanDérsal (1974) gives some good general rules about listening, including relaxing so you can listen patiently, and hearing the speaker out before commenting or seeking clarification.

Motivating the primary nursing group requires listening to what staff members say motivates them. Primary nursing in itself will only motivate a staff that wants to try it or has just begun it. The positive qualities of primary nursing are only as powerful as the motivational status that they are given by the group.

The nurse-manager controls the motivators, because the nurse-manager controls the environment. Managing group process rather than people is the best way to reinforce the characteristics of a productive, professional milieu.

PEER SUPPORT IN PRIMARY NURSING

A primary nurse's support of and by other staff nurses is the most sustaining and rewarding aspect of working in a professional milieu. The greater the quantity and quality of interactions among primary nurses, the greater the possibility that the staff group will be in the constructive stage of group development. Optimal primary nursing cannot exist in an environment that lacks the following characteristics of peer support:

- Belief that each person is needed by the group because of professional skills and personality strengths.
- Toleration for individual personality weaknesses as long as they do not interfere with work or the esteem of the group's members.
- Demonstrated willingness to listen, speak, and be heard.
- Personal acceptance that no one person is all-knowing, all-caring, or all-powerful (Adler, 1972).
- Desire to achieve one's own objectives while allowing others to achieve theirs.
- Willingness to question fairly and disagree if the motivation is good patient care.

The nurse-manager who recognizes the need for mutual support among primary nurses will be able to help create an atmosphere which is conducive to the characteristics of positive peer relationships. Opportunities for improving the quantity and quality of staff interactions are plentiful, even in the most frantic nursing situations. Obstacles to peer support must be overcome by everyone so that the rewards of group problem solving can be felt and ultimately transferred to primary patients.

The Need for Peer Support

Primary nursing requires interdependency between all nursing staff members, which requires that everyone be willing to allow others to have specific areas of authority. The primary nurse should be the authority on assigned primary patients, but should bow to the authority of other primary nurses in regard to their own patients.

Primary nurses need the group's permission to design and recommend nursing approaches and treatments for primary patients that will be followed by everyone. Such responsibility and authority can only be delegated by the group itself. In a way, the primary nurse becomes a facilitator for the rest of the staff's work with that nurse's primary patients. The primary nurse is the translator of the patient's needs to the nursing staff and of the nursing staff's system to the patient (See Figure 5-1).

Figure 5-1 The Primary Nurse as Translator/Facilitator

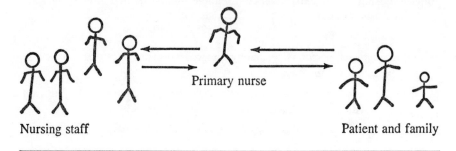

Nursing staff   Patient and family

However, because most of the nursing staff will have contact with each primary patient, they will also have opinions about that patient's needs and the best way to meet them. How this shared territory (such as working with the same patient) is handled characterizes the nature of peer support in primary nursing.

Decreasing Isolation

Primary nursing is a complex role for any registered nurse, and the work can seem excessively demanding without a primary nurse's belief that "I'm not alone." If a nurse knows that other nurses are willing to identify immediately with the variety of experiences in the nurse-patient relationships, the nurse will feel a bond with the other nurses. Bonds create allegiance to the larger group, which results in an "enlarging" of each member. Thus, individuals feel a little larger or more capable than they would by themselves.

Staff-Generated Rewards

When professional nursing peers support each other, they do not have to rely on patients for positive reinforcement or good feelings about themselves. They do not have to rely solely on "the boss" (nurse-manager) for every morsel of praise or suggestion. A staff that can nurture itself is a strong staff with a lot of energy reserved for patient care, if the nurse-manager sets up a good structure and environment.

Teaching

Primary nurses who feel supported by other primary nurses agree that they have learned important things from each other. Peer support implies that the peer is worthy of new information or thinking through former information to arrive at a new understanding. Often, the gift of a new thought is worth more to a primary nurse if it is given by another staff nurse rather than the nurse-manager because the feelings about authority figures do not detract from the teaching. Coteaching is an important part of a staff group's professional growth.

Safeguards of Practice

As primary nurses discuss their patients with each other, they need to feel comfortable in order to ask potentially difficult questions or even to disagree with one another. Open debate is much safer than subtle or covert disagreements. Without overt argument, staff members will behave according to their own unspoken ideas about patient care. If there is no attempt at consensus about approaches to patient or staff predicaments, members are left completely on their own, which often results in confusion, omission of vital information and activities, and loss of control over standards of care. Well-meaning arguments about patient care issues are the best system of checks and balances a staff can have because disagreements stimulate critical thinking.

Continuity of Care

The accountability of primary nurses for the outcomes of nursing care directed and given to primary patients necessitates concrete peer support. Every member of a nursing staff is constantly obligated to carry out approaches and treatments ordered by primary nurses. They are also obligated to hold primary nurses' orders temporarily if they feel that they are not appropriate or safe at a given moment—just as they should do with physicians' orders. In either event, primary nurses need to be kept informed of new developments concerning primary patients. Each staff primary nurse needs the assurance that primary patients will receive continuous quality care, even when the primary nurse is not present. Policies and procedures regarding continuity of care can never replace the positive atmosphere of a nursing staff that respects one another and is proud of its combined efforts.

Obstacles to Peer Support

Unfortunately, the obstacles to peer support are many. The obstacles probably outnumber the advantages because genuine peer support takes a long time to grow, while the obstacles are always present due to the constant stress of nursing staffs.

> We ask the nurse to exercise judgement, set priorities, make choices, and deal with considerable frustrations—and we expect her to do it happily, accepting all the inconsistencies and failures of the modern organization. Not surprisingly, she often fails to cope, and she and her work group cease to function effectively (Oberst, 1973, p. 1917).

Peer Equals Twin

If primary nurses were asked who their peers are, they would probably say other primary nurses. However, on closer scrutiny they would probably admit that their personal idea of a peer is someone who shares values and characteristics with them. Thus, the more like a twin another person is, the closer is the perception of "peership".

Even though the idea of a staff of clones is absurd, the differences between individuals often cause a lack of peer support. If a person is too different from most group members, the group will try to decrease the differences or to maximize the similarities. There is always a delicate balance between individual aims (chaos on one extreme) and superficial group togetherness (robotism on the other). As shown in Figure 5-2 the recognized task or mission of the staff is what transcends differences and unites similarities, like the fulcrum of a teeter-totter.

Primary nursing accentuates the differences of nurses by individualizing nurses in the same way that it individualizes patients. Because primary nursing is likely to tip the balance of peer perceptions of each other, the nurse-manager should make the task greater than the personality differences. "Avoid interpersonal confrontations. Don't let people focus on each others personalities rather than the ideas" (Wong et al., 1975, p. 39).

As long as primary nurses are completing their responsibilities, the style in which they work should not be open to doubt or criticism. Safe and therapeutic nursing care rather than personality change should be the priority of a primary nursing staff.

Unhealthy Competition

Primary nurses who compete with each other to be the best to the exclusion of all others set up an unhealthy work environment. Individual differences become a source of judgment rather than professional stimulation and enjoyment. In healthy competition primary nurses strive to grow beyond yesterday's limitations, attaining skill and knowledge in new areas of the primary nursing process. Healthy competition occurs because the nurse-manager respects individual staff members for their strengths and takes care not to play favorites. The competition learned through the educational system has to be unlearned if primary nurses intend to work well together.

Fear of Retaliation

Anyone in a group tends to be reluctant to speak on an issue when they fear losing face or suffering retaliation. If supporting one peer means losing the support

---

Figure 5-2 Balance of Peer Perceptions of Each Other

Absolute individualization		Absolute nondifferentiation
(Chaos)	The task	(Robots)

of another, primary nurses will tend to be silent and avoid each other. Cliques will become the sole source of support instead of the total group, including the nurse-manager.

Primary nurses may also be fearful that if other staff members disapprove of actions or ideas, their primary patients may be mistreated or neglected. Indeed, primary nurses need expertise in interpersonal relations with fellow staff members to deal with some of the conflicts that arise in a day's work. Otherwise, primary nurses will feel isolated and uninvolved.

The nurse-manager can decrease the fear of retaliation by using the following guides:

- Devise protocols that fairly delegate the workload and provide for numerous contingencies, in particular, clear and realistic arrangements for follow-through of a primary nurse's plans that are upheld by the nurse-manager.
- Hold staff meetings in which everyone is encouraged to participate in order to decrease isolation and increase consensus.
- Allow time at nursing conferences for primary nurses to develop and present the rationale for decisions they have made or plans they are considering.
- Encourage self-evaluations by primary nurses to learn their perceptions of themselves and help correct any distortions by determining areas for growth together.

Instability of Staffing

Despite the group legacy, "turnover and frequent (shift) rotation are not conducive to establishment of an interacting group that is mutually supportive. While the repertoire of resources may be quite wide there may be little consensus on coping mechanisms which are successful for the group" (Oberst, 1973, p. 1918).

However, once a solid base of peer support has been developed, it is very contagious. New members of the staff will immediately see and feel that "this is a place where people can be honest adults." The drawbacks to peer support created under unstable staffing patterns can be overcome by positive group momentum.

Conflict Resolution and Group Problem Solving

Peer support is not a stable quality that one staff possesses and another does not. Every staff has the seeds of peer support which grow if staff conflicts are resolved as they occur and if the staff group unites around problem solving to provide better patient care through good staff relationships. The nurse-manager has a key role in resolving conflicts so that the staff group can pursue problem solving energetically.

Although there are many methods for conflict resolution, there are similar elements contained in them all which stem from how the group treats each member's work and ideas:

> Because we see our work and ideas as extensions of ourselves, a response to what we have done or suggested carries a dual message. One message conveys information about the problem or decision we happen to be working on, the other message tells us something about ourselves. And if we perceive that our work is being called into question, we will begin to devote our talents and energies to protecting and defending ourselves. Our motivation shifts allegiance, from the group's task objective to the personal objective. . . what is needed are. . . ways of interacting that can satisfy both the personal and the task objective (Chopra, 1973, p. 57).

Suggestions for Conflict Resolution

- Listen carefully without interruptions.
- Focus on the issue not the personalities involved.
- Allow enough time for all concerned with the issue to participate if they wish.
- Define the conflict or problem in workable, adjustable segments.
- Get facts in order to mediate opinions.
- "Accept incomplete ideas. If the group members are thinking in disorganized fragments, let them do it for a while; see if they're able to pull their thoughts together" (Wong et al., 1975, p. 39).
- Allow silences if people are using them to contemplate the issues.
- Use the question and answer teaching technique to help the staff move along to the broader subject at hand.
- Admit lack of knowledge or lack of opinion when appropriate.
- Use humor if it will help people gain objectivity on the issue.
- Stick to one conflict at a time.
- Avoid kidding people during meetings in which there is a high degree of tension.
- If the conflict cannot be resolved in one meeting, set a date and time for the discussion to be continued.
- Make sure that if someone receives feedback, including the leader, the feedback is fully understood.
- Avoid the scapegoating that arises when a group under stress needs to "deny responsibility by blaming others. . . . Determining the transactional level (Parent, Adult, Child) underlying scapegoating behavior is one way to break out of the scapegoating pattern" (Wachter-Shikora, 1977, pp. 408-409).
- Don't force a premature resolution to a problem. Some problems have been so long in brewing that a 30-minute discussion may just begin to touch the issue.

- Become familiar with the specific roles people take in meetings that might interfere with conflict resolution. Outside of the discussion at hand, help people learn how their actions are perceived by and influence others.

> The goal in any conflict situation is achievement of a satisfactory disposition of the issues involved. . . . As people become aware of their responsibility in a conflict situation and learn to accept it, commitment to achieving effective resolution increases. . . . Exploration of what they think needs to be changed, what they can do and what they are willing to do, aids in developing an awareness of their responsibility in a given situation (Thurkettle & Jones, 1978, pp. 42-43).

An example of conflict resolution follows in which the nurse-manager facilitates acceptance of current policy.

The setting is a weekly staff meeting with the nurse-manager. A staff nurse in the psychiatry unit questioned a patient's boyfriend about whether he had a gun and then took it from him. The policy is that no guns are allowed on the unit. The topic was not discussed for five minutes until an unrelated comment was made by another staff nurse about guns.

NM: Since you brought it up, I don't understand. What happened last night with Mr. X and the gun? (Honestly asking for clarification of behavior)

RN 1: I asked him if he had a gun and he said yes. He said he'd give it to me on the unit because he didn't want security to have it. I'd never seen a gun before—it was terrible! He took out the bullets and gave me the gun to lock up while he visited. He was very nice about it.

RN 2: Weren't you scared?

RN 1: Yes.

NM: What do you *each* understand is the policy?

RN 1: No guns are allowed on the unit.

RN 3 (orientee): Or we call security and they either escort the person out or take the gun. (Everyone shakes head) Of course, I just found that out today! (Laughter)

NM: I can understand that you wanted to solve the problem as easily as possible, but the policy is there to protect us and the patients. (Promotes peer support)

RN 1: Did I set myself up for a dangerous situation? (Everyone nods)

NM (to everyone): How could it have been done differently? (Encouraging problem solving)

RN 2: When we knew he had a gun, we shouldn't have said anything to him but gone straight to call security.

NM: Right. We've all been trying to do a lot for people lately, but we have to be careful not to go overboard. (Discussion goes on to other areas in which the nurses felt stressed)

The nurse-manager of primary nursing should realize that conflict can be a useful part of a staff's life. Conflict indicates that people are thinking and evaluating, and therefore it should be worked with rather than avoided. The more respect that the staff feels toward each other, the more easily and quickly conflicts will be voiced and resolved. Just as primary nurses enjoy seeing the results of their work with patients, they enjoy seeing changes that they have fostered in the way the staff works together.

Peer support is the interpersonal glue that binds without smothering a constructive, energetic staff group. "The greatest reward of primary nursing is improved morale and personal growth among nurses who work in an atmosphere which promotes expression of the full breadth and depth of their professional skills" (Bartels, Good, & Lampe, 1977, p. 29). Given effective management, primary nursing is synonymous with a professional milieu.

REFERENCES

Adler, G. Helplessness in the helpers. *British Journal of Medical Psychology*, 1972, *45*, 315-325.

Bartels, D., Good, V. & Lampe, S. The role of the head nurse in primary nursing. *Canadian Nurse*, March 1977, *73*(3), 26-30.

Chopra, A. Motivation in task-oriented groups. *Journal of Nursing Administration*, January-February 1973, *3*(1), 55-60.

Clark, C. *The nurse as group leader*. New York: Springer Publishing, 1977.

Davey, J. The employee's meaning of supervision. *Supervisor Nurse*, May 1978, *9*(5), 93-94.

Davis, D. Informal organization. In G. Labovitz (Ed.), *Motivational dynamics*. Minneapolis: Control Data, 1975, 2-21-2-42.

Ganong, J. & Ganong, W. *Nursing management*. Germantown, Md.: Aspen Systems, 1976.

Labovitz, G. *Motivational dynamics*. Minneapolis: Control Data, 1975.

Maslow, A.H. *Motivation and personality*. New York: Harper and Row, 1954.

Oberst, M. The crisis-prone staff nurse. *American Journal of Nursing*, November 1973, *73*(11), 1917-1921.

Thurkettle, M., & Jones, S. Conflict as a systems process: Theory and management. *Journal of Nursing Administration*, January 1978, *8*(1), 39-43.

VanDérsal, W. How to be a good communicator—And a better nurse. *Nursing 74*, December 1974, *4*(12), 57-64.

Wachter-Shikora, N. Scapegoating among professionals. *American Journal of Nursing*, March 1977, *77*(3), 408-409.

Wong, P., Doyle, M. & Straus, D. Problem-solving through process management. *Journal of Nursing Administration*, January 1975, *5*(1), 37-39.

Chapter 6

Managing Toward Collaboration of Energies

The role of the nurse-manager is to ensure that primary nurses spend the time not devoted to direct care as productively as possible. The nurse-manager must monitor the way energies of nurses are spent while away from patients. In fact, primary nurses may spend a large part of their time in dealings about primary patients rather than in interactions with them. Collaboration among primary nurses and other health care providers who work with primary patients is a hallmark of a professional milieu. Collaboration is part of patient advocacy, and each primary nurse must become actively involved in daily discussions and decisions about patients.

Depending on the professional climate and the ease with which patient outcomes are achieved, the nurse-manager needs to adjust the way primary nurses relate to the system. Some of the nurse-manager's interventions are with individual nurses and nonnursing staff, while others necessitate involvement in the policies and politics of the institution. The head nurse of a surgical unit appropriately described the role changes the nurse-manager must make to pursue collaboration in primary nursing:

> In the conventional setting as head nurse, I was the advocate for thirty patients. In the primary nursing model, it is the primary nurses who are the advocates for their primary patients. As head nurse, I am now the advocate for the staff on my unit, facilitating their personal and professional growth and supporting them in their pursuit of excellence in providing nursing care for patients (Garber, 1977, p. 31).

In primary nursing, the nurse-manager must be able to take a back seat in much of the discussion about patient admissions. The nurse-manager is more like the director of a play, working hard behind the scenes by teaching primary nurses the principles of effective collaboration and by giving them the confidence to pursue what they think is best for their patients. In contrast, however, the nurse-manager must be able to take a front-seat position when the actions or position of primary nurses need support. The nurse-manager must have political savvy to know when and how to intervene in order to prevent interdisciplinary collaboration from grinding to a halt.

Collaboration with others is the best way for patients to acquire professional resources. Indeed, people are admitted to clinics and hospitals in order to benefit from the collective skills of the agency's personnel.

Of the many situations that require collaboration of energies, there are two areas that have the most implications for primary nursing and the nurse-manager. The first area is the ever challenging physician-primary nurse relationship, and the second is primary nursing in specialized clinical settings. Although neither area can be covered thoroughly, the discussion that follows offers a synthesis of information about collaboration.

COLLEGIAL RELATIONSHIPS WITH PHYSICIANS

Are primary nurses really the colleagues of physicians? Surely the last century of nursing history does not legally or traditionally support the idea that nurses are in equal partnership with physicians in matters of patient care. Nurse practice acts and the lack of clear definition between nursing and medical practice add to the role confusion of primary nurses and undermine their confidence. In turn, this lack of confidence fosters a lack of assertiveness, and to be a colleague, a person must feel confident enough to be assertive.

To use energies most effectively in the patient's behalf, primary nurses must have the self-image of a colleague in partnership with the physician. Primary nursing makes individual nurses more visible and hence less anonymous. But primary nursing in itself does not convince nurses that they have something valuable to offer their patients and their patients' physicians.

In primary nursing, two conflicts are painfully apparent: (1) "The authority/subordinate relationship between physicians and nurses reinforces the male/female societal role" (Menikheim, 1979, p. 138) and (2) curing and curers have higher status and societal rewards than those for whom prevention, protection, restoration, and provision of comfort are the major professional orientation. The more that primary nurses and their managers are aware of these societal values and the more effective they feel in their own roles, the more conflict will occur in daily interactions within the health care delivery system.

Primary nursing brings to light the realization that "nurses are in the midst of an inequitable health delivery system in which care is dictated by physicians, hospital administrators, university administrators, and insurance companies" (Bush & Kjervik, 1979, p. 47). Perhaps it is this inequality that makes nurses hesitant to implement primary nursing or so ready to abandon it if it does not bring them the equality of status and influence they deserve. Indeed, primary nursing uncovers many chronic problems in health care settings, one of the greatest being collaboration of energies. However, with astute planning and negotiating on the part of nurse-managers and their administrations, many of these old problems can be gradually alleviated. Rather than arbitrarily criticizing other professionals, the task is to develop competent, confident primary nurses.

Nurse-managers and primary nurses need to respond to the conflicts of the physician-nurse relationship with new approaches. Some strategies that work and should become part of the repertoire of the nurse-manager include:

- clarifying the role of nursing in a given setting
- giving primary nurses the confidence to collaborate with physicians
- teaching primary nurses the skills and politics of collaboration in that system
- becoming involved in policy making on a senior level with physician colleagues

The Primary Nurse's Territory

Any nurse-manager continually defines the nature of nursing for the staff. When making assignments, dealing with tasks, encouraging nurses to question orders, or putting a priority on teaching patients, the nurse-manager is defining nursing. The definition naturally is influenced by the nurse-manager's education and experience. It is also strongly affected by the department of nursing. There are many forces inside and outside of nursing that will work to confuse the definition. Revisions can be a positive experience if the nurse-manager feels that values are not compromised by putting a new idea into operation.

The content of the nurse-manager's definition is only as valuable as the consistency with which it is applied in everyday practice. No nurse would ever say, "I didn't have a chance to give all the medications today," but how often do nurses say, "I didn't have a chance to do pre-op teaching today"? The activities that the nurse-manager sanctions are quickly woven into the staff's, patients', and physicians' perceptions of nursing. Just as nursing takes place within the interpersonal processes of the primary nurse-patient relationship, nursing is defined within the interpersonal processes between primary nurses and other health care disciplines. Of the nonnurses, nurses grapple the most over perceived territory with physicians.

Historically, physicians have been considered to know more than nurses about every aspect of medical practice. Since it is logical for decision making responsibility to reside with the most knowledgeable individual, the physician has traditionally held such authority without challenge.

> Now, nursing specialists, whose training and experience may give
> them more clinical insight than some physicians to whom they are
> nominally subordinate, have emerged. In some circumstances, the
> nurse's relatively superior understanding may become obvious to both
> parties. In such situations, an anomaly occurs—the physician has the
> power to make decisions, but the nurse has the superior knowledge
> (Budassi & Rockwell, 1978, p. i).

This is the case with more senior primary nurses and nursing specialists: they
know the totality of the health-related difficulties of their primary patients because
it is their business to know. Primary nurses are expected to plan and give nursing
care based on a complete assessment of the individual patient. With the dwindling
number of general practitioners and the increase of medical specialties, the
primary nurse is often the only person in the health care system whose role is
defined by an ability to form a relationship and to effectively intervene at any point
in the continuum of an individual's needs. This certainly has implications for the
primary nurse-physician relationship.

Primary nurses and physicians need each other's knowledge, if for no other
reason than that they share the same territory—the patient. There is certainly
enough work for each of them, but the work is usually quite different. Although
specific functions or the way patients perceive those functions often overlap, the
territory of each discipline can be defined. Physicians are responsible for diagnosing the disease entity and etiology during disease and for the medical and drug
management of symptoms. Primary nurses are responsible for provision of comfort from the symptoms of disease, detection and prevention of complications,
protection of human and legal rights, and restoration of lost physical and mental
functions to previous or realistic levels.

It would seem that the more strictly nurses function in the caring domain and
physicians in the curing domain, the greater the possibility and need for collaboration. With definite territories or jurisdictions, border clashes are infrequent and
mild because no one's control is threatened. Although complete division of labor
does not necessitate collaboration, in health care certain realities make complete
division of labor impossible. These realities are more apparent with primary
nursing.

Nurses are constantly carrying out orders from the physician, but they lack
ownership of the decision and knowledge of how the decision was made. Thus they
are in the uncomfortable middle-man position. For instance, a nurse may think that
a bowel specimen is being collected for occult blood when actually the physician is
ruling out ova and parasites; or a nurse may assume that a confused patient is being
checked on every 15 minutes to keep the patient oriented, when the physician is
worried about a reaction to medication, but does not want to formalize it in the
chart. However, primary nurses know enough about the patient not to need to

assume and enough to ask why certain things are being ordered. Thus, primary nurses force explanations. Traditionally, nurses could allow themselves to follow orders blindly, especially those that were not glaringly life threatening. However, in primary nursing, the nurse must understand what significance the orders have for the patient's total status.

Collaboration increases the chance for quality care. Using the first example, once the primary nurse understands that the stool specimen is for ova and parasites, other signs of parasitic infection, such as diarrhea, weight loss, and thirst can be watched for. The primary nurse may elaborate on the treatment plan by instituting daily weights. In the second example the primary nurse could give the physician some new clinical data to substantiate or allay fears about a reaction to medication. Strict division of labor would not be needed for the treatment of either patient, but they could benefit if their physician and primary nurse function as colleagues.

When the processes—"a series of actions, changes or functions that bring about a particular result"—of medical and nursing models of patient care are compared, the importance of collaboration becomes evident (Ganong & Ganong 1976, p. 37). (See Table 6-1.) In fact, the fundamental tasks, or system elements, of physician and nurses are identical. Equal tasks should indicate an equal collegial relationship.

The roles of physicians and primary nurses differ in how fundamental tasks and priorities are accomplished. Disagreement at any stage of the system elements often causes breakdown of collaboration. An analysis of the system elements in relation to primary nursing should help the nurse-manager.

Preadmission Procedures

Nurses are usually not part of preadmission routines, although as primary nurses they may find themselves more involved in getting patients into the health care system. As nurses become established in more outpatient positions, such as screening clinics and specialty areas, the phenomenon of a primary nurse contacting another primary nurse may occur more frequently. Examples include the rehabilitation nurse practitioner informing a former rehabilitation primary nurse that a patient is returning to the hospital for a bladder training program; a nurse from a triage unit of a health maintenance organization (HMO) asking for the primary nurse of a hospital unit when there is specific information that may affect the newly admitted patient's nursing care; or a private nurse psychotherapist, needing to admit a delusional teenager to an inpatient unit, explaining the possible meaning of the delusions to the future primary nurse to speed up acceptance of the patient by the nursing staff. Thus, primary nursing may be increasingly included in collaboration that occurs prior to admissions. In this stage, the nurse-manager can assert the importance of primary nursing in preadmissions through staffing patterns. Priority can be put on the planning phase of health care by establishing nurses as gatekeepers to agencies and units along with physicians.

Table 6-1 The Patient Care Process: Comparison of Medical and Nursing Models of Patient Care

Medical Model	System Elements	Nursing Model
1. Assess patient, write initial orders	1. Patient preadmission procedures	1. Preadmission procedures
2. Write additional orders	2. Admission	2. Admit
3. History and physical exam	3. Assessment of patient	3. Initial patient interview & observation
4. Problem list	4. Problem identification	4. Problem list
5. Medical plan	5. Plan of care	5. Initial nursing plan & nursing directives
6. Order Rx, medications, record	6. Implementation of care plan	6. Give care, Rx, meds, teach, listen, observe, record, initiate discharge planning
7. Rounds, observe, confer	7. Evaluate problems & progress	7. Give care, rounds, observe, confer, coordinate
8. Write new orders, document on progress notes, Rx, medications, rounds, observe, confer	8. Identify new problems, adjust plan, implement adjusted plan, evaluate problems and progress	8. Revise care plan, write new nursing directives, modify care appropriately & document on patient record, give care, rounds, observe, confer, coordinate

REPEAT SEQUENCE 1 THROUGH 7

Medical Model	System Elements	Nursing Model
9. Order	9. Discharge	9. Finalize discharge plans, write discharge summary, discharge
10. Write order, fill in referral forms	10. Referral	10. Write nursing directives, fill in referral forms
	11. Initial visit and assessment	11. Initial interview, observation, examination

REPEAT SEQUENCE 1 THROUGH 7 AS REQUIRED

Source: Nursing Management by J. Ganong and W. Ganong, 1976. Copyright 1976 by Aspen Systems Corporation. Reprinted by permission.

Admission and Assessment

Primary nurses make formal assessments on the day of admission or, if someone else was assigned, must show accountability for the information by cosigning the assessment. Division of labor between physicians and primary nurses starts to get fuzzy at the assessment stage because both disciplines focus on the immediate crisis; what constitutes care and cure are as yet undetermined. Disagreements between physicians and primary nurses usually begin at this stage, because both feel the pressure of rescuing the patient from the condition which is victimizing him.

> Games begin when members of the helping professions . . . start jockeying for the position of rescuer. Maneuvers are probably the result of the injunction that only one person should be in charge of the care of the patient. Since the physician has more authority than a nurse, he almost always wins the rescuer slot if he wants it (Levin & Berne, 1972, p. 484).

The positions of primary nurses and physicians usually become polarized: the nurse wants to give the patient something immediate and tangible, and the physician wants to investigate the causes of the presenting problems. Often, nurses tend to get more emotionally involved while physicians tend to withdraw into scientific rationale and tests. Both sides are valid, but without collegial respect avoidance rather than collaboration occurs. The nurse-manager can aide collaboration at this stage by periodically reviewing categories which nurses or physicians should assess and being aware of protocols for action. For instance, the nurse-manager may suggest to the chief of a noncardiac service that all patients over a certain age should be given electrocardiograms. When this becomes common practice, they have collaborated successfully around the value of health screening. At another time, the chief physician may request that any admitting nurse record all medications that the patient is currently taking. When this practice is institutionalized, they have collaborated successfully around the value of thorough assessments. An overall perspective of how a unit functions within an agency helps each discipline to understand and respect the other and prevents polarization of attitudes and behavior.

Problem Identification

Problem identification probably disrupts consensus between primary nurses and physicians more than other problems because of the differences in conceptual training. Physicians and primary nurses look at the same problems from the view of their own disciplines, which enables each to define the problem in workable terms. Traditionally, nurses define problems in terms of symptoms, and physicians, in terms of underlying diagnoses:

- RN: High blood pressure
  MD: Hypertension

- RN: Cardiac arrhythmias
  MD: Hypokalemia

- RN: Immobilization
  MD: Congenital hip disease

- RN: Lack of knowledge
  MD: Noncompliance

- RN: Lack of self-esteem as a woman
  MD: Oedipal conflict

- RN: Anurea
  MD: Chronic renal failure

The division of labor between professionals is straightforward in the way problems are defined. The use of nursing diagnosis clarifies what a nurse can do about patients' problems within the jurisdiction of nursing. To make collaboration possible, primary nurses and physicians must respect the conceptual framework in which each has been socialized to function. There must be an acknowledgment of the sameness of intelligence but the difference in vision. Mutual respect results from frequent discussions that begin with the day of admission. Collaborative energies are wasted if each of these professionals fails to realize that the other is viewing the patient from a different perspective.

The nurse-manager can promote collaboration by helping primary nurses to identify the various levels on which patients' symptoms and needs can be understood. For instance, a quadriplegic with a spinal cord lesion at the T-5 or T-6 level is prone to autonomic dysreflexia. The nurse-manager helps the primary nurse to identify the symptoms, relate them to autonomic dysreflexia, validate assumptions, and coordinate appropriate intervention. The physician becomes involved "if removal of the source of stimulation has little or no effect on reducing blood pressure, or the blood pressure is dangerously high and any increase in stimulation by checking the source (skin stimuli, bowel impaction, bladder distention or obstruction) could prove threatening" (Zander, K., Bower, K., Foster, S., Townson, L., Wermuth, M., Woldum, K., 1978, p. 330). Long-term management by the primary nurse includes prevention of the problem by an effective bowel and bladder program and instruction to the patient about how to manage the treatment. The physician is involved if adrenergic or cholinergic blocking agents are required. Physician and primary nurse are interdependent on each other's knowledge of the patient.

It should be noted that it takes time for primary nurses to become sophisticated in their nursing territory. Knowledgeable nursing care is very complex and continually growing. The nurse-manager must be skilled in teaching about each level of patient needs, including symptoms, pathophysiology, and interventions. This requires an ability to teach concepts as well as bedside techniques.

To be an effective collaborator, a primary nurse must be able to integrate and converse about all levels of patient needs, i.e., ask the aides to take the patient's blood pressure, irrigate a catheter, and discuss medication management with the physician. The primary nurse is a colleague to everyone with whom collaboration is essential.

Plan of Care

A plan of care for a patient includes the problem, the desired resolution, or goal, and the prescribed nursing actions to alleviate the problem. Traditionally, a plan of care usually meant following the doctor's orders and giving support to the patient. Although primary nurses now have many alternatives with which to determine a plan of care for primary patients, it is quite common for care plans merely to repeat the treatments ordered by the physician. This indicates the problem of clarity about nursing territory; nurses are not sure what nursing is. Problem identification through nursing diagnosis is the first step in making an overall plan of care. In addition, the plan must contain specific goals for each nursing diagnosis and the proposed interventions to achieve those goals.

By listening, watching, and reading documentation, the nurse-manager can determine how clearly primary nurses perceive their territory. The nurse-manager will probably have to strengthen the three areas of problem identification, goal setting, and interventions. The clearer the problem and the more descriptive the goal, the better the plans for intervention. Although caring is harder to define than curing, it can be done.

Implementation of Care Plan

Implementation of the care plan is the most exciting and gratifying aspect of primary nursing. Because nursing can be defined as providing direct service to people who cannot care for themselves in certain areas and helping the remainder learn to care for themselves, there is a wide variety of nursing interventions that go beyond physician orders. The nurse-manager can help the nursing staff to devise ways of implementing nursing-ordered care. This can be facilitated by allowing primary nurses to apply their personal style to well thought out short-term goals.

Evaluate Problems and Progress

Both physicians and nurses are attentive to progress or the lack of it. However, each discipline has a particular way of determining the presence of a problem, judging potential resolution of the problem, and deciding when progress has been made. The greatest area of conflict between nurses and physicians—especially physicians who have not been the long-time general practitioner for a patient—is the way the patient as a person is viewed. The same lines are drawn once again: nursing = the holistic approach = caring, and doctoring = the focused approach = curing. Although individuals in each discipline understand and even support each other's viewpoints, stress and conflict can push the most flexible nurses and physicians into their traditional camps.

Primary nurses must have a strong identification with the meaning of comprehensive nursing care. Evaluating patients in the psychosocial as well as physical areas can easily be taught, but must also be structured into the primary nurse role through goal-directed practice which is monitored in documentation and primary nurse conferences. Equally as important, primary nurses need the flexibility to accept and assist the more focused approach of physicians. Nursing and doctoring are not mutually exclusive, but it is essential that each respect the other's way of conceptualizing a problem in order to obtain realistic outcomes and honest evaluation of the results of their mutual labors.

Such collaborative work can be carried on in any forum where the patient is the center of professional attention on a staff level, such as teaching conferences, walk rounds, discharge rounds, and outside consultations. The nurse-manager must be sure that nursing is always represented, even if it increases everyone's workload for a few hours. Attendance at interdisciplinary conferences about primary patients should be a major part of a primary nurse's role. The primary nurse must be prepared to discuss the assessment of problems and the status of resolutions, which preferably should be written down ahead of time. Primary patients need this type of advocacy so that problems are presented in a comprehensive manner to those who can take action.

Differences of opinion about proper patient management are not in themselves bad but should be discussed until at least a temporary resolution is planned. Everyone benefits when mutual understanding is actively sought.

> Nurses who understand why physicians have chosen a particular course of action will almost certainly provide more effective care. The inefficiencies in patient care which occur when a patient's nurses don't understand the general rationale for therapy probably will ultimately take more of the physician's time than would be required to discuss controversial decisions (Budassi & Rockwell, 1978, p. iii).

Identify New Problems, Adjust Plan, Implement Adjusted Plan, Evaluate Problems and Progress

The process of evaluation for both disciplines repeats itself until the patient's health is no longer within the jurisdiction of the physician or primary nurse. Until the patient leaves, with or without medical advice, or dies, the nurse is most often the first person to spot new problems. Identifying subtle changes in condition is the nurse's forte. The majority of physicians' orders are written after nurses have reported the need and described all the details of a current problem. Most nurses usually know what kind of order the patient needs before they contact the physician. At this juncture the nurse's ability to collaborate is crucial to get the necessary work accomplished.

Discharge and Referral

Discharge is foremost on the patient's mind and should be as important to physicians and primary nurses. However, planning around the patient's discharge can be very nerve-racking for nurses. While the physician's role in discharge may be merely to write an order and prescribe take-home medication, the primary nurse's role involves helping the patient to finalize plans to leave and finding out what the patient needs for home care. Too often the pressure on the physician to clear bed space and the pressure on the primary nurse to do a complete job become mutually exclusive. Examples are seen daily: the child sent home with a tracheostomy before the primary nurse has a chance to teach the parents how to care for the trach, or the immobile patient who is discharged without proper equipment in the home. When primary nurses participate in patient discharge in a clearly defined way, the role of the physician is clarified as well.

Another element should be added to those in Figure 6-1, expected death. Although most of the system elements also apply to terminally ill patients, discharge is no longer the goal of care. Primary nurses have a crucial role with terminally ill patients. Although the physician's moral support and orders are important, the curing is over. The nurse-manager becomes the advocate for the primary nurse, who is in an emotionally strained position. The nurse-manager can help by encouraging discussion of feelings, assigning other nurses to serve as substitutes when necessary, and discussing death and dying and administrative policies regarding terminally ill patients, such as private rooms, family rooms, and code status, at staff meetings.

The Confidence to Collaborate

A nurse-manager needs to build the confidence of nurses without tearing down the abilities of professionals in other disciplines. Valuing oneself by devaluing others is not firm ground for collaboration. The nurse-manager has a difficult task because society overvalues physicians and undervalues nurses. Nurses are often listed as paraprofessionals or referred to as physician extenders! The nurse-manager must have the attitude that nurses are not paraprofessionals, but that the input and perspective of primary nurses is as valuable as that of physicians.

Confidence requires trust in your own judgment, and primary nurses must have the confidence to check out perceptions of clinical situations with the nurse-manager. They must feel that their needs are important enough to request attention, even when it means interrupting the nurse-manager's other duties. They must realize that the nurse-manager is working for them, not that they are working for the nurse-manager. Primary nurses learn to trust their own clinical judgment as they validate areas of uncertainty with the nurse-manager. If nurse-managers listen carefully, they find that many statements made by primary nurses are actually requests for confidence building. Comments such as "I don't think there's anything more I can add to the care plan" or "that long-term goal is not realistic now" are openings for feedback from the nurse-manager.

The nurse-manager must strive to create an atmosphere in which primary nurses feel that they have their own resources and those of others to act as checks and balances. The less the nurse-manager assumes the role of clinical expert regarding questions and statements, the more confidence is built. The nurse-manager can do this by using a questioning style similar to that employed in primary nurse conferences.

> PN: Mrs. S's BP goes up when she faints, and she's been fainting twice a day.
>
> NM: What is your understanding about why she faints?
>
> PN: Dr. P is still checking with the neurologists who think it's all emotional. (Lack of data and confidence)
>
> NM: What do *you* think is happening?
>
> PN: I think she's been fainting more and the situation is getting serious because the last time her BP was 180/110 and she had a nosebleed. Now because her electrolytes are off, Dr. P is taking her off antihypertensives. (Has a tentative formulation of the problem)
>
> NM: I'm not knowledgeable about the connections between antihypertensives and electrolytes. Do you know? (Uses own lack of knowledge to help nurse to clarify)
>
> PN: No. I think I'd better ask Dr. P because I think she needs to stay on antihypertensives. I don't think I told him about the nosebleed she had last night. (Gains confidence to question MD as the area needing collaboration is defined)
>
> NM: I'm interested in the outcome; let me know what he says. We should have a clear plan for people working over the weekend. (Reinforces PN's decision to collaborate by showing interest in results and provides a monitor for potentially negative resolutions)

In this example, the nurse-manager not only encouraged the primary nurse to solve the problem, but also encouraged autonomy by avoiding the task of speaking to the doctor. If the nurse-manager had offered to do this, the primary nurse may have felt too stupid, weak, or without status to collaborate.

In every conversation with a primary nurse, there are critical points at which the nurse-manager can contribute to or detract from a primary nurse's confidence. If a nurse-manager is not accustomed to the question-asking method of clinical teaching, it is a mandatory area for development. The nurse-manager should practice turning statements into questions, always being aware of reversion to statements. Usually, statements are used at times of clinical crisis, personal competition, or exasperation with a particular nurse.

Directives at times of clinical crises are perfectly acceptable, but there are times when the nurse-manager needs to take clinical action and collaborate with physicians in place of the primary nurse. Such instances usually occur when the primary nurse is not readily available and the patient's clinical status demands an immediate response. Although problems sometimes can be deferred to another nurse, often, however, the nurse-manager has the necessary information and contacts to intervene quickly. When the nurse-manager takes over, it is important that the primary nurse is acquainted with the actions and decisions, as any other colleague would do.

There are also times in clinical crises when the nurse-manager must force a primary nurse to speak with appropriate professionals about a patient. The nurse-manager should stay with the nurse to act as interpreter/clarifier during the discussion, but should not become involved in content. In this way, the primary nurse is given the support needed to endure the uncertain moments of collaboration, but is allowed to conduct the effort alone.

The nurse-manager can easily undermine the confidence of primary nurses by making subtle, unintentional, devaluing remarks. Statements such as "you're just new, you'll learn" or "you can try it, but I've never seen it work" indicate a lack of confidence that can only decrease the primary nurse's willingness to problem solve and intervene. Nurse-managers should learn to censor the reactions that arise from their own defensiveness. Otherwise, energy that is needed for collaboration is spent on vying with the nurse-manager.

It is very difficult to support nurses who refuse to take the risk of collaborating. The nurse-manager learns quickly which primary nurses take a passive stance toward the larger system. Repeated statements such as "I didn't have time" or "what good does it do anyway" indicate that a nurse's energies are going in the wrong direction. The lack of confidence displayed is probably entwined with a long-standing pattern of passivity. These nurses can be helped by catching them up in the staff group's activity. It is difficult to maintain a passive position if there are no rewards and no company. Although such nurses may never be the epitome of wholehearted collaboration, they can develop basic skills in that area.

The nurse-manager is the person behind the scenes who gives primary nurses the confidence to collaborate as successful attempts begin to outnumber disheartening ones. The following statement was made by a confident primary nurse engaged in purposeful interaction.

> I have found repeated satisfaction in approaching the physician (with a thorough knowledge of the status of our patient) with requests for alternate means of meeting all patient needs. I find myself analyzing which approach would accomplish my purpose best when I approach the physician with suggestions for ways to provide better care, or with discovery of a previously unknown variable which indicates a change in care. Thus, a professional collaboration between doctor and nurse is fostered with the patient's welfare at its center (Grover & Golback, 1977, p. 24).

The Politics of Collaboration

"That we (nurses) have not influenced the health care system in proportion to our potential strength may be due to our inability to attract an audience, to be granted credibility or to express ourselves forcefully" (LeRoux, 1978, p. 52). The politics of collaboration refers to the ability of nurses, individually and collectively, to influence people in other disciplines, as well as other nurses, so that a different attitude or action is produced. Politics can imply self-interest, but in nursing it often means that the nurse is collaborating with the interest of the patient in mind.

Although there are many occasions for friendly collaboration, primary nurses are literally forced into collaborating with physicians when they seek changes that can only be made through the physician's legal authority. Without the primary nurse's initiation of strategic interactions, the lack of collaboration can interfere with safe patient care.

As primary nurses become more capable in their roles, they are ready to enter the politics of collaboration. Therefore, primary nurses should learn some principles of working with others, especially physicians, toward the benefit of patients. Collaboration involves a degree of intuitive bargaining, but it also involves ten basic truths.

Truth 1: Collaboration is easier when the desire for communication is abandoned.

Communicate and *communication* have been overused as concepts to the point where they do not mean anything. They imply more than the exchange of information, and cover a wide range of interrelationships between two or more individuals. People tend to define communication as an attempt to perceive something in exactly the same way as someone else, resulting in identical actions. Although mutuality of perceptions is an admirable goal, chances of this happening in the medical-nursing world are slim. Perhaps it is better that doctors and nurses do not perceive situations the same way; otherwise, the clinical checks and balances would be lost!

When the desire for communication is given up, primary nurses begin real collaboration. Collaboration requires primary nurses to decide ahead of time what and how facts and opinions will be presented to appropriate persons. When primary nurses put aside the desire for communication, they can collaborate more scientifically. Principles of collaboration must also extend beyond those seen in typical interactions between nurses and physicians:

> I'd be very concerned if the nurse's capabilities were recognized and her skills used only because of personal relationships, because the doctor knows and likes me, the nurse. What about me when I don't know the doctor but have a problem with a patient? (Bernstein, Hinton, & Taylor, 1972, p. 34)

Truth 2: Collaboration is more effective in face-to-face contact than in medical charts or over the phone.

Personal contact is always best because body language adds honesty to the interaction. It is also easier to keep a person's attention. However, face-to-face discourse is less controlled than written messages:

> The receivers tend to respond more holistically and subjectively. There is little time to critically analyze, to review the message, to dissect it. The speaker's voice, manner and personality may enhance or distract from what is being said. Substance and style are both important for maintaining the listener's attention and interest (LeRoux, 1978, p. 53).

Primary nurses need to be aware of the way they present themselves and their issues. The nurse-manager can be very instructive in this regard.

Truth 3. Collaboration works best when personal issues are omitted and egos are put aside.

Nurse-physician discussions should be patient-oriented and should not regress into territorial struggles or personal remarks. People can work together better if they do not feel that they are fighting for their esteem and their identity. Both parties must be able to save face and not to lose pride in themselves because of a professional interaction.

Truth 4. Primary nurses can facilitate collaboration if they inform the physician of the pressures that are motivating them to collaborate.

This information should not be presented as an excuse or apology, but in an attempt to increase professional understanding. Too often, nurses are expected, and expect themselves, to understand the pressures on physician. This is especially true in residency training programs where nurses learn that to get what they want for patients, they have to gratify a resident's narcissism by couching approaches in ways that will not threaten the resident. Nurses end up mentally writing care plans for the idiosyncrasies of each physician. Although nurses are experts at nursing physicians in this way, it is condescending because it assumes that physicians are too delicate to be approached as equals.

Nurses appreciate the pressures that physicians are under, but they should expect physicians to understand their pressures too. "I try to remember what influences, education, and training [the physician has] had, and how it's contributed to his view of himself. But at the same time, I'm always keeping in mind why I'm there, so that I don't let myself be intimidated" (Bernstein et al., 1972, p. 35).

Truth 5. Intimidation is the surest way to halt collaboration.

Intimidation is the social way of putting someone in their place, and it is the most prevalent disease in the hospital. Next to the patient, the nurse feels intimidated most often. Common signs of intimidation are power plays, orders written without planning or consulting nurses, and innuendos about the intellectual or scholastic deficits of nurses. The problem is compounded in psychiatry by physicians' pseudopsychological interpretations of nurses' motivations.

Intimidation occurs when a person or group assumes that it is better, more knowledgeable, and more powerful than another. Before primary nursing, it was easy for physicians to assume that they were dictating patient care, because nurses did not make a practice of knowing individual patients in depth. With primary nursing, however, nurses are as much if not more intimately involved with the patient's situation than the physician, thus putting the nurse on a separate but equal basis with the physician on a case. The basis for intimidation, by its definition, is thus reduced. However, as long as nurses feel subordinate to physicians, they are easily intimidated. After nurses have assimilated the nursing process and have the self-assurance of support from the nurse-manager and the nursing department, they are less likely to be intimidated.

Nurses need to recognize the first signs of intimidation and be able to change course during the interaction. A physician's intimidation usually indicates defensiveness, stemming from a sense of being cornered. The following statement about psychiatric residents is probably true for most physicians:

> Much of these adjustment difficulties grow out of the resident's assumption that they must solve all problems or answer all questions that nurses (or patients) bring to them. Perhaps such attitudes grow out of medical training or the physician's locus high on the formal hierarchical ladder. Whatever their origin, once residents learn that they need not be omniscient or omnipotent, such defenses tend to lessen (Westermeyer, Labeck, & Pisani, 1977, p. 78).

Truth 6. The most productive collaboration occurs before a crisis in the planning and replanning phases of patient care.

When physicians and primary nurses are not in the crunch of a crisis situation, collaboration is more likely and may even prevent crises. Frequent planning meetings between nurse and physician are useful, and physicians will learn that formal authority can be shared with nurses, thus lightening the burden of decision making. Planning ahead minimizes the mutually exclusive pressures that develop in each discipline. For example, when residents take cases for educational rather than patient care motives, a collaborative situation allows them to feel that they can learn about their patients from a primary nurse. Most of this kind of teaching by nurses is unrecognized in the medical world, but is an integral aspect of collaboration.

Planning ahead also allows for identification of separate and mutual goals for patients. Clarification of desired outcomes and the ways to achieve them is a hallmark of collaboration. Requesting counsel before action is required is the best way to avoid power plays.

Nurses have never been powerless in clinical situations. Unfortunately, the nurse's power is often the negative control of omission. Nurses alone or in conjuction with other nursing staff can "accidentally on purpose" obstruct the physician's orders. It is not uncommon for nurses to forget treatments, to make medication errors, or to respond to a patient less than adequately in response to their feelings about the patient's physician. Nurses and physicians are in a tenuous balance of power and subterfuge.

Nurses need to experience the positive power that comes from confidence in the nurse-physician partnership for patient care. "Such decision making by consensus, whenever possible, enables the doctor to abandon unilateral fiat as his sole repertoire for exercising leadership and enables the nurse to abandon sabotage as a defense against fiat" (Westermeyer et al., 1977, p. 78).

Truth 7. Although ideal collaboration takes place as a style of planning, patient care situations require collaboration during crises.

In crisis situations, the guidelines developed by Bernstein et al. (1972), will be helpful to primary nurses:

1. Before contacting the doctor, do a conscientious job of assessing the patient's condition.
2. Then give him specific details.
3. When in doubt, call him. Don't wait, wondering.
4. Believe your own judgment, and don't be dissuaded if the doctor at first doubts it.
5. Use common sense in assessment, and try to correlate your findings.
6. Convey your belief that your role is important in patient care.

7. Keep your notes complete.
8. Don't be intimidated by the doctor. When it's vital, insist he listen.
9. Realize sometimes you may have to put yourself on the line; do it when you feel you should.
10. If you don't know the doctor's plans, ask him.
11. If you think his inaction is causing you problems, tell him (p. 36).

Truth 8. Not all problems and certainly not all feelings can be worked out through collaboration.

Sometimes primary nurses have to call in the nurse-manager, supervisor, or the next in power above the physician with whom they are working. Primary nurses should be encouraged to use this avenue when certain problems arise, usually in emergency situations. Otherwise the following statement is applicable: "Once the resident surrenders the need for omnipotent solutions and the nurse admits that all of the ward problems cannot be solved, they are both in a better position to deal with one another" (Westermeyer et al., 1977, p. 79).

Truth 9. Not all difficulties in the nurse-physician relationship are based on female-male role stereotypes, but many are.

Although it is unproductive to blame all the faults in collaborative efforts on traditional male-female clashes, some female nurses tend to revert to behavior patterns which bog them down when they are dealing with male physicians.

- Asking permission: "is it all right if . . . ?" or "would you mind if . . . ?"
- Giving opinions and intuitive feelings rather than factual or prepared information.
- Disowning the motivation or content of an interaction: "I wouldn't be asking this except . . ." or "I'm not sure why we're here, but. . . . " Disowning stems from the nurse's need to avoid blame. "Blame avoidance is characterized by a fear of being wrong which is so strong that the person can *never* be responsible for a wrong act; the individual *always* has to be right. There is an extreme desire to be safe and correct" (Menikheim, 1979, p. 138).
- Asking approval and avoiding commitment by using tag questions as identified by Lakoff. These turn a statement into a question that the recipient has to validate: "Don't you think the family should. . . ?" or "Billy is getting worse, isn't he?" "A tag-question is midway between an outright statement and a yes/no question: It is less assertive than the former, but more confident than the latter" (Lakoff in Menikheim, 1979, p. 136).
- Getting emotional, hysterical, and vague which causes the man to get tight, rigid, and nonempathic. To show rage, concern, or love is not in itself bad, but the intensity can deter a male.

It would be very valuable if typically female and male perspectives could be given equal value. Nurses need to maintain their objectivity and scientific approach to problems, and physicians need to admit their more nurturing and emotional characteristics. Such cultural exchanges make up an important aspect of effective collaboration.

It is also quite feasible that some of these patterns occur in interactions other than those with a female nurse and a male physician. In all situations, the person who is least sure of himself will retreat to nonassertive behaviors rather than take the risk of admitting uncertainty or asking for information. A health care provider cannot hide for long behind either gender or role because patients will not gain the benefits that are derived from professionals who collaborate.

None of these patterns are completely avoidable, especially in the intense environment of a hospital or clinic. Some of them are highly appropriate in some circumstances. However, they should not be the only collaboration techniques in the primary nurse's repertoire, because they require too much energy to go into pretense rather than problem solving.

Truth 10. New patterns of collaboration can be learned, though changes involve personal risk taking.

The nurse-manager's values and style of collaboration greatly influence the motivation of primary nurses to broaden their approaches. *Broaden* is a better term to use than *change,* because as primary nurses find new techniques that work well, they gradually give up the less effective patterns. One good example of the gradual shift in approach can be seen in the sequence:

a) "There is nothing to be done about the situation" to
b) "What can be done about the situation?" to
c) "This is what can be done about the situation" (Menikheim, 1979, p. 139).

Policy Making and Collaboration

Too often in nursing we are reactive rather than proactive. Too often the system controls us rather than our controlling the system. Often when we try to influence the system and do not meet with complete success, we think we have lost the total war rather than just one of many battles (LeRoux, 1978, p. 51).

The nurse-manager has the role of effecting policies that allow primary nurses to collaborate with physicians and other health team members as easily as possible. The nurse-manager's goal should be the establishment of organizational structures that are well illustrated in the following description given by Milton Weinberg, Jr., Department of Cardiovascular and Thoracic Surgery and president of the medical staff, Rush-Presbyterian-St. Luke's Medical Center, Chicago:

> The relationship with the medical staff is infinitely better than it was before primary nursing. Doctors no longer find it difficult to find someone who can answer questions about the care their patients receive. They are assured that one nurse has responsibility for the overall care of the patient and will be able to assess any changes in a patient's condition that the physician should be aware of (Pryma, 1978, p. 16).

The nurse-manager can gain this goal by involvement in agency politics, overcoming personal inertia, and assuming a position of influence. This involves actively dealing with health care issues as they revolve around certain personalities.

The nurse-manager must identify the level of the physician hierarchy on which unit policies and decisions are made. The physicians at this level are those with whom the nurse-manager needs to collaborate consistently. Collaboration begins with the way the primary nursing is introduced and continues with regular meetings and general policies that are part of primary nursing.

Introducing Primary Nursing

Physicians should be informed about the decision of a unit or department to introduce primary nursing. They should not be asked for permission because primary nursing is not a medical matter—it is well within the jurisdiction of nursing to define how nursing care will be delivered.

Once this is clear, physicians deserve explanations to clarify the way primary nurses will be functioning with patients and with physicians. The nurse-manager is most often asked for information and explanations about primary nursing. This role will seem less threatening and frustrating if nurse-managers view themselves as translators and educators for the physicians about nursing matters. Physician cooperation is not mandatory for primary nursing, but it certainly makes work more enjoyable and effective.

> The development of the colleague relationship took time, but I feel it met with little resistance. There were some raised eyebrows and startled looks as questions from nurses directed to physicians regarding goals and discharge planning were posed, but our commitment was always so obvious that it was part of the growth process that took place. The recognition by the physician of the primary nurse became apparent. As is the custom today, the attending physician would seek out the primary nurse before making his rounds, and a common sight at the patient's bedside was his doctor and his primary nurse (Esposito, 1977, p. 22).

The Benefit of Regular Meetings

Policies that improve a nurse's abilities and opportunities to collaborate with physicians take several years to develop. It is impossible to work out everything before the transition to primary nursing.

The surest guarantee for policy making is the nurse-manager's insistence on regular, frequent (weekly is ideal) meetings with lateral partners in the physician hierarchy. For instance, in a medical center the nurse-manager should have regular policy meetings with the chief resident, the chief of the service, or both.

A nurse-manager's meetings with physicians are for collaboration about policies and should not be used for evaluative supervision. The nurse-manager's supervision must have a secure base with the nursing administration so that the nurse-manager is not dependent on the physicians for paychecks, evaluations, or moral support. The nurse-manager must be free from any relationship with physicians that would prejudice collegial interaction.

Meetings can cover a wide range of topics bearing on primary nursing, and the content need not always be directed at specific policies. As time goes on, both nurse-manager and physician-manager find that sharing perceptions is invaluable. Information that seems vaguely related one month may begin to form a policy the next month. Some suggested areas of discussion that the nurse-manager may want to include in collaboration are:

- specific patient cases, including diagnoses, treatments, and related literature
- instructional needs of nurses and physicians as groups or individuals
- problems with the physical environment or equipment
- interdepartmental liaison work
- ideas about rounds, conferences, documentation, and other shared territory
- clarification of the rationale for decisions made in the previous week
- staffing, personnel changes, vacation coverage
- aspects of the collegial relationship

Policies result from collaboration, such as the physician-manager requesting a more senior primary nurse for cases with medical students to increase safety; the nurse-manager asking that new equipment be requisitioned; or the nurse-manager and physician-manager realizing that too many patients developed complications postoperatively. The meetings provide an opportunity for problems to be identified and addressed rationally, and the results are felt by all primary nurses.

The nurse- and physician-managers need to present a united front to upper level hospital administration when trying to change policies that may affect other clinical areas. Examples may include changes needed about direct admissions from the emergency room or about family visiting hours. The request for such changes may come from primary nurses who are affected by the collaborative work done by the nurse- and physician-managers.

The nurse-manager needs to use leverage as well as maintain the equality of collaboration. In addition to the influence that personal attitudes about nursing's role in a clinical area have on the staff, the nurse-manager has the leverage to ensure quality care.

A reputation for quality care directly affects the amount and kinds of referrals a hospital and physicians receive. For instance, Kenneth T. Swanson, president of the Bayfront Medical Center in St. Petersburg, Florida, reported that:

> Primary nursing care has changed the image of our hospital with the professionals in the community and with the laymen. The improved care has made our regular staff admit more patients to the hospital, has brought some of the members of the staff who were not a part of the active staff back to the hospital, and has also helped to attract new physicians moving into the community. Today, patients who have to be readmitted for hospital care are not only specifying our hospital, but also the actual floor and station they had been on previously (Swanson, 1977, p. 6).

Physician-Nurse Policies for Primary Nursing

1. Nurses should be included in all rounds, conferences, and planning sessions about current patients.

2. Plans for discharge should be discussed well in advance, giving the primary nurse a chance to help the patient and family make appropriate plans based on accurate knowledge of the health situation.

3. The professional development of nurses should be a priority. They should be included in as many teaching conferences and seminars as possible and should be notified ahead of time so that schedules can accommodate attendance.

4. Documentation in the medical record should be integrated into one set of progress notes.

5. Primary nurses should have access to the physician-manager when collaboration breaks down. Likewise, primary physicians should have access to the nurse-manager regarding the work of primary nurses.

6. If physician assistants are present, their role should be carefully delineated from that of primary nurses and other health care providers.

7. The discrepancies in priorities between residency training programs and patient care should be adjusted frequently.

8. Criteria for optimal patient care outcomes should be formulated and given priority through nurse-physician collaboration.

By actively collaborating with the physician-manager, the nurse-manager sets an example for the primary nurse to follow. Furthermore, the nurse-manager's actions have other positive results:

1. Patients are spared some red tape when their needs demand response. If nurses and physicians collaborate on admissions, patients and their families are less overwhelmed and frustrated with the health care system.

2. The nurse-manager is viewed as an important force in the clinical area. Physicians learn that collaboration is expected not just of themselves, but of their manager. The cycle continues when they become managers.

3. If the staff sees the nurse-manager pursuing policy making, they feel hopeful that their ideas will be addressed seriously at the appropriate administrative level. The nurse-manager needs to keep the primary nursing staff informed about the progress of their contributions.

4. Primary nurses understand the origin of policies because they have participated in formulating some of them, and therefore they are more confident in upholding policies. They also have backup from both disciplines if they are questioned.

A nurse-manager's collaborative projects are longer term than those of a primary nurse because a competent primary nursing staff which is respected by all disciplines takes several years to develop. Similarly, effective collaboration is a management goal which needs continual effort. "We should not expect immediate results, but . . . many messages delivered over an extended period of time, will inevitably produce a subtle awareness of issues, arouse public opinion, reinforce attitudes, and cause attitude change" (LeRoux, 1978, p. 57).

PRIMARY NURSING IN SPECIALTY AREAS

As primary nursing is actualized, old problems are resolved and new situations develop because of professional growth and variations in clinical settings. Nurse-managers benefit greatly from the experiences of others in similar clinical areas. Although the primary nursing process is the same in every agency and clinic, different diagnoses and levels of care require emphasis on different aspects of the primary nurse's role. In turn, the nurse-manager in differing clinical areas have differing focuses in directing efforts toward maximum outcomes of patient care.

A comparison of primary nursing in various clinical settings can be made with two types of measurements: the hierarchy of needs (Maslow, 1954) and the length of the primary nurse-patient/family relationship. Both can be used to analyze primary nursing management needs.

Figure 6-1 shows selected specialty areas in relation to Maslow's hierarchy. It illustrates that primary nurses need a wide range of skills to meet multiple needs.

Figure 6-1 Maslow's Hierarchy of Needs in Relation to Primary Nursing Specialty Areas

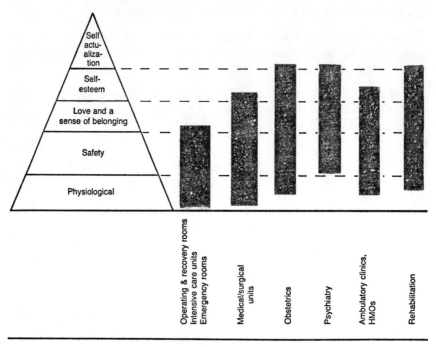

It also demonstrates that one level is no more important than another, but that each specialty area has its own predictable range of priorities.

Many times we hear nurses in the intensive care unit say they do not feel like primary nurses because they are not carrying out patient education programs. This indicates a misunderstanding that primary nursing is only for higher level needs, which is certainly a restrictive definition for nurses and patients. Nurse-managers can do a great deal to correct this fallacy among a staff group. Indeed, primary nurses move up and down the hierarchy, depending on the condition of patients. That is the exciting part of primary nursing—to accurately assess the type and level of need and to accurately respond to it.

Figure 6-2 presents a model of the length of primary nurse-patient/family relationships and representative specialty areas. It helps to understand the primary nurse's role in the areas of:

- influence of the primary nurse as balanced by influences from the rest of the patient's world
- patient dependence

Figure 6-2 Length of Primary Nurse-Patient/Family Relationships in Representative Speciality Areas

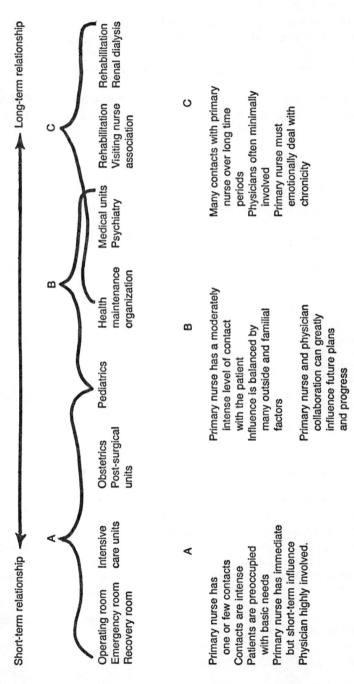

Short-term relationship ⟵⟶ Long-term relationship

A

Operating room	Obstetrics	Pediatrics	Health	Medical units	Rehabilitation	Rehabilitation
Emergency room	Post-surgical		maintenance	Psychiatry	Visiting nurse	Renal dialysis
Recovery room	units		organization		association	

A

Primary nurse has
  one or few contacts
Contacts are intense
Patients are preoccupied
  with basic needs
Primary nurse has immediate
  but short-term influence
Physician highly involved.

B

Primary nurse has a moderately
  intense level of contact
  with the patient
Influence is balanced by
  many outside and familial
  factors

Primary nurse and physician
  collaboration can greatly
  influence future plans
  and progress

C

Many contacts with primary
  nurse over long time
  periods
Physicians often minimally
  involved
Primary nurse must
  emotionally deal with
  chronicity

- relationship between primary nursing and primary care
- time frame in which primary nurses function
- implications of transferring patients to new specialty areas
- future career pathways
- prospective roles in areas of the health care delivery system

The experiences of managers and primary nurses in a variety of specialty areas are presented in the following chapters. They further elaborate on the similarities and differences of role enactment that occur when the first exciting days of primary nursing are over.

REFERENCES

Bernstein, S., Hinton, A., & Taylor, P. Trouble communicating with doctors. *Nursing 72*, January 1972, *2*(1), 30-36.

Budassi, S., & Rockwell, M. Who should be in charge here? *Critical Care Quarterly*, May 1978, *1*(1), i-v.

Bush M.A., & Kjervik, D. The nurse's self-image. In D. Kjervik & I. Martinson, *Women in stress: A nursing perspective*. New York: Appleton-Century-Crofts, 1979.

Esposito, N. In The Evanston story: Primary nursing comes alive. *Nursing Administration Quarterly*, Winter 1977, *1*(2), 20-23.

Ganong, J., & Ganong, W. *Nursing management*. Germantown, Md.: Aspen Systems, 1976.

Garber, R. In The Evanston story: Primary nursing comes alive. *Nursing Administration Quarterly*, Winter 1977, *1*(2), 30-31.

Grover, L., & Golback, J. In The Evanston story: Primary nursing comes alive. *Nursing Administration Quarterly*, Winter 1977, *1*(2), 23-25.

LeRoux, R. Communication and influence in nursing. *Nursing Administration Quarterly*, Spring 1978, *2*(1), 51-57.

Levin, P., & Berne, E. Games nurses play. *American Journal of Nursing*, March 1972, *72*(3), 483-487.

Maslow, A. *Motivation and personality*. New York: Harper and Row, 1954.

Menikheim, M. Communication patterns of women and nurses. In D. Kjervik & I. Martinson, *Women in stress: A nursing perspective*. New York: Appleton-Century-Crofts, 1979.

Pryma, R. Primary nursing—A working philosophy—An organizational style. *The Magazine* (Rush-Presbyterian-St. Luke's Medical Center, Chicago) Spring 1978, 3-17.

Rockmore, M. Are doctors stifling better nursing care? *Chicago Tribune*, January 6, 1979.

Smith, C. Primary nursing care—A substantive nursing care delivery system. *Nursing Administration Quarterly*, Winter 1977, *1*(2), 1-8.

Swanson, K. Primary nursing care as a management tool. In C. Smith, Primary nursing care—A substantive nursing care delivery system. *Nursing Administration Quarterly*, Winter 1977, *1*(2), 6-7.

Westermeyer, J., Labeck, L., & Pisani, S. Dynamics of the resident-nurse alliance in psychiatry *Journal of Operational Psychiatry*, 1977, *8*(1), 75-79.

Zander, K., Bower, K., Foster, S., Towson, L., Wermuth, M., & Woldum, K. *Practical manual for patient-teaching*. St. Louis: C.V. Mosby, 1978.

Chapter 7

Primary Nursing in the Critical Care Areas

by Arlene Schiro

IS CRITICAL CARE PRIMARY NURSING A NEW CONCEPT?

We are approaching a stage when the status of inpatient populations in our hospitals is becoming more acute. Why is this so hospital administrators ask. One explanation could be recent scientific and medical advances. Patients are being treated for diseases and conditions that probably would have resulted in death not long ago. Trauma, respiratory failures, abdominal aneurysms are among the diagnoses that now have improved survival rates because of the quality of the personnel and equipment. Critical care teams have been trained to assess quickly and act appropriately in order to stabilize patients.

As integral members of such teams, critical care nurses have assumed additional responsibilities. The nurse working in a critical care unit is faced with tremendous pressures and emotional stresses. The critical care nurse must be able to apply the concepts of the nursing process and nursing diagnosis directly to the acutely ill patient. Because these nurses are taught to assume a holistic approach in administering patient care, they see each patient as a whole, not as a series of systems and parts. Critical care nurses assess, organize, distribute medications, deliver basic care, and coordinate other services for patients within an atmosphere of crisis intervention.

Usually in the critical care unit one nurse is accountable for providing total, comprehensive, patient-centered care for the duration of a single shift. Coordination and communication of all aspects of the patient's progress to the physician and other staff members is essential for nursing accountability. It can be argued that critical care nurses have always performed primary nursing during their eight-hour shift. In primary nursing, however, the objective is to provide optimum patient care through comprehensive and continuous accountability throughout the patient's stay in that unit.

229

PREPARATIONS TO IMPLEMENT PRIMARY NURSING

Several bridges must be crossed before primary nursing can be fully implemented in critical care units. First, the concept of primary nursing as a standard of care for acute care must be defined. Questions, problems, and needs must be evaluated before the decision is made to implement such a change. In order to accomplish this, critical care nurse-managers must:

1. Define primary nursing in critical care areas and the need for flexibility in these specialized areas
2. Discuss goal setting as the means to introduce planned change
3. Acknowledge the importance of improved relationships by the critical care nurse in primary nursing
4. Identify problems that must be continually evaluated during the process of change

Definition of Primary Nursing in Critical Care Settings

The dynamics of specialized critical care units are a function of the interaction between the patient and the critical care team. The nature and intensity of this interaction is the most important factor in the critical care environment. In specialized units input and output are continuous. "The system receives energy from the environment, uses it when needed, then loses it via output to the environment, where it is exchanged again" (Roberts, 1976, p. 47). From this perspective, the critically ill patient and the critical care unit exchange energy continually with each other. Each unit, however, sets energy patterns in a specific way. By understanding the patterns and organization of each type of specialized unit, nurses can establish goals that are specific to the setting.

Dynamics of a Surgical Intensive Care Unit

This critical care area is often described as a beehive of activity. The nursing staff is geared to act, change surgical dressings, evaluate fluid balance postoperatively, and promote immediate pulmonary toilet. Generally, the causes of patient problems are visible, such as thoracic suture lines, abdominal dressings, and the open wounds of trauma cases. The pain of the patient can be attributed to a particular operative site or invasive procedure. The nursing staff knows the actions of pain medication and the mechanics of third spacing and uses this knowledge to plan short-term goals for the patient. Because the patient stay is generally short, the primary nurses only see patients approach homeostasis before they are transferred to a general unit. Critical care nurses expend a great deal of personal energy to restore the patient's status through collaboration with all of the unit's personnel. There are situations, however, when feedback from the patient's vital signs and diagnostic laboratory values indicate a poor prognosis. This creates a stressful environment and difficulties for the nurse's own intake system. How can nursing reduce this stress?

Primary nursing in a surgical intensive care unit is an approach to patient care that promotes patient and staff satisfaction. Personal and professional development of the staff should be an outgrowth of the nursing care modality in the unit. By visiting patients prior to an invasive surgical procedure, the primary nurse can see the whole person before the patient becomes a vehicle for tubes and machines. This alone can benefit the postsurgical nurse-patient relationship. The primary nurse must also be aware of the importance of meeting the patient's family. This decreases the fear that the family might experience, and it helps the nurse to obtain information needed to complete the patient assessment form. This is important because patients often remain intubated and on a respirator and are unable to represent themselves.

In the early stages of primary nursing, it is advisable to use the day staff. In this way, the nurse-manager is available for consultation and evaluation. When the day staff is comfortable with the major concepts of primary nursing, it can be introduced to the evening shift. The evening hours offer special opportunities. Surgical rounds, family visits, and quiet late evening hours give the critical care nurse a chance to talk to doctors, families, and patients. Primary nursing can be incorporated into this shift very smoothly for the benefit of all involved.

The manner in which primary nurses and associate nurses are assigned must be set by the nurse-manager. In the surgical intensive care unit nurses may be assigned in advance in order to allow the primary nurse to choose and regulate the workload and the type of patient case.

The flexibility with which each unit adapts primary nursing objectives depends on the tone, pace, and values of the unit. Emphasis in the surgical unit should be placed on the use of preoperative visits and family interviews, along with sound principles of surgical nursing to perform assessments. In so doing, primary nursing can be utilized to the benefit of the entire staff.

Dynamics of a Medical Intensive Care Unit

The type of patients in the medical intensive care unit varies. In general they represent most of the medical emergencies that are seen in any acute care setting. The degree and kinds of nursing skills required are equally as varied. For the most part, patients are dependent on respirators or dialysis for survival. Nursing care is geared toward maintenance of optimum function of all body systems and avoidance of problems of immobility. Patients may simply require prompt emergency treatment for a metabolic crisis or may remain in crisis over a longer period of time.

Because diseases, acid-base disturbances, and hemolytic conditions are not visible to the naked eye, the nurses rely on patient responses and laboratory results for signs of clinical improvement. Often patients are unconscious and cannot offer information about their life style. Nurses must rely solely on the family for clues to the history of the patient. Assessment skills are crucial for the evaluation of change in clinical status, and nurses must have an established baseline in order to set up a care plan based on the individual needs of the patient. Due to the amount of physical care and emotional support needed during a long patient stay, it is advisable to assign two primary nurses to one patient. The nurse-manager can thus promote communication and sharing of ideas to reduce the input stress on each primary nurse.

Primary nursing in medical intensive care units has an impact in the delivery of crisis intervention to the family, and it creates a professional atmosphere that lends itself to continuous evaluation and professional challenge.

Dynamics of a Neurosurgical Intensive Care Unit

The neurosurgical nurse possesses specialized skills that help the acutely ill to achieve their maximum health potential. These patients have often lost their ability to think clearly, to move their extremities, to speak, or any combination of the three. Patient improvement is routinely measured by hourly neurochecks. The age of patients ranges from the young adolescent to the elderly, with tragic diagnoses of spinal cord injury and a cerebral vascular accident. These diagnoses represent sudden catastrophes that are often irreversible. The goal of the nursing staff is not total cure, and therefore treatment and action revolve around maintenance of a steady state for that patient. Changes in intercranial pressure are subtle but are picked up by astute nurses. Primary nurses have a definite advantage in this setting, and the nurse-patient relationship can enhance the fulfillment of both nurse and client. Primary nurses must get to know the patient's personality and then recognize mild changes in levels of consciousness that signal a potentially serious change in condition. By learning about the patient's life style prior to admission, primary nurses can incorporate aspects that may be useful in setting long-term goals. There are specific areas within a neurosurgical intensive care unit that increase stress and that a nurse-manager must be aware of. For example, the nurse whose primary patient remains in the subarachnoid room may require a change of assignment periodically. In this situation two primary nurses should probably be assigned to one patient. This is also true when patients display difficult personality syndromes secondary to brain damage. Primary nurses must not feel that time and energy is wasted on hostile patients. The nurse-manager must be aware of and try to reduce high frustration levels in the staff. Primary nurses should follow patients after discharge to the general floor or the rehabilitation unit in order to see the patient improving and carrying out activities of daily living.

Dynamics of a Cardiac Care Unit

Nurses in a cardiac care unit work with patients who have the diagnosis of myocardial infarction. This critical care area incorporates a nurse-patient relationship within a generally quiet environment. Patients can verbalize their frustrations and question their care, and nurses use advanced equipment to judge the clinical status of the patient. Cardiac monitors are used to assess immediate changes in the status of the cardiac system, and a changing pattern on the scope alerts the nurse to begin immediate action. Nursing care extends from the treatment of cardiogenic shock to relief of the fears of a young person awaiting the possible diagnosis of a heart attack.

The role of the primary nurse in the cardiac care unit can be very challenging. The teaching plan uses information such as risk factor reduction and medication therapy. Because nurses and patients share information, primary nurses learn how patients have accepted their condition or what stage of grief they are suffering. When patients are transferred out of the unit, the primary nurse can visit the patient and continue their relationship. This is also a perfect time for the primary nurse on the floor to discuss goal planning with the primary nurse from the cardiac care unit. The expanded primary nurse role has many advantages for patient care in the CCU.

Dynamics of a Pediatric Intensive Care Unit

Pediatric intensive nursing care involves working with children, understanding their needs, and providing for their requirements. The physical and behavioral characteristics of each age group must be taken into consideration during acute crises. Primary nursing, therefore, must be incorporated into this system using child development therapy and family dynamics.

Critical care nurses in the pediatric area are faced with children whose lives are severely threatened. The nursing process is built upon observation, assessment, and also the inclusion of the family interview. Primary nurses must interpret children's needs, as well as those of the parents. This provides the foundation upon which specific nursing interventions are planned and implemented.

Primary nurses become the surrogate parents to acutely ill children in the hospital. They are given the opportunity to maintain personal rapport with a specific group of nursing staff. When parents realize that the primary nurses are surrogate parents, they seek out familiar faces—nurses who are there when they themselves cannot be at the hospital. The parents should feel that they can call on the telephone and get a personal response about their child's progress.

Although in the pediatric areas nurses fulfill the needs of the children and their families, in the acute areas nurses should not be overburdened with healing the relationships of family members. This is not a requirement of primary nurses who are already under stress due to the situation. Acute disease, potential death, and parents' responses can be very difficult for some nurses to deal with.

Here the nurse-manager can guide staff nurses by listening to their feelings and supporting their needs. The nurse-manager must give primary nurses the independence that is required for primary nursing to work, but must also be aware of the limits that are needed to maintain realistic responsibilities. This support is crucial to the functioning of primary nursing in pediatric acute care areas.

Pediatric areas are an ideal environment for primary nursing care. The subtle aspects of nurse-patient family relationships are always present, which provides an ideal atmosphere for a continuous approach to patient care with the primary nursing modality.

Goal Setting for Planned Change

The scope of the primary nursing concept requires total commitment from the nurse-manager. The nurse-manager usually selects the form of care delivery, because the nurse-manager is the person who determines the unit's climate. The manner in which the nurse-manager introduces planned changes into the critical care unit depends upon the philosophy and needs of the staff and their patients. The commitment of staff nurses is, therefore, of importance. They must be well versed in the principles of the nursing process and convinced that primary nursing will improve patient care for critically ill patients and their families. The nurses working in these units are faced with tremendous pressures, responsibilities, and emotional stresses. They are professionals who are knowledgeable, decisive, and objective. They are continually faced with advancing technology and treatments. These nurses must decide the best approach to foster quality patient care, and primary nursing is the perfect vehicle to approach that high level of care delivery.

Critical care nurses need time to discuss their feelings about the change to primary nursing. Staff conferences to define how it fits into their value system provide such opportunities. Supportive group discussions facilitate awareness of the primary nursing role, and input from staff nurses helps the nurse-manager to formalize an implementation plan. This is a challenging job for the nurse-manager who can use the experiences of other nurse-managers as a guide.

The results of a critical care nurse-manager seminar in a medical center setting illustrates the use of planned change to introduce primary nursing. The nurses who had recently initiated primary nursing in their respective units met monthly to share their progress and concerns with the hospital's Primary Nursing Committee. The nurse-managers represented different areas of acute care nursing, and the diversity of expertise was apparent in discussions of the dynamics of their approaches to planned care. Even though primary nursing was introduced simultaneously, the nurse-managers found that their units were at different stages of development. There was, however, a striking similarity in the positive aspects that evolved from the use of primary nursing. (See Table 7-1.) These elements were:

Table 7-1 Primary Nursing after One Year

Intensive care unit	Strengths	Weaknesses
Medical	Staff is trying hard(motivated and committed) Improvement in assessment sheets Care plans show continuity of care	Need resources on how primary nursing is utilized in an intensive care setting Require more time for completion of nursing care plans by staff
Surgical	Same as above	Patients can't talk and difficult to relate to Not enough time during patient stay to learn about patient and family
Coronary	Patient gets to know the primary nurse, especially since coronary care patients are usually able to talk Strong documentation	Staff unsure that they are doing proper primary nursing Need to relate more with patients after they are transferred to floor
Neurosurgical	Updated assessments Inclusion of family in planning long-term goals	Coping with long-term patient problems and needs
Pediatric	Increased family orientation Associate nurse gives relief to primary nurse if the primary patient is long term	Coping with patient over period of time

- willingness and enthusiasm of the staff to participate
- promotion of documentation in medical records
- promotion of documentation using the principles of continuity
- collaboration in planning nursing care with the medical staff
- interest in participating in staff conferences
- follow-up on patients after transfer to the floor

By evaluating the points that were presented at the seminar, other nurse-managers of critical care units can see the evidence needed to say that primary care has a place in critical care units. Through discussion of the concerns that each unit had, the nurse-managers at the seminar shared their mutual satisfaction in an initial evaluation of how primary nursing was working. Although they could not claim complete transition to primary nursing in such a short period of time, they had set the groundwork.

Critical care nurse-managers ask where to begin. Start by setting long- and short-term goals for the unit. To do this, however, strong leadership, positive motivation, and continual evaluation must be provided. After analyzing the environment of the unit's dynamics, the nurse-manager will be able to use the nursing process to design planned change. The flexibility with which primary nursing can be adapted will allow the nurse-managers the freedom needed to implement the change.

Improved Relationships Through Primary Nursing

Environmental assessment is an aspect of primary care that is frequently forgotten. To nurses working in the critical care unit, the environment may provide an overabundance of stimulations. As a result, critical care nurses may be unable to systematically set priorities. This is found in statements such as "what am I doing this for, no one listens to me anyway?" Nurses in a critical care unit can become increasingly alone although they are surrounded by other people. Critical care nurses and other members of the health team must be cognizant of each other's verbal clues. During the course of patient assignments, primary nurses must be aware of the interdependency between nurses and others in an intensive care unit. Energy should be focused on these throughout the day. Primary nursing can focus on verbal communications with patients, the peers, physicians, and families. As problems in personal relationships are removed, the frustration level of primary nurses decreases. The nurse-manager must strive for positive outcomes that can be directed toward improving unit dynamics.

Nurse-Patient Relationship

Patients in a critical care area lose the freedom of choice and come in contact with a variety of other forces, such as, nurses, doctors, technicians, therapists, and machinery. Because of the nature of their illnesses, another person, the nurse, assumes responsibility for their well-being and has, possibly, the greatest influence over them. The role of primary nurses as patient advocates is crucial for dependent patients. The nurse-patient relationship is established when patients are admitted to the unit. Upon entering the room, the primary nurse connects the patient to the monitor, starts an intravenous line, and places the bedrails up before leaving. In essence, patients lose control over their environment, as well as the supportive assistance of the family and familiar surroundings. This causes patients to experience psychological immobility. Critical care nurses can move the patients toward psychological mobility by providing an environment in which patients feel secure because a primary nurse is representing them. Primary nurses can influence the environment by minimizing noises, explaining procedures and unit protocols, and providing family and supportive contact. By using the nursing process, primary nurses formulate care plans that decide the direction of care.

Primary nurses are responsible for identifying the negative coping mechanisms that patients use and helping them to adapt in a more useful manner. There are many reasons why patients are unable to cope. The postsurgery patient is afraid to cough for fear of opening the wound. The patient receiving peritoneal dialysis fluid into the stomach does not want to move because the fluid might become displaced. Primary nurses must notice these behaviors and formalize a care plan to be acted upon over a 24-hour period. Empathy is the element that enables primary nurses to move toward an open relationship between nurse and patient and to achieve personalized care.

Nurse-Nurse Relationship

In adopting primary nursing, critical care nurses are faced with heightened expectations regarding their professional function. To achieve this professionalism, peer support is crucial. Because critical care nurses pride themselves on their ability to make independent decisions, competition among staff is developed, which forces each nurse to maintain knowledge and skill levels. It can create, however, a distance between staff members. Nurses develop with past experience, and gain individual repertoires of nursing approaches. Often these individual approaches alienate one nurse from another. This is detrimental to the growth of the primary nurse. The nurse-manager must provide unit conferences where the staff can openly discuss and share their ideas. This not only decreases competitiveness within the unit, but promotes group cohesion. Since critical care nurses face many situations that are emotionally and physically draining, peer support is necessary to reduce the stress. Rotating shifts, terminally ill patients, and difficult physicians can wear down the nurses' confidence. Discussion among nurses offers a chance to share these feelings of frustration.

Before primary nursing is initiated, the nurse-manager should evaluate the interrelationships of the nurses. Critical care nurses derive support from other staff members in the unit, on one hand, while assimilating the anxieties of patients, families, and physicians on the other. These nurses more than any others need to emphasize what expectations they have from primary nursing. It is the immediate goal of nurses to save the lives of critically ill patients; however, if they take the patients as primary, this may not be possible. The truth is that many patients will die despite the efforts of the health team. This is extremely dissatisfying and discouraging. Nonetheless, death must be accepted as the last stage of a patient's life, not as a failure. All that can be done to keep patients alive is done.

This points out the value of assigning associate primary nurses. Not only does this decrease the stress on primary nurses, but it also increases the consultation process. Implementation and evaluation of a care plan can be a mutual effort between the primary and the associate nurses. Under the unpredictable conditions of a critical care setting, nurses should be relieved of responsibilities for difficult patients if they wish. The associate can take over temporarily. Thus, both nurses have shared their skills and interest with each other and will decide the future care of that patient.

The change to the role of primary nurse has interesting implications for the attitudes of nurses toward professionalism. The entire team of nurses on each unit must be inspired by their nurse-manager to share their ideas and expertise. This is essential for maintaining mutual respect among a professional group.

Nurse-Physician Relationship

The health team implies a group of professionals working together for the purpose of improving patient care. There are times in the critical care unit that there does not appear to be smooth communication between nurses and physicians. This can be detrimental to the delivery of primary nursing and, therefore, must be evaluated. As the relationship between the nurse and the patient becomes more cohesive, the physician is less likely to be considered the principal provider of care. In this sense, primary nursing may be considered a threat to physicians. Critical care nurses try to increase nursing accountability by improving decision-making abilities and physicians may find this difficult to accept.

Since most nurses are women and most physicians are men, social structure has conditioned nurses and physicians to relate in stereotyped patterns. Traditionally, nurses have accepted their unequal status and have been reluctant to become patient advocates. If primary nursing is to survive in the critical care areas, nurses must identify the need for collaboration with physicians. Although critical care nurses are not to be portrayed as minidoctors, they are independent practitioners who are complementary to the role of the physician. Nurses are not in a critical care unit simply to carry out doctors' orders and perform housekeeping chores. The prime goal of critical care nurses is to assess and evaluate patient responses. They use nursing diagnoses and the nursing process to carry out optimal patient care. For example, the critical care nurse is the best person to diagnose disseminated intervascular coagulation (DIC) from the clinical symptoms, because nurses can pick up slight changes in the patient's responses, such as hematuria, increased clotting time after drawing blood, and hemoptysis. When these symptoms are identified the critical care nurse must then notify the physician and communicate the findings.

Despite the existence of symptoms, physicians may react with intimidation or anger to the nurse on the phone. Let us look at this problem further. In an acute care setting, patients are like children without the ability to make their own decisions. The nurse is the mother who feeds, cares for, and stays with the patient-child all day. The physician takes the role of the father as the strong, demanding provider.

There is no place for primary nursing in this structure. To attain primary nursing, nurses and physicians must be part of a team working for the benefit of critically ill patients. There is a special patient-physician-nurse relationship. Primary nurses act for the welfare of patients as advocates, not as surrogate mothers. Physicians are colleagues who realize that nurses have important input that they need. There must be trust and respect between the two professions. Games must be put aside, and doctors and nurses must listen to each other for the sake of patient care.

Listening and being heard are skills that are learned by using assertive communication principles. How does one suddenly become assertive in a critical care unit? Many nurses are victims of the team of doctors who briefly enter the unit, write orders, and then leave. Many nurses find that this produces anxiety when they have something important to discuss. Nurses then become angry and frustrated with physicians in a passively aggressive manner. Primary nurses must overcome this problem in critical care units by developing a definite plan of action. Since the responsibility of nurses is to the patient, input must be given to physicians. Peer support is not enough in this instance; assertiveness skills are also necessary. Using eye-to-eye contact and a voice that reflects confidence, physicians should be given information as mutual professionals.

The regard of physicians for primary nursing will grow as they become more familiar with this new modality of nursing care. The nurse-manager must remember that the house staff that works on the unit also needs instruction on the dynamics of primary nursing. This is not an easy job. Most members of the house staff retain the grabbing reflex, where doctors grab any nurse in the area and ask questions concerning a patient's status. When this occurs, the physician should be referred to the primary nurse. The name of the primary nurse should be placed on the patient's chart for easy reference. Many units have a blackboard which contains the names of patients, their primary doctors (usually interns or residents), and their primary nurses. The nurse-manager should anticipate the need to instruct new house staff each time the rotation schedule changes. The relationship between physicians and the nurses in the critical care unit must be maintained as a colleagueship, because collaboration as a team is for the benefit of patients.

Nurse-Family Relationship

The nuclear family is faced with the problems common to all social groups, including task performance, goal satisfaction, and pattern and organization. Like other systems it is characterized by an equilibrium tendency; a change in one part of the system is followed by a compensatory change in other parts. These principles can be related to patient/family crises in the critical care unit. The circumstances surrounding the hospitalization of one family member ultimately affect the emotional state of the others. Primary nurses in critical care units must be attuned to family theory when the care plan is designed. Families react individually to crisis situations. Serious illness causes stresses from social loss in financial status and role changes. Critical care nurses' responsibilities extend far beyond simply caring for the acutely ill patient. Supportive care for the family is also needed. Critical care nurses are informed individuals who should be easily accessible to the family. Nurses are the main providers of care in the family's eyes, because of the amount of time that the nurse spends with the patient.

Primary nurses play a vital role by helping the family to understand the treatment and care that is given to the patient. To do this they must understand the family's behavior. This provides the family with support in coping with the crisis and in relieving their anxieties. Due to the hectic schedule of critical care nurses, the family is often forgotten, and the only time the nurse, patient, and family get together is during the five-minute visits.

How can primary nurses fulfill this responsibility to the family? Begin with a proper introduction. The best way to do this is to take the family aside and state, "I am the primary nurse working with your family member. If there are any questions I will be glad to help you." The family should know the names of the nurses working with the patient during other shifts. This gives the family a sense of security in the crisis that has befallen them.

The primary nurse-family relationship begins on admission of the patient to the unit. Families can make valuable contributions to the history and physical aspects of the assessment. This is especially true when the patient is unable to speak. Nurses can find out what patients were like before the change. Patient likes and dislikes, idiosyncrasies and preferences can all be obtained from the family for inclusion in the care plan. The personality that nurses see may result from a change caused by the illness and may not represent the patient's normal personality. Only the family can give the nurse clues about this.

In regard to visiting hours, primary nurses may find that the unit rule of five minutes is too short for particular patients. Critically ill patients may need more time with their families. Critical care primary nurses must decide whether increased visiting time will help patients and their families. Although it may be helpful to patients, the sight of a loved one under tubes and bottles may be quite disturbing to the family. Nurses must be aware of this and try to prepare the family for what to expect. Unfortunately, in the daily routine not much time is available to talk to families individually. Critical care nurses must realize that primary nursing does not obligate them to solve family or financial problems. However, the family could be referred to social services, a patient omsbudsman, or the psychiatric department for consultation. This is especially helpful when the family needs the objective viewpoint of someone who is not a direct member of the health team.

THE REALITIES OF PRIMARY NURSING IN CRITICAL CARE UNITS

To prepare for the change to primary nursing, the nurse-manager must broach problem areas that make change difficult. The realities of critical care units force consideration of actions that will facilitate a smooth transition. Although other areas of the hospital have similar complaints, they are more pronounced in the critical care areas: heavy workload, insufficient time for documentation and attendance at meetings, rapid turnover of patients, emotional stress of caring for critically ill patients, and departmental floating when staffing is maximum. The nurse-manager must devise means to overcome these problems. If not properly assessed, they are serious deterrents to the functioning of primary care.

The nurse-manager can decrease these hazards by acknowledging these hazards as inherent in the critical care unit and clearly defining goals for the staff. Primary nursing is a tool that will help to decrease staff frustration and increase patient health care. The positive aspects of primary care should give the nurse-manager the incentive to continue. Staff satisfaction will increase after primary nursing has been instituted. By staging the introduction, shock that the unit might experience if it were introduced all at once is eliminated. (See Table 7-2.) Each stage must have a means for implementation in every unit. A time limit for each stage will allow the nurse-manager to evaluate progress of each.

During the evaluation, if the nurse-manager finds decreased morale or enthusiasm among the staff, a new plan of action should be made after the causes of discontent are identified through staff conferences.

Critical care nurses should be reminded that because they are trained to set priorities, they have a basic skill that is central to primary nursing. Due to the unpredictability of the patient load, nurses should be prepared for days when the unit "falls apart." When the patient load is heavy or staffing is inadequate, disequilibrium results. In these instances the nurse-manager must use a day-by-day problem-solving approach. Because patient care is the prime concern, the nurse-manager must meet patient needs with the available staff. Optimal primary nursing may have to be postponed until the unit returns to its equilibrium again. Once the unit approaches normal, the change to primary nursing can resume.

Future Expectations

Increasing changes in society and science indicate new expectations for critical care nursing. Professional practice requires knowledge, judgment, and compassion. The tools of practice are numerous and increasingly complex. Critical care nurses are independent practitioners who must work in collaboration with many

Table 7-2 Planned Change: Primary Nursing in the Intensive Care Setting

Goals	Plan
Short-term:	
Increase assessment documentation on critically ill patients by primary nurse	Complete assessment sheet within 24 hours of admission
	Review assessment skills on the critically ill
	Review interview skills
Improve master problem list on primary nursing care plan	Review concepts of nursing diagnosis as applied to critically ill
Improve primary nursing care plan on Kardex	Pertinent changes in patient status noted on primary nursing care plan as guide for associate nurse
	Collaboration between primary and associate nurses in setting short- and long-term patient goals
Improve peer support	Promote communication skills among staff
	Organize weekly staff conference
	Associate nurses assigned with a primary nurse
Improve collaboration of health team	Organize team conferences
	Reinforce primary nursing concept among health team members
Long term:	
Define primary nursing concept to nursing staff	Acknowledge need to change to primary nursing by nurse-manager and staff
	Define role of primary and associate nurses in critical care unit
	Define administrative support and expectations
	Nurse-manager should share expectations and goals according to unit values
	Set time limit for each stage (short-term goal) and evaluate outcome
	Begin selection of primary patients on day shift
	Include primary nursing consultant in planning and supervising unit goals
Encourage primary nursing to the medical team	Introduce concept of primary care to physicians in charge and assigned to units, paraprofessionals, and representatives of other departments
	Refer physicians to the primary nurse when questions are asked
	Encourage primary nurses to use physicians as planning care resources
	Encourage primary nurse-health team conferences to discuss care plan

Table 7-2 continued

Implementation	Evaluation
Admitting nurse should pick up patient as a primary	Admission interview, history, and physical completed by primary nurse within 24 hours using available resources
Use family for information on life style if patient is unable to supply it	
Provide classes on assessment and interviewing skills	
Provide classes on principles of nursing diagnosis	Master problem list adjusted to nursing problems
Ask primary nursing committee to act as consultant if unable to incorporate nursing vs medical diagnosis principles	Master problem list reflects changes in patient status
Indicate patient-centered conferences	Care plans reflect changes in patient conditions
Associate nurse continues primary nurse's care plan	Time to complete care plans
	Incorporating assessment skills and nursing process in care plans
Weekly meetings for staff and nurse-manager discussion	Decrease competition
Set unit goals evaluation by staff at meetings	Decrease frustration
Promote primary and associate nurse conferences	Increase morale
Direct physicians to primary nurse for patient questions	Increase stability of nursing care with the same nurse for physician's patient daily
Provide assertiveness training to improve communication skills	Decrease anxiety in questioning physician
Have one member from each team attend conference if possible	Decrease threat of primary nurse to physician
	Improve climate at work
	Question physician's opinion or attitude of primary nursing
Introduce research and literature defining primary nursing	Schedule discussions to review literature
Nurse-manager sets unit conferences about the adaptability of primary nursing in the critical care units	Adequate staffing patterns for primary nursing
Nurse-manager coordinates objectives and policies using the specialized unit's objectives and policies	Evaluate effectiveness of short-term goals during staff conferences
Nurse-manager offers direction to staff and learns individual capabilities and limitations	

Table 7-2 continued

Implementation	Evaluation
Nurse-manager collaborates and communicates with supervisor on progress	
Unit manager sets minimum staffing patterns	
Nurse-manager initiates selection of primary patients	
Nurse-manager initiates selection of associate nurses	
Nurse-manager supports staff during heavy patient loads	
Nurse-manager holds conferences with individuals to evaluate strengths and weaknesses	
Nurse-manager and chief of department discuss the planned change	Physicians ask for patient's primary nurse
Put primary nurse's name on chart so team knows who to ask about patient status	Physicians understand nurse's ability to plan, problem solve, and make decisions
Encourage primary nurse to use pertinent data and observations when reporting to physicians	Decrease threat of the primary nurse to primary physician in planning care
State time for weekly team conferences so house officers will be present if patients are being presented	Decrease grabbing reflex by physicians to nurse-managers when information about patient is needed
Post blackboard or chart for names of patients and their primary physician and nurse	
Nurse-manager will repeat concept to new house officers when they rotate on service	

other members of the health team. Human relationships, thus, are integral to the function of the job, which is to support patients in such a way that their dignity and well-being are maintained.

Primary nursing is consistent with the responsibilities of critical care units. To deal with such a wide range of problems, nurses must devise a continuous care plan. Primary nurses in critical care units collect data and determine immediate short-term goals for patients and their families. Within the framework of this dynamic role, nurses must be committed to critical care nursing.

The most efficient way to introduce primary nursing into acute care areas is to utilize the nursing process. This means that the nurse-manager is responsible for the evaluation of each stage of implementation. It is imperative that continual and systematic research is carried out.

Perhaps the most critical aspect of evaluating primary nursing is the effectiveness of time. By observing the organizational skills of nurses, the nurse-manager can find answers to many questions. Can nurses complete their morning duties before attending team conferences? Is overtime required for the completion of adequate written care plans? If there is a problem, the nurse-manager can discuss potential solutions with the supervisor. In some institutions, the 10-hour day provides overlap time that is used for conferences and care planning.

The decision of the nurse-manager to develop primary nursing is a challenging one. When primary nursing is implemented nurses will discover that it is a rewarding way to practice. After all, it is the function of critical care nurses to continually assess and evaluate. Thus the development of primary nursing in intensive care units is secondary only to the promotion of the nursing process. Furthermore, the resultant accountability is a primary goal of the nursing profession.

REFERENCES

Marram, G., Schlegel, M., & Bevis, E. *Primary nursing–A model for individualized care*. St. Louis: C.V. Mosby, 1974.

Roberts, S. *Behavioral concepts and the critically ill*. Englewood Cliffs, N.J.: Prentice-Hall, 1976.

Rogers, M. *An introduction to the theoretical basis of nursing*. Philadelphia: F.A. Davis, 1970.

Chapter 8

The Family's Nurse*

There are smiles everywhere on the seventh floor of Presbyterian-St. Luke's Hospital — on new mothers, proud fathers, happy grandparents, excited brothers and sisters. It is, of course, the maternity floor, where the Family-Centered Care Unit (FCCU) is located.

Several years back, as at most other hospitals, things were different. Mothers and babies were separated shortly after birth. Babies went to the nursery; mothers went to their rooms and saw their babies only at scheduled times of the day, usually only for feeding. Occasionally, they could walk down the hall to peer into the nursery, waiting until the nurse announced, "Mothers, here come your babies."

Fathers were outsiders then. Visiting privileges were limited to only a few hours a day. If the father worked an evening shift, or was unable to be at the hospital during visiting hours, he might not see his baby at all.

There were other problems. Mothers and fathers got little or no instruction on how to care for their infant at home. Different nurses cared for mothers and their babies; mothers couldn't ask their own nurses such things as how their baby was sleeping or if he was crying very much.

In 1975, a committee of maternity nurses at Presbyterian-St. Luke's got together to talk about the state of obstetrical nursing practice and needs for growth. Their recommendations were implemented by the Department of Obstetrical and Gynecological Nursing and included utilization of primary nursing, which gave mother and child the same primary nurse. Other changes included a rooming-in option that put the baby at the mother's bedside for most of the day, extended visiting hours for fathers, visiting privileges for siblings of newborns, and an active program of instruction for mothers and fathers.

---

*From *The Magazine,* Spring 1978, pp. 8-11. Copyright 1978 by Rush-Presbyterian-St. Luke's Medical Center (Chicago). Reprinted by permission.

"All these changes enable us to live up to our name—Family-Centered Care Unit," says Carol Olson, R.N., Head Nurse on the FCCU. "After all, a child is not born to the mother only, but into a family. We try to gear the hospital experience toward the family."

Giving newborns to their mothers immediately after birth and allowing them to make physical and eye contact provides maternal-infant bonding. "Since the first few days after birth are so crucial to bonding, we encourage this process by allowing babies in the mother's room for as much of the day as possible and as the mother's health permits," says Myra Ringuette, M.S.N., Acting Associate Chairman in the Department of Obstetrical and Gynecological Nursing. Increased visiting privileges and rooming-in involves fathers in the bonding process as well and brings them into closer contact with their children.

Sibling visitation privileges enhance the family-oriented nature of the unit; having a new baby effects children in a family as well as parents, and being separated from their mother can be unsettling for them.

"Letting the brothers and sisters join in the experience of the first few days reduces their fears about their mother's well-being and makes them feel a part of the family experience," says Ms. Olson. "We try to encourage this feeling by letting the little ones come and see that their mother is fine, and even look into the nursery at their new baby." A lounge area directly adjacent to the FCCU is reserved for visits by children.

Primary nursing has made these changes possible. It puts the care of the patient under the direct supervision of one nurse and eliminates fragmentation of care. Primary nursing on the FCCU is similar to primary nursing in other areas of the hospital, with a twist—the mother's primary nurse is also her baby's primary nurse. When a mother speaks to her nurse, she is now also speaking to her baby's nurse.

"This has meant a great deal to our patients," says Ms. Olson. "The one-to-one relationship between mother and nurse reinforces the family orientation of the unit. Mothers no longer feel isolated from those who are watching over the care of their child."

Nurses are now more actively involved in teaching their patients. "There is so much that the mothers and fathers want to learn," says Ms. Ringuette, "that this is one area where instruction is so important *during* hospitalization." Nurses on the FCCU provide instruction in breast-feeding, bottle-feeding, postpartum exercises, bathing the baby, birth control, and hygiene.

"We also try to educate the parents as to what to expect when they get the baby home," says Gloria Herrera, R.N., Assistant Head Nurse. "Much of what they learn from us is the result of the barrage of questions we get throughout the hospitalization, but it is also important to have some formalized instruction on child development, so that parents don't panic when the baby does something they otherwise might be unprepared for."

One of the biggest advantages to the parents is having the father participate in the instruction; nurses on the unit usually try to arrange instruction sessions when the father can be there. "Even fathers who have other children get excited about this, because sometimes they were virtually excluded when their other children were born," says Ms. Ringuette.

Teaching mothers and fathers, encouraging bonding between parent and child, and making the birth of the baby a family event—these are the goals of the Family-Centered Care Unit.

Says Ms. Olson, "We're continually working toward making the first few days after birth the wonderful family experience that it should be."

Chapter 9

The Primary Nurse in Hemodialysis: A Long-Term Relationship*

End-stage renal disease, which requires more than weekly dialysis for the patient to live, produces special needs for patients and families, primary nurses and colleagues, and the nurse-manager.

THE PATIENTS

Hemodialysis unit nurses dialyze the more acute or unstable patients during the day shift and chronic patients during the evening shift. A dialysis takes an average of five hours of intimate contact between nurse and patient. The staffing ratio is one nurse for every two patients. The average length of stay of patients is six months to two and a half years. The unit has accepted patients for chronic dialysis since May 1977, when the second shift was opened.

Patients are sent to the dialysis unit with both acute and chronic renal failure. Patients with acute renal failure have an abrupt decrease in the quantity of urine output coinciding with the rapid increase and retention of metabolic waste products in the body. Most often this is caused by an acute insult to the kidney, such as ingestion of toxins or inadequate perfusion of the kidneys. Renal failure following injection of intravenous pyelogram (IVP) dye, which can be nephrotoxic, or postoperative renal failure where hypotonicity leads to acute renal failure (ARF) are examples of this. Such patients are referred to the renal unit from the ward, intensive care units (ICUs), or other hospitals.

If patients are unstable, dialysis is initiated in the ICU. Causes of ARF associated with surgery and trauma have the highest mortality rate, about 60 to 80 percent. Those causes associated with medical complications have a mortality rate of about 30 percent with postpartum renal failure at 10 to 15 percent.

---

*This chapter is based on an interview with Jean Mortarelli-McCorry, Assistant Nurse Leader of the Hemodialysis Unit, Tufts-New England Medical Center Hospital, Boston.

The typical pathway for chronic renal failure (CRF) is:

- In-house patients with abnormal laboratory values are referred to the renal staff physician for consultation.
- Local physicians refer the patients to medical center's renal clinic.
- Depending on the cause of renal failure, the patients may eventually need dialysis.
- As the renal failure itself is controlled with dialysis, patient deaths usually result from other medical problems, such as myocardial infarction or cerebral vascular accident (CVA).

PRIMARY NURSES

The unit is staffed by nurses who have had ICU or dialysis experience. In interviewing primary nurses, the nurse-manager should ask:

- Have you ever experienced being assigned to one patient from admission to discharge?
- What kind of patients do you like and work best with?
- Describe how you have involved patients' families and assessed home situations.

The nurse-manager needs to know if prospective nurses are interested in patients beyond the tasks involved. Nurses who have worked previously in an ICU or other dialysis unit need to show evidence that they can follow the nursing process. If they can do it in an acute situation, they can do it more easily in dialysis. The nurse-manager will find that nurses who are comfortable with technical skills can more readily make emotional and professional commitments to patients. Also, primary nurses must be people who seek information by initiating questions.

Patients are assigned to primary nurses collaboratively by the staff nurse and the nurse-manager. The assignment entails a long-range commitment which includes:

- introducing patients to machines
- initiating and individualizing dialysis treatments in conjunction with the physician
- staying full time with patients until they are stable on the machine
- developing, initiating, and modifying patient teaching plans in accordance with assessed needs
- continually assessing the patients' compliance with the prescribed medical and dietary regime

THE NURSE-MANAGER

The primary nurses consult the nurse-manager for matters requiring advanced clinical expertise, scheduling, evaluations, moral support, and liaison between the unit, physicians, the hospital, and agencies, such as other dialysis units and the End Stage Renal Disease Commission.

The nurse-manager must regularly review the how's and why's of care planning and documenting with the primary nurses, because they tend to neglect updating their documentation due to the lack of dramatic change with long-term contact.

The nurse-manager also develops support systems for primary nurses by:

- Encouraging peers to discuss patients' personalities and nurses' reactions to them.
- Involving the consultant from the primary nursing committee.
- Initiating weekly psychiatric rounds so that primary nurses can present a case to a psychiatrist and psychiatric social worker. This was requested because nurses were counseling patients without a theoretical framework for the relationship between the body and mind.
- Finding support from the immediate clinical supervisor, especially in gaining perspective on the differing styles that primary nurses have with patients.

THE DECISION TO LIVE

Primary nurses in hemodialysis know that their role is crucial to sustaining the lives of patients. They are involved not only in providing adequate dialysis treatment but in humanizing the experience as much as possible.

Here is how one primary nurse individualized care through understanding the patient's personality. Mary, who was very unstable on dialysis, was a chronic dialysis patient with a long history of cardiac problems. Cardiac catheterization revealed severe and life-threatening mitral valve disease, and the patient was advised to undergo mitral valve replacement, to which she consented. After the operation was scheduled, the primary nurse noticed an increase in somatic complaints that could not be medically supported: diarrhea started just after the visiting nurse left; nausea and vomiting occurred just before the visiting nurse arrived; a nagging cough kept Mary awake at night, but was not present during her dialysis hours. The primary nurse also found that the patient, who was usually quite compliant about taking her medications, began to confuse them.

The primary nurse reported these observations to the physician, but resultant medical evaluations were all negative. The primary nurse was still not satisfied with the progress, because she felt there was a message in the patient's behavior pattern. Mary said that she was not afraid of surgery and was even looking forward to it as a way of returning her to a better state of health. The primary nurse initiated a referral to psychiatry, because cardiac surgery is so stressful that it is beneficial to talk to someone prior to surgery and contact would already be made if Mary needed help afterwards.

Through interviews with Mary and her husband, the psychiatrist helped her to verbalize her tremendous anxiety about the impending surgery and her overwhelming fear of death. The patient was greatly relieved by these sessions and her somatic complaints diminished. The primary nurse was instrumental in assessing the behavior change and in initiating steps to deal with the change. These interactions helped make Mary's preoperative period less stressful.

In another case a primary patient showed a failure to thrive on dialysis. The patient was withdrawn, had fistula pain, developed repeated shunt infections, and blood pressure was very labile on the machine. The patient had been tissue typed with her brother and sister and was found to have an identical kidney match. However, she was unable to make the decision to have a transplant. The primary nurse assessed that the patient was afraid of dying but could not verbalize this fear. The primary nurse increased contact by staying with the patient for all dialysis treatments, except on days off. The patient responded to this and confided fears about dying. Subsequently, the patient began to take better care of herself. She complied with her medication regime, stabilized her blood pressure, and began to take better care of her shunt, which reduced the problem of repeated infection.

On a troublesome note, the primary nurse also found that the patient was abusing Percocett, a pain medication. Although the nurse reported this to the physician and social worker, the patient manipulated prescriptions. Eventually, the patient had to be put on a methadone program which was less harmful than Percocett. The primary nurse felt that if other colleagues had collaborated, this could have been prevented.

In a final example, a 25-year old man, Jack, benefited from the skills of his primary nurse and nurse-manager. Jack experienced a rejection episode after his second transplant, and he was on support dialysis. He had believed that the new kidney would make him whole. On one Friday, he started acting differently than usual and by his Monday evening treatment, Jack was quite agitated, talking about guns and sexual impulses. His primary nurse was not in charge of that shift, but took the responsibility of telling Jack that he could not go home. The primary nurse immediately called a psychiatrist in to see him, but the psychiatrist said that Jack could go home.

Meanwhile, the primary nurse had left a message for the nurse-manager stating that Jack should not be dialyzed on evenings for a variety of reasons: limited availability of medical personnel and increased ratio of patients per nurse; Jack had difficulty controlling his emotions while on steroid medications and did not seem able to control his reactions to simple stresses; and possible overstimulation by the presence of some pregnant nurses (kidneys seem to hold some pregnancy symbolism—waiting, living, aborting). The decision made sense, and the nurse-manager agreed that he should be scheduled on days. The nurse-manager's validation of the primary nurse's plans was crucial at this juncture. If the nurse-manager had not respected the primary nurse's assessment, the nurse-manager would have implied that the nurse intentionally provoked Jack, that the nurse had misinterpreted Jack's behavior, or perhaps would have said only "acutes" can be dialyzed during the day shift.

It was also the primary nurse's suggestion to give him more supervision than usual during his treatments. By Wednesday he was more in control but by Friday he was psychotic, hallucinating, and defecating on the floor. He was admitted to a medical unit where it was determined that the rejection of the transplant was not reversible. Psychiatry supported that prolonged steroid therapy was dangerous and contributing to his symptoms. A nephrectomy of the transplanted kidney revealed that the kidney was septic and necrotic. The primary nurse was too upset to visit Jack immediately in the medical unit, but was able to discuss his needs with the unit's staff.

THE RESULTS OF PRIMARY NURSING

When a staff is committed to primary nursing, it is committed to analyzing and solving the difficulties that arise. Some of the problems that have been identified in this dialysis unit are discussed below.

1. Sometimes primary nurses can be too smothering and controlling. By being excessively concerned and overprotective, primary nurses can try to run patients' lives inside and outside of the unit. Primary nurses who always nag patients about diets or weight gain do not allow any latitude. They may begin to interpret noncompliance with diet or fluid regimes as a personal affront. This personal reaction may cause dialysis patients to rebel and jeopardize their health or to become very dependent on their primary nurses. It is difficult to maintain therapeutic relationships if patients put their nurses in a mother or child role.

2. Sometimes sympathy is a paralyzing emotion—when you know people so well, you can feel the needles and the injustice of end-stage renal failure. Primary nurses need to strive for empathy, not sympathy. Some of the personal intensity of a relationship can be diffused if primary nurses do a maximum of one dialysis per primary patient each week. Teaching self-care dialysis when indicated may also help nurses and patients to develop a less symbiotic way of dealing with each other.

3. Some primary nurses and renal physicians become aggravated because other nurses do not dialyze patients in exactly the same way. Arguments about the quality or the length of time of the dialysis in relation to patients' toleration of it are common. The nurse-manager should usually intervene in these discussions to bring about a resolution of the conflict. Communication between primary nurses

and peers is essential in interpreting the behavior of patients. Is the patient manipulating to cut down dialysis time or are the complaints real? The patient has been eating better, dry weight is increasing and must be reevaluated.

4. The nurse-manager should direct physicians to the primary nurse with questions regarding specific patients. In a fast-paced multipolicy unit, the nurse-manager is often the prime mover for all disciplines.

5. Primary nurses are most anxious about patients who are extremely unstable on the machine either emotionally or physically, such as postmyocardial infarction or acute emotional breakdown. Primary nurses most enjoy working with perceptive patients, regardless of the length of the relationship.

Primary nursing can be readily implemented on a dialysis unit, especially with the guidance of a skilled yet compassionate nurse-manager. Already primary nursing has changed this dialysis unit, because primary nurses feel more prestige when patients and families identify them as "my nurse." Some patients express pride and gratitude in having a primary nurse. Primary nurses are better able to determine teaching needs by the assessment and evaluation of patients' behavior. They are more aggressive in pursuing independent study and researching unfamiliar medical problems. They feel personally responsible for communicating patients' idiosyncrasies to the floor nurses, should the patient require in-hospital admission. And the primary nurses are able to apply both their technical and interpersonal skills in long-term relationships with patients and families.

SUGGESTED READINGS

Jones, K. Study documents effect of primary nursing on renal transplant patients. *Hospitals, J.A.H.A.,* December 16, 1975, *49,* 85-89.

Dixon, S. The Evanston story: Primary nursing comes alive. *Nursing Administration Quarterly,* Winter 1977, *1*(2), 37-38.

Chapter 10

Psychiatric-Mental Health Primary Nursing

The components of the primary nursing process (Figure 4-2) are the same in psychiatric-mental health nursing as in any other clinical area. The differences that do arise as psychiatric nursing staffs implement primary nursing lie in the control and selection of interventions at the disposal of primary nurses.

In psychiatric nursing the selection of approaches is influenced by factors such as:

- personal beliefs about mental illness and health
- agency attitudes about what constitutes treatment, including medications, supportive counseling, crisis intervention, therapeutic alliance, catharsis of intense emotion, abreaction, and family involvement
- physical aspects of the agency, such as proximity to the patient's home, degree of freedom allowed the patient, and surrounding grounds
- ability of the nurse-manager to provide case supervision that integrates a sound formulation (premorbid personality, precipitants inducing present condition and symptomatology, description of alteration in defense mechanisms) with a nursing treatment plan

Each agency is so individual that this section does not attempt to say how primary nursing in psychiatry should be performed but addresses the typical issues that have been identified through consultation.

WHAT IS THE UNIVERSAL INGREDIENT?

The universal ingredient of nursing in psychiatry is the use of the self, "which implies an in-depth understanding of that tool and the theories which govern it in order to use it meaningfully in a therapeutic relationship" (Rutledge, 1974, p. 82). Although the concept of professional closeness (see Chapter 2) applies to all areas of nursing, in psychiatric-mental health nursing it takes on expanded meaning. In fact, the relationship with patients is the only vehicle by which nurses can make a difference in their conditions. Even a task like giving a medication or requiring a patient to get out of bed is an interpersonal process.

The difference in the use of self in primary nursing is the intensity of transference and countertransference reactions between nurses and patients. With the permanent pairing of primary nurses with patients, the relationship which is supposed to help the patients get well is a reliable but always changing part of their clinical course. The changes occur as primary nurses and patients are exposed to each other over a period of time during which they try to exert influence over each other. For example, a primary nurse beginning with a suicidal woman may interact in this way:

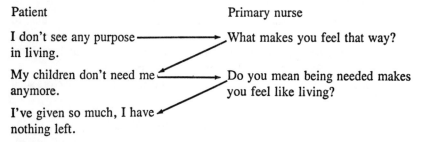

Patient	Primary nurse
I don't see any purpose in living.	What makes you feel that way?
My children don't need me anymore.	Do you mean being needed makes you feel like living?
I've given so much, I have nothing left.	

Once the patient learns that the nurse is not going to agree that death is the best option and once the nurse identifies that the patient cannot label emotions, which subsequently are enacted in a passive fashion, a new chapter in the relationship emerges:

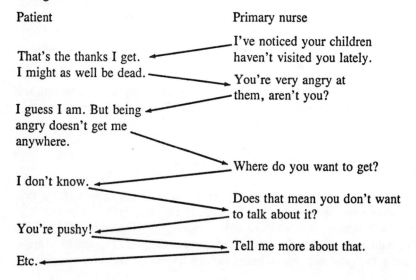

Patient	Primary nurse
	I've noticed your children haven't visited you lately.
That's the thanks I get. I might as well be dead.	You're very angry at them, aren't you?
I guess I am. But being angry doesn't get me anywhere.	
	Where do you want to get?
I don't know.	
	Does that mean you don't want to talk about it?
You're pushy!	
	Tell me more about that.
Etc.	

Eventually, the patient learns that the perceived pushiness of the primary nurse makes her label and actively become involved in the consequences of her own feelings. The primary nurse also confronts the patient about the ways in which she makes it difficult for her children to visit or show their love. The primary nurse is able to help the woman acknowledge that her approach to solving problems is not useful and to help her adopt a more gratifying and mature solution.

The effectiveness of psychiatric nurses is increased by primary nursing because the consistency of assignment really allows the nurse to use the nurse-patient relationship toward healthier resolution of problems. Many other providers interact with patients, but each relationship has different characteristics, transferences, and opportunities for alternatives to the life crises of patients.

IS THE PRIMARY NURSE A SURROGATE MOTHER?

There are many kinds of mothers: mothers of growth, mothers of abuse, mothers of separation, biological mothers, and father-mothers, to name a few. Which of these, if any, is the primary nurse? Psychiatric primary nurses have the role of an ego-integrator, because they help primary patients of any diagnostic category to gain control and esteem in nonfunctioning areas of their lives. There is an endless list of the types of interventions that primary nurses can use to help patients restore their abilities. Ego-integrator interventions include:

- assisting reality testing
- encouraging activities of daily living
- expecting behavior which is not harmful to the patient or others
- expecting participation in life plans
- encouraging and teaching socialization skills
- identifying emotional changes in interpersonal situations
- helping patients learn about the connection between their emotions and their bodies
- helping patients adopt healthier defense mechanisms, such as humor, anticipation, and sublimation
- gaining some objectivity or distance from intense emotions
- teaching patients how to turn passivity and/or aggression into assertive behavior in order to meet their own needs

The role of psychiatric primary nurses is similar to that of a process consultant. The focus "is on the client's ability, learning to identify problems and to share in and be actively involved in formulating solutions or remedies. The objective is promotion of the client's ability, knowledge, interest, and experience in diagnosing and solving his own problems" (Sedgwick, 1973, p. 773). In effect, psychiatric primary nurses are mothers of education. The classroom is the clinical setting and the texts are the patients' experiences. The homework is what primary nurses have, overtly or not, encouraged patients to think about or try to do.

Primary nurses should be far more than sounding boards for feelings—there is so much more to offer patients! By engaging in active relationships with primary nurses, patients learn how to own their feelings and their actions. Patients initially take a more constructive interest in their welfare because their primary nurses reinforce that behavior. Ultimately, with repeated successes patients grow in control and self-esteem.

> It is not enough to understand [patients] nor is it enough to talk to the patient in his own language. Doing only that may even keep him anchored in his pathological state. What we need to learn—and this skill does not come overnight—is to develop hunches as to how his messages that come directly from the unconscious are related to his life. An understanding of these messages may help us to reach the eventual goal, which again is to help the patient to evaluate and restructure his life in such a way that a balance can be achieved between his unconscious forces and his consciousness (Ujhely, 1969, p. 324).

The question of the surrogate mother also involves underlying concerns of staff who work in psychiatry, the greatest being that of dependency. If a specific role behavior is expected of a nurse, what becomes the nature of the relationship between that nurse and the primary patient? Will identifying one nurse on a staff as a patient's primary nurse change the nature and intensity of the patient's expectations?

As with the other issues, the answers largely depend on the agency's view of its role to patients. Agencies that tend to provide custodial care may define the primary nurse-patient relationship differently than an agency that provides short-term hospitalization or crisis intervention. In both cases, patients are dependent on the nursing staff for certain essentials, such as provision of safety and meeting of basic physiological needs, if patients are not able to meet their own.

The concern about dependency, however, centers around the provision of the social needs of love and belonging. It is in this realm that psychiatric primary nurses often feel the most valuable and comfortable, because nurses encourage patients to feel more accepted, to grow in ability to trust, or to socialize beyond the emotional level they were in when they entered the agency. Indeed, it is dysfunction in this social realm that causes many people to become unlikable enough to themselves and to others that they end up in mental health facilities as patients.

When patients for whom loss of love and a sense of belonging are the major problems have primary nurses, they make demands on a single nurse that they previously spread around the whole staff. Although the focused, one-to-one dynamic is initially quite uncomfortable for primary nurses, there are several advantages to knowing a patient on this level which facilitate:

- identification of needs previously distributed to the nursing staff
- opportunity to understand these needs and their subtle variations and the process by which the patient enacts or demonstrates them
- opportunity to work out some of the needs by stimulating patients to find alternate ways to meet them through control, gratification, friends, and work
- integration of data from many sources, including therapist, milieu behavior, and mental health workers, that aids understanding of the patients' view of their place in the world
- recommendations for appropriate aftercare, therapy, and support systems

Thus, primary nurses have several ways to be useful to patients within the nurse-patient relationship. The more of the categories in the list above that nurses can do, the more chances there are that the patient will be responded to in a mature, respectful way that does not induce further regression to the dependency which the nurse fears. Thus, the consistency of the primary nurse-patient relationship can provide a way to deal with dependency, rather than being an opportunity for the patient to let go of all personal motivation and responsibility.

WHERE DOES PRIMARY NURSING WORK BEST?

Primary nursing works best in agencies that have an effective nursing management system that espouses the attainment of the optimum use of the therapeutic self through the primary nursing system of care. Thus, it does not matter if the agency is a state or private hospital, as long as the components of the primary nursing process can be initiated.

An important aspect of the psychiatric setting which is conducive to primary nursing is the opportunity for primary nurses to provide continuity of care on the various levels of need for a specific patient. Some examples of the advantages of interventions at several levels follow:

1. The patient who somaticizes needs a primary nurse to see the pain, to believe how painful the psychological component of the physical pain is, and to respond appropriately. Eventually, a primary nurse may be able to help such patients discuss the mental pain without becoming incapacitated in a bodily location.

2. A primary nurse is very useful to an acutely psychotic patient if the nurse appreciates the defensive constellation of psychosis (such as denial, distortion, and projection) and adjusts approaches as needed. For instance, decreasing stimulation and giving medication may help the patient to recompensate quickly. Over

time, the primary nurse may be able to help the patient recognize what precipitates the acute episodes and prevent them.

3. The patient who is terrified of discharge may be helped to make the transition if accompanied home several times by the primary nurse before discharge.

4. The patient who is on long-term antipsychotics is helped by the primary nurse who suggests drug holidays, periods of no medication, to the physician to decrease the likelihood of tardive dyskensia (Shader, 1975).

5. Primary nurses who can conduct mental status exams (see Bates, 1972) are a great help to a treatment team in determining the more subtle changes in the condition of patients. The ability to perform and interpret a mental status exam can be one of the primary nurse's most valuable skills.

Primary nursing works well in either acute or chronic care settings, because the primary nursing process remains the same. What differs is the level of interventions, which also differs with each patient within the same setting. If primary nurses can assess the level of patient ego integration and respond accordingly, primary nursing can be adapted to any setting.

HOW SHOULD STAFFING BE ARRANGED?

This question requires a great deal of attention from agencies in order to prevent primary nursing that exists in name only. In fact, a mental health agency should only attempt primary nursing if it has enough nurses and support systems to enable primary nurses to make and follow through on their commitments: "Hello, I'm your primary nurse, and I will be responsible for the outcomes of the nursing care you receive while here. I will work with the staff on your behalf (and I will use my experience with you to evaluate the consequences of primary nursing)."

The number of nurses necessary for primary nursing depends on the level of care required by the patients, and the types of programs which the patients attend. For example, a primary nurse can carry more clients in a day hospital where both nurse and patient are present during the same hours with more chances for contact than an inpatient primary nurse who must rotate to shifts. A primary nurse on a hectic unit for disturbed children may have fewer primary patients at one time than a primary nurse on an adult unit with the same census, because the needs of the patient population require different functions and involvement from the nurse, depending on the developmental levels of the patients.

When assessing staff requirements, avoid setting up unrealistic expectations for recruitment or the primary nursing program. Asking two psychogeriatric unit nurses, who have defined their roles as passing medications and doing treatments, to divide up the patients and call themselves primary nurses is doomed to failure. Staffing should not be rearranged until the administration has agreed that primary nursing is a long-range goal involving far more than a new title (see Chapter 14).

WHAT IS THE NURSE-MANAGER'S ROLE?

The nurse-manager of a psychiatric primary nursing staff has the same challenges and rewards found in other primary nursing units. However, there are some pitfalls of which the psychiatric nurse-manager must be keenly aware. These include primary nurses who:

- compete with each other for the most meaningful relationships with their patients
- become excessively involved in their patients' troubles
- value talk and mental activity to the near exclusion of physical needs
- are unable to set firm but caring limits on patients' behaviors
- interpret each other rather than being direct about interpersonal staff relationships
- value what they conceive as therapy more than providing safety; "he'd be humiliated to have someone ask him if he's suicidal"
- avoid supervision, not wanting to disclose their work with patients for fear of exposing their own imperfections
- expect patients to lead lives that nurses approve of, requiring compliance and imitation rather than genuine growth

The nurse-manager can help the staff avoid or resolve these problems through frequent staff groupings in seminars, meetings, and case presentations. Frequent meetings increase group cohesiveness and respect for individual styles.

It is very important that the staff group has a unified understanding and approach to patients because in many ways the milieu is the treatment. Because primary nursing involves more individual work and interaction with all patients, there is a greater need to share data and assessments of primary patients with the staff group. A cohesive nursing staff decreases staff splits which are so common, especially in the hospital treatment of borderline patients: "The staff members, when they are the recipients of projected parts of patients, tend to act like those projected parts . . . an internal drama within the patient can become a battleground among the staff" (Adler, 1973, p. 33). Staff splits can create a destructive milieu.

The nurse-manager must have the attitude that building staff cohesion and knowledge will benefit patients because splits will be minimized. In addition, important patient information will not be forgotten, and nurses will be able to have their own needs for love and belonging met by the staff rather than by the patients. Development of these attitudes should be the goal of the nurse-manager.

WHAT ABOUT OTHER PROVIDERS?

The trend toward primary nursing puts the role of other mental health providers into serious debate. Because other providers are less expensive for the institution and because the value of psychiatric nurses has not been precisely defined, nurses have gradually lost ground while the mental health movement has expanded. Consequently, nurses are seen as part of the hierarchical, task-oriented medical model. Nurses are given—and accept—the least creative roles in psychiatry: medications, first aid, provision of credentialing legitimacy for institutions. They take a back seat to enthusiastic and often intimidating paraprofessionals. Nurses have no answer to the common belief that a nurse is a glorified mental health worker who gives medications.

An important consideration in the problem of professionals versus paraprofessionals is that often paraprofessionals are males who have had more formal education than female nurses. This combination intimidates those nurses, who are already insecure in their roles and cannot find reassurance from their own clinical and administrative leaders.

In response to their own frustrations and the demands of patient care needs, nurses have allowed paraprofessionals to reap the rewards, such as one-to-one relationships with patients, leading groups, and going to conferences. Consequently, paraprofessionals tend to be a very demanding, entitled group, which is accentuated by their low paying, deadend position. They often leave for further education, although they rarely go into nursing.

Primary nursing turns the mental health system upside down, no matter how wisely and gradually it is implemented. As mental health workers and others leave, some of their vacant positions could be filled by nurses in order to increase the ratio of nurses to patients.

There is usually a need for some nonprofessional staff, but the scope of nursing practice should be determined before delegating responsibilities. Nurses have an important place in providing direct care to patients, and that position should be maintained.

WHERE DO PRIMARY NURSES FIT?

Interdisciplinary is probably the most commonly used word around psychiatric services, although it usually stands for an ideal rather than a reality. Interdisciplinary teamwork is very rewarding, but extremely difficult to attain. Once it is reached, the components of a professional milieu are in place and the work of everyone is needed to maintain it.

Primary nurses contribute to every aspect of a professional milieu, by virtue of their clinical overview of the total person, especially strengths. Psychiatric nurses tend to value restoring, caring, and curing equally, which is useful because curing in psychiatry is a vague goal at best. Psychiatric nurses also emphasize the practical aspects of a treatment team's approach and because of this often find themselves in the position of patient advocate.

Primary nurses potentially fit into the hub of the patient's hospitalization, although their skill and personality greatly influence the use that they make of this key position. In some ways, the roles of each discipline are equal. Because self can be used therapeutically by anyone having contact with a patient, much of the clinical territory is shared. There is great potential for skills to be equalized, and because everyone in mental health is constantly interpreting everyone else, gender and character style rather than strict professional discipline lines are drawn. However, personalities are equal only in that all have their strengths and weaknesses. Because of this strangely egalitarian situation, mature and skilled primary nurses stand just as much chance as members of other disciplines to contribute to the welfare of patients.

Another factor that has a bearing on primary nursing is the decrease of inpatient hospitalization time, largely due to legislation and limits on third-party reimbursement. With these changes, patients cannot afford to stay in an institution forever, even when it would be the best treatment. Thus, hospitals have to gear their financial resources and personnel to rapid assessments, client and family involvement in objectives for hospitalization, efficient treatment modalities, and thoughtful dispositions and referrals. The days of tennis courts and swimming pools in private mental hospitals are limited for all but the very wealthy, as are the days of lifetime institutional care for the underprivileged. Thus, comprehensive nursing care for acutely ill patients becomes the focus of primary nursing.

Through basic nursing education primary nurses also have the best of what other disciplines have learned over the years. Nursing has gained professional expertise by its generalistic, nonspecific background and its integration of theory and techniques developed in other disciplines. Thus, a primary nurse is in a unique position to offer the team skills at integrating:

- growth and development
- epidemiology and community health
- family dynamics in health and illness
- crisis theory
- learning theory and patient education
- mind-body continuum
- pathophysiology
- pharmacology
- theories of Maslow, Erikson, Freud, and other psychological scientists

In addition, nurses have a high tolerance for dependency and regression which, when knowledgeably exercised (i.e. when dependency and regression do not serve to meet the nurses' needs), is very useful in the treatment of primitive hysterics, borderlines, and schizophrenics.

By combining physical and psychological theory with a tolerance for patients who require the collective skills of an interdisciplinary team, the primary nurse is very much the hub of treatment. More specific techniques used for collaborating with an interdisciplinary treatment team include:

- having frequent meetings to share and compare historical and clinical data
- helping the team define realistic goals for new patients
- being prepared with a written assessment of the patients' current status, including a mental status exam, the chart with results of psychological testing or a medical consultation, patients' poetry, etc.
- being cognizant of patients' current problems in conjunction with their total life situation
- helping the team talk with, not at, each other
- being sure that meetings do not end until there is a tentative plan or agreement to disagree
- not leaving a meeting feeling that you should have said something
- not letting people interpret your motives or counter-transferences—save that for your supervisor
- seeking information, thus promoting consciousness, about what the patient perceives is going on (for example, "Does Danny know we're having this meeting?" or "What does Mr. N say about his therapy?")
- having team meetings with the patient and family
- using terms properly, aiming at a meaning that the whole team understands (for example, "suicidal ideation", "firm limits", "manipulative")
- using factual descriptions of patients' statements or behavior when in doubt of the proper term or when trying to make a strong point

Far too often, even in teaching hospitals, primary nurses find that they learn more from other disciplines than they do from their own. Although this might be termed interdisciplinary, it is deceptive because primary nurses can lose identity with their own profession. Primary nurses need one foot strongly in nursing so they have a base on which to expand their knowledge and skills. However, primary nurses may have the opportunity to do things that are not typically within nursing practice, such as casework with a family or group work with a certain population. These new areas can enrich the staff and will certainly give them an appreciation of other people's work.

Anything that augments skill or creativity increases the effectiveness of nurses with primary patients. For instance, knowledge about art therapy or vocational counseling expands the intervention repertoire. Primary nurses may not have chosen art therapy as a career, but they may be able to use some aspects to form a relationship with borderline or schizoid patients. Similarly, primary nurses can learn to identify that certain types of drawings indicate organicity. In this way, the drawings function like a clinical sign which can be used to revise opinions and approaches to patients.

In general, primary nurses can make more clinical use of an expanded therapeutic repertoire than someone from any of the other disciplines. Nursing's traditional roots in the medical model insure that nurses will be used at least minimally for inpatient staffing. When choices are made about what kind of professional staffing to use, it should be kept in mind that a creative nurse offers more versatility than persons whose disciplines afford them little access to or rigid role behaviors with patients.

HOW DO PSYCHOTHERAPISTS DIFFER?

Primary nurses do not try to be mini-psychotherapists, which would entail the promotion of transference and the patient's reenactment and working through of a transference neurosis. Of course, nurses who are trained as psychotherapists can and should do this type of work with appropriate patients. Rather than promoting transference, which is a psychic regression to infantile patterns, primary nurses strive to decrease transference reactions. The primary nurse's goal is to help patients strengthen their egos by acquiring the skills to cope with external realities.

Both approaches have their own value and are not mutually exclusive. Primary nurses often help patients to adjust their immediate reactions to external facts. Likewise, creative psychotherapists listen with careful attention to the realities of a patient's experiences. These psychiatric approaches can and should overlap.

The differences between psychotherapists and primary nurses lie in the focus and tasks related to their work rather than in the goals. Just as a repaired motor will not move a car with a flat tire, a resolved narcissistic injury will not help a person who has no place to live after discharge. The more fragile the ego, the more attention is needed at all levels.

People enter psychiatric hospitals because they lack, have rejected, or are at an impasse in their psychotherapy. They need nursing care, or they would be outpatients. When the hospital supplies nursing care in the form of primary nursing, the chance is increased for individualized care based on the empathic formulation of a patient's life experience, because primary nurses can assess and intervene at the immediate level of need when the need is real.

Primary nurses participate in experiences with patients because they are part of patients' everyday lives. This provides an opportunity to help because the immediate response of patients to milieu or ward occurrences that arouse internal conflict can be understood and occasionally modified with the primary nurse's assistance.

Primary nursing does not replace or detract from psychotherapy. On the contrary, the work of patients with skilled primary nurses and nursing colleagues accelerates psychotherapy because it provides ego-integrator activities.

WHO HAS POWER ON A TREATMENT TEAM?

Power in psychiatric settings is always an ingredient in primary nursing care. According to *Webster's New International Dictionary,* third edition, *power* "refers to the ability of a person, group or system to use their concerted strategies, energy, or strength to influence the behavior or action of others." Each member of a treatment team has specific formal roles: for instance, physicians sign commitment papers, nurses observe the patient in the milieu, and social workers speak to the family about financial coverage for long-term planning. Likewise, each person on the team has an informal role that is either delegated to them or taken outside of the strict line of authority. Primary nurses are no more or less powerful on a team than anyone else, but they may feel more confused or pressured if anxieties about patient care situations are not answered.

Patients in psychiatric settings are unconsciously giving up power over their own lives, whether with hysterical seizures, psychotic thoughts and bizarre actions, or extreme passivity. Ironically, patients are constantly using nonconstructive means to gain control and power over their surroundings, including over their treatment team. Patients with anorexia nervosa, catatonia, and passive-dependent personalities are just a few examples of this phenomenon.

Thus, a treatment team can best assist patients toward healthier goals by encouraging the patients, rather than the team, to feel and cope with their conflicts. Otherwise, the treatment team becomes anxious while the patients remain comfortably protected from living through their own lives. The team that finds itself fighting over the proper referral for a patient would do well to expect the patient and family to participate in planning meetings.

The nurse-manager can help the nursing staff to be less confused and pressured about teamwork by helping primary nurses to predict areas of team stagnation and to prepare for team meetings. The nurse-manager can also teach and emphasize techniques of cognitive dissonance relief. These are techniques that primary nurses can use to alleviate the frustration and guilt that arise when everyone on the team is trying to do their best but no solution is adequate.

Cognitive dissonance is relieved with creative but reasonable solutions that get the treatment team off the hook. This can be achieved by clarifying the predicament at hand as well as by discussing the team's desired outcomes. Sometimes it helps to review all possible pathways to the outcome, even the most unrealistic. It also helps to review the past behavior of patients in regard to problems. Chances are that the problem is not a new pattern for the patient and family. However, the team has the advantages of objectivity, predictive ability, and collective problem solving. Often primary nurses have a great deal of data and suggestions to offer the team as a result of clinical observations and contacts with a patient, as well as experiences with similar patients.

The person who has ultimate power on a treatment team is the one who can (1) encourage the team members to clarify the stress they are feeling, (2) understand its connection to the patient's psychodynamics, and (3) develop a plan which is reasonable and facilitates giving control to the patient in manageable doses. The primary nurse can certainly contribute to, if not conduct, discussions which lead to conflict resolution.

WHAT IS THE FUTURE OF PRIMARY NURSING IN PSYCHIATRY?

Primary nursing in psychiatric settings must be clearly defined in relation to other professional and paraprofessional disciplines. Primary nurses must maintain their role in medication administration and evaluation, while asserting expertise in the areas of:

- the mind-body continuum
- work with families and groups
- mental health system planning
- home visits
- activity therapy
- crisis intervention
- discharge planning

Primary nurses should continually expand their intervention repertoires and strive to make their intervention delivery efficient yet appropriate to the patients' levels of functioning.

Primary nurses are particularly valuable in short-term hospitals and aftercare clinics. Aftercare is an excellent area for psychiatric nurses, because it offers the opportunity for extension of their primary nursing skills into primary care.

Likewise, primary nurses who have experience in helping patients to integrate the way their bodies respond to emotional conflicts are the perfect professionals to deal with patients who somaticize in order to gain the caring protection of a stronger person. Nurses can easily learn to evaluate the physical complaints of patients and to address the concern that underlies the complaint. The role of primary nursing is also invaluable for nurses who want to become psychotherapists. The experiences of making professional commitments, being professionally close to patients, and presenting one's work to a supervisor are good practice for future career development.

Primary nurses can use their individual and group therapeutic skills to offer leadership and consultation to medical-surgical nursing staffs, geriatric facilities, and other agencies. Most importantly, psychiatric primary nurses need to use their knowledge of behavior to build their professional image. Many psychiatric principles used with patients can be applied equally to staffs and organizations.

REFERENCES

Adler, G. Hospital treatment of borderline patients. *American Journal of Psychiatry*, January 1973, *130*(1),

Bates, B. Mental status. In *A Guide to Physical Examination*. Philadelphia: J.B. Lippincott, 1972.

Rutledge, K. The professional nurse as primary therapist: Background, perspective, and opinion. *Journal of Operational Psychiatry*, Spring-Summer 1974, 76-83.

Sedgwick, R. The role of the process consultant. *Nursing Outlook*, December 1973, *21*(12), 773-775.

Shader, R. (Ed.). *Manual of Psychiatric Therapeutics*. Boston: Little, Brown, 1975.

Ujhely, G. Nursing intervention with the acutely ill psychiatric patient. *Nursing Forum*, 1969, *8*(3), 311-325.

Chapter 11

Discharge Planning by Primary Nurses

by Patricia A. Miodonka

Because the interaction between primary nurses and primary patients is close and continual, primary nurses have more responsibility for planning discharge. With a given framework, clear communication, and resources to draw upon, primary nurses can be effective in coordinating this task.

THE PATIENTS

Mrs. K was a middle-aged, widowed female hospitalized with symptoms of shortness of breath secondary to advancing chronic obstructive lung disease. Due to several episodes of increased anxiety and decompensating respiratory status, she had short stays in the intensive care unit, and then returned to the floor. Most of her belongings sat by her side in bed, and her widely opened eyes looked testingly at everyone who entered her room. When anxious, she became tachycardic, increasingly short of breath, and yelled to have her oxygen increased. She continually asked, "Am I going to die? . . . You're not telling me the truth." She had been an active, healthy accountant until her lung disease was diagnosed two years before. She lived alone in a small apartment and was fearful that her sister and brother-in-law would gain all of her possessions. They were her only family. She was not compliant with the program of care instituted by her visiting nurses.

Mr. R. was an intelligent, adolescent male admitted for his first treatment of acute leukemia. According to him, he was hospitalized for treatment to correct his blood. A pale child of small stature, he spent most of his day in bed sleeping, building models, painting, and refusing most of the food he was offered. He continually asked direct and explicit questions such as "exactly what does this treatment do to my blood?" and "how many days will this IV stay in?" His parents were divorced, and he lived with his mother, sister, grandmother, and grandaunt. The grandmother and grandqunt took turn spending two or three-day intervals with the patient. At times they were difficult to deal with because they would question nursing judgment and nursing plans. Mr. R's mother worked full-time and visited daily. However, she had difficulty accepting that her son had leukemia and seeing the grandmother and grandaunt in the active mothering roles.

Mrs. C was an elderly widowed female hospitalized with complaints of back and hip pain. Her medical history included sarcoma, diabetes mellitus with foot ulcers, hypertension, degenerative joint disease, and depression. Initially she was very verbal and explicit about how she wanted her care performed. Despite her back pain, she could ambulate with a walker for short distances and use a commode. Her pain was thought to be advanced joint disease. She was fitted for a corset and had pain medication available. She became less talkative, refused food, refused to get out of bed to ambulate or to participate in physical therapy. She needed close guarding when walking with the walker and when wearing her corset. Her daughter, who was most involved in her care and saw her daily, began to question whether Mrs. C could be managed at home. Mrs. C lived alone in the same apartment building as her daughter. A visiting nurse saw Mrs. C twice weekly. She evaluated Mrs. C's ulcer care and monitored the effects of the chemotherapy for sarcoma. A volunteer from the Golden Agers visited her several times a week.

How would you as a primary nurse begin planning for discharge? And when?

How could members of the health team be of assistance?

How could you coordinate their efforts for an effective discharge?

PRIMARY NURSES

In hospital settings where primary nursing is fully implemented, primary nurses should be responsible for coordinating discharge planning. Discharge planning is a continuous process necessary for helping patients meet their health care needs as they move from the hospital into the community. Assessment of the continuing health care needs of patients should be made early in hospitalization (Johnson, 1976). Implementation of plans to fulfill patient needs should be carried out by a coordinated, communicating health team (Phillips cited in Bristow, 1976). In hospital settings discharge planning has been coordinated by health team members, including social workers, designated discharge planning coordinators (Isler, 1975), public health nurses (Lamontagne & McKeehan, 1975), and staff nurses (Moreland & Schmidt, 1974).

EVALUATION OF DISCHARGE PLANNING

As a staff primary nurse in a 24-bed, medical unit in a teaching hospital, I was involved in many patient discharges. When discharge planning was continuous and coordinated, patients left us informed and confident with community follow-up already arranged. When discharge planning was coordinated the day of discharge, patients usually seemed confused and the staff frustrated. During my experience primary nursing replaced team nursing, and I began to feel responsible for my patients' discharge planning. My continual, close contact with patients made my plans work, and I began to communicate effectively with appropriate health team members and to use them as resources for solving problems.

Because I felt that my experiences had implications for other primary nurses and their patients, I decided to evaluate the discharge planning done by primary nurses in the unit. With the support of staff nurses and the nursing administration, I formulated the goal to implement better discharge planning. To meet this goal involved the completion of several behaviorally defined objectives.

1. I examined the problem-oriented charts of primary patients for evidence of discharge plans. I looked for evidence of explicit discharge planning, documentation of teaching with or without patient teaching plans (Zander et al., 1978), and documentation of discharge problems on the patient master problem list.

2. I examined nursing care plans for evidence of discharge plans. There was a category for "plans for discharge" and a more specific discharge planning sheet added to the formal care plan. I also looked for lists of short- and long-term expected outcomes used in the nursing care plan. Mayers (1972) states that this measurable patient behavior should be used as criteria for patient discharge or health maintenance.

3. I asked primary nurses what they thought about the process of discharge planning. Questions included, "define discharge planning" and "when do you begin planning for discharge?"

4. I met individually with representatives of the hospital departments that I identified as the resources for discharge planning. I asked for their suggestions about what information they had to offer primary nurses. Representatives included physicians, social workers, community services, continuing care, dietary, pharmacy, unit coordination, visiting nurse liaison, and clinics.

The documentation of 24 patients was examined and 12 primary nurses were interviewed about discharge planning over a two-month period. The evaluation of charts revealed that 8 percent had teaching documented, none had documentation of discharge planning, and 20 percent used the patient master problem list for discharge problems. In the nursing care plans 50 percent had notations in the plans for discharge category, 38 percent used the specific discharge planning sheets, and 58 percent had expected outcomes listed.

The meetings with primary nurses revealed several predominant attitudes. Most first think of discharge planning when patients are admitted. They felt it should be considered when completing the assessment and listed it as a problem in the care plan. They felt that the specific discharge planning sheet should be used as part of the care plan. They also felt that they were consistently doing patient teaching but not always providing documentation. Some suggested that physicians should take part in the weekly patient rounds attended by primary nurses, social workers, the continuing care coordinator, and the dietitian. As a result, all health team members would know of a patient's total needs and programs. Most felt that patient needs must be individualized when planning discharge and that the family should be used more.

The departmental representatives who were interviewed provided useful information for coordinating patient discharge. For example, the continuing care section provided help in how to evaluate patient and family for return to home and outlined types of nursing home facilities, patient needs for each, and type of payment. The visiting nurse section explained its liaison with the hospital, its coordinated care programs, points to consider when completing a referral, and insurance coverage for different home health care services.

RECOMMENDATIONS FOR IMPROVEMENT

1. *Charting:* Thoroughly assess the patient's home situation or alternative care facilities during the admission assessment to provide information when plans for posthospital care are made. Document all teaching with appropriate plans from the teaching plan book or the general discharge teaching plan (Zander et al., 1978). Specific discharge instructions should be written for the patient as deemed necessary by the primary nurse. Steagall (1977) advocates written discharge plans that are sent home with the patient. Patients felt more secure going home with written instructions, and some used them as a source of reference for subsequent care.

2. *Nursing Care Plans:* The discharge planning checklist was revised and included on the nursing care plan. A quick glance shows the status of the patient's discharge. The upper section provides information that needs to be known several days before discharge or for nurses who cover a primary nurse's patient. It is important to know where patients are going, how they will get there, and what equipment will be needed. This allows others besides the primary nurse to know what has been done and what needs to be done. The lower half of the section indicates which health team members are involved in discharge planning needs and how involved they are. Using this form, primary nurses can document up-to-date discharge plans in charts at any point during hospitalization. Cucuzzo (1976) supports the problem-oriented form of charting which her hospital initiated to improve discharge planning documentation. She used the *method* form in which each letter defines specific discharge criteria and the charting indicates how certain criteria were met. Use of expected outcomes stated in measurable patient behavior in care plans should be continued. Having fulfilled short-term goals, patients move closer to discharge; having fulfilled long-term goals, patients are ready for discharge.

3. *Resources within the Hospital:* As a result of requests that physicians attend weekly patient rounds, several physicians became part of these meetings. Based on the information obtained from departmental representatives, a discharge planning resource booklet was compiled which lists each department, its representative, and information important for the primary nurse coordinating discharge. If the information the nurse seeks is not in the booklet, the appropriate representative can be contacted. The format of the booklet complements the discharge planning sheet with the idea that used together, they would be more effective than used separately. The booklet is located at the nursing station along with other resource materials. Based upon the recommendations, primary nurses in the unit began using resources in their discharge planning. New staff nurses are oriented to all of the resources available for making discharge plans.

USING DISCHARGE PLANNING

Given the framework recommended for improved discharge planning, the following cases show how primary nurses coordinated the discharge of three patients.

For Mrs. K, the primary nurse established a close working relationship with the physician and social worker early in hospitalization. The three met daily to discuss her medical, nursing, emotional, and social status, and to plan for consistent and complete care. As Mrs. K's respiratory status improved, her primary nurse assessed her home situation. The social worker provided more information, and the visiting nurse liaison informed the team of her home care status. In the nursing care plan, the discharge planning checklist was kept up-to-date (see Exhibit 11-1), and expected outcomes were stated in the care plan. An example of a short-term goal: Patient will walk from bed to door without oxygen. An example of a long-term goal: Patient will identify medications by name and purpose of taking medication. Charting was based upon the patient's behavior and clinical status. As Mrs. K's status stabilized further, the continuing care coordinator was notified to assess posthospital care. The coordinator suggested that the patient be transferred to an interim facility before returning home. Mrs. K vacillated between wanting to return home and feeling she needed more time and support to recuperate. Staff members were aware of Mrs.K's feelings. The discharge planning checklist was kept up-to-date, and Mrs. K's case was presented at weekly patient care rounds. After being evaluated by a rehabilitation facility, she was accepted. Because there was a lapse of time between notification of her acceptance and the actual transfer, her primary nurse was able to complete all teaching and coordinate all plans. Suitable medication dosages and regimes were finalized, and Mrs. K understood her inhalation therapy regime. The dietitian, who had been working with Mrs. K on eating a nutritious, high calorie diet, evaluated her knowledge. When notifica-

Exhibit 11-1 Discharge Planning Checklist: Mrs. K

Patient___Mrs. K_____Primary Nurse __Pat M.___

Expected Date of Discharge: 5/20

Where to:__Mass. Rehab. Institute_____

Travel:__ambulance_____

Family Participation:
           none-sister and brother-in-law
           have minimal contact with pt.

Equipment:
           None

Nursing/Medical Follow-up
     By Whom:__Dr. B._____
     Where:__NEMCH_____

Intrahospital Resources	Date Contacted	Comments
Physicians	5/1	-conference daily with both due to
Social Service		increas. pt. anxiet. which worsens med. status
"Community Serv." of NEMCH	X	-? medicaid applic.
Continuing Care	5/10	-working on placemnt needs interim care
Dietary	X	before home -sees pt. daily for
Pharmacy		compli. of hi-cal diet
Unit Coordination		
VNA of Boston	X	pt's former PHN provided info on
Clinic		pt noncompli. in home care rx
Other:		

*Specific Discharge Teaching Plans in chart include:

tion of her transfer came, Mrs. K's primary nurse consulted the unit coordination section of the resource booklet and arranged for ambulance service. Mrs. K's former visiting nurse was informed of the transfer, and a patient care referral was completed by physician, primary nurse, dietitian, and social worker. Suggestions for writing referrals in the visiting nurse liaison section of the resource booklet were helpful.

Discharge planning for Mr. R began soon after admission (see Exhibit 11-2). Contact was made with the member of the physician team primarily responsible for the patient's care. The primary nurse explained her role and requested that ample information be communicated to her frequently. She needed to know what the physician had told the family and patient in order to care for the patient effectively. The primary nurse also discussed with the physician what should be taught to the patient about his disease and its treatment. The teaching plan for the home care of the leukemia patient was used as a guide in teaching Mr. R (Zander et al., 1978). To help in teaching, the primary nurse consulted the clinic section of the resource booklet. There the hematology clinic nurse urged primary nurses to start teaching early and to document it, because it would be valuable to the clinic nurses who would follow the patient in the hematology clinic after discharge. As a result, all teaching done with Mr. R was explicitly charted.

During weekly patient rounds members of the health team updated others on their involvement with Mr. R. At this time the discharge planning checklist was also updated. The dietitian noted efforts to have Mr. R eat high calorie foods. The social worker noted the results of meetings with Mr. R's mother. The primary nurse commented on some teaching problems. The parent was not there consistently, and the grandmother and grandaunt, who seemed to fulfill the mothering role. questioned nursing intervention. After meeting with health team members about the matter, it was decided to direct all instruction and information to patient and mother. Therefore, about one week before discharge, the primary nurse reviewed with patient and mother precautions the patient should take, symptoms for which he should consult his physician, and medications. On the day of discharge he was given these instructions in writing. As he went home in a taxi with his grandaunt, the primary nurse phoned his mother to review instructions and answer any questions.

When initially assessing Mrs. C's home situation for potential discharge planning, it appeared that discharge would be a smooth transition back to the home. She had appropriate equipment and community and family support. However, when she became less talkative, less active, and refused many things, her daughter and her primary nurse talked about the possibility of placement in an extended care facility. The continuing care coordinator evaluated Mrs. C and supported returning her home. These events were discussed in patient care rounds and noted in her progress notes; the discharge planning checklist was used as a guide to arrange for a complete discharge plan (Exhibit 11-3). Expected outcomes were revised in the

Exhibit 11-2 Discharge Planning Checklist: Mr. R

Patient _____Mr. R_____ Primary Nurse ___Sue B.___

Expected Date of Discharge: 4/3

Where to: _____home_____

Travel: _____taxi with family_____

Family Participation:

        will be at home with mother, sister,
        grandmother, grandaunt

Equipment:

        may need supplies for maintenance
        chemotherapy at home at a later date

Nursing/Medical Follow-up

    By Whom: ____hematology clinic next week_____

    Where: ____NEMCH_____

Intrahospital Resources	Date Contacted	Comments
Physicians	X	-working closely with HO re: pt. teaching
Social Service	X	-mother being seen q week by Ms. R
"Community Serv." of NEMCH		
Continuing Care		
Dietary	X	-helping pt in choice of hi-cal, hi-protein foods
Pharmacy	4/2	-pt. given written instruc. re: meds
Unit Coordination		
VNA		
Clinic	4/1	-clinic nurse to visit pt. before dc
Other:		

*Specific Discharge Teaching Plans in chart include:

    home care for leukemia pt. — pt. given handwritten sheet with instructions

Exhibit 11-3 Discharge Planning Checklist: Mrs. C

Patient   Mrs. C   Primary Nurse Mary J.
Expected Date of Discharge: 5/5
Where to: home
Travel: ambulance
Family Participation:
                 daughter lives in adjoining apartment
Equipment:
                 commode
                 hospital bed
                 dsg supplies — 2x2 gauze pads, normal saline
Nursing/Medical Follow-up
    By Whom: VNA by 5/7   medical clinic in 2 weeks
    Where: at home   NEMCH

Intrahospital Resources	Date	Contacted Comments
Physicians	4/20	-ongoing contact with HO re:pt's progress
Social Service	X	-presented in rounds not currently seen
"Community Serv." of NEMCH		-? if pt. may need to apply for medicaid
Continuing Care	4/20	-after being seen for poss. ECF placement,
Dietary		support curr. given for return home
Pharmacy		
Unit Coordination	5/1	-arranging for commode, bed, dsg supplies
VNA of Boston	5/4	referral sent, will see for dsgs, PT
Clinic		
Other:		

*Specific Discharge Teaching Plans in chart include:

care plan. They were stated: Patient will ambulate with corset to door, patient will sit in chair for one-half hour. Through unit coordination, equipment and supplies were arranged. Mrs. C's visiting nurse was contacted regarding the findings of her hospital stay and her new needs. Nursing and dietary referrals were sent.

CONCLUSIONS

Primary nurses need to develop a continuous system for improving discharge planning which should include:

1. Documentation of detailed discharge plans in charts monitored by retrospective audits.
2. Pertinent and complete discharge planning checklists preprinted in nursing care plans monitored by concurrent audits.
3. Reference material in the unit which includes intrahospital resources and representatives helpful for discharge planning and information provided by intrahospital resources which is pertinent to discharge planning.
4. The responsibility of primary nurses to be familiar with intrahospital resource material and to utilize it when necessary.
5. Emphasis by the nurse-manager on making discharge planning a priority.

REFERENCES

Bristow, O., Stickney, C., & Thompson, S. *Discharge planning for continuity of care.* New York: National League of Nursing, 1976.

Cucuzzo, R.A. Method discharge planning. *Supervisor Nurse,* January 1976, 7:43-45.

Isler, C. Helping hospital patients out. *RN,* November 1975, 38:43-44+.

Johnson, J.A.R. Discharge planning. *Texas Nursing,* November 1976, 50:9-10.

Lamontagne, M.E., & McKeehan, K.M. Profile of a continuing care program emphasizing discharge planning . . . Continuing care program of the Boston Hospital for Women. *Journal of Nursing Administration,* October 1975, 5:23-33.

Mayers, M.G. *Systematic approach to the nursing care plan.* New York: Appleton-Century-Crofts, 1972.

Moreland, H., & Schmidt, V. Making referrals is everybody's business. *American Journal of Nursing,* January 1974, 74:96-97.

Steagall, B. How to prepare your patient for discharge. *Nursing '77.* November 1977, 7:14-16.

Zander, K., Bower, K., Foster, S., Towson, L., Wermuth, M., & Woldum, K. *Practical manual for patient teaching.* St. Louis: C.V. Mosby, 1978.

Chapter 12

Primary Care: The Extension of Primary Nursing

by Joan Gluck

The nurse-manager in specialized clinical areas has the task of refining the general role of primary nursing. Although the definition of primary nursing remains constant, the way in which nursing is operationalized is adapted to the setting and type of institution. An emerging role for nurses is the delivery of primary health care in an ambulatory setting, such as a health maintenance organization (HMO). On comparison, the primary nursing role differs little from the primary care nursing role. Primary care is the logical extension of primary nursing, and primary nursing is a vital part of primary care.

Nurse practitioners and clinicians in primary care nursing are involved in the assessment and management of a wide range of acute and chronic illnesses in collaboration with a physician or other health professional and as defined in a set of written guidelines. Activities include the assessment and treatment of acute illness, the management of patients with stable chronic illness, health screening, patient and health education, quality assurance, and research activities. This nursing role brings an added dimension to the commitment and accountability inherent in primary nursing and adds many unique problems. It is the responsibility of the nurse-manager to understand the problems of nurses in the clinical area in order to channel their energies most productively for the benefit of the health care team and the consumer.

Institutions specializing in primary health care are becoming more prevalent as the cost of health care rises and as consumer access to care becomes more difficult. The HMO offers an alternative to traditional health insurance coverage by combining health insurance and health care delivery in a comprehensive package that is based on cost containment and quality care. The HMO concept is not new, but stems from prepaid group practices which have been in business since the late 1940s. In 1973 Congress passed the Health Maintenance Organization Act to define how such organizations should be organized and operated to be eligible for federal funding and, thus, to promote the development of comprehensive, prepaid

281

health care (Haendel, Sinclair, & D'Erasmo, 1978, p. 25). According to the 1973 law, a prepaid group practice becomes federally qualified as an HMO by meeting several strict organizational requirements. Once qualified as an HMO, the group practice may implement its own system of health care delivery. Many HMOs were developed to serve as models for the provision of quality comprehensive health care at an affordable price through the creative use of all members of the health care team. Professional roles can be creatively defined to maximize the capabilities of all members of the health care team in the delivery of comprehensive health services. Services include 24-hour emergency care, primary care, health screening for early detection and treatment of illness, preventive health care, specialty services, and inpatient care. Because they have a defined membership and are committed to intervention on an ambulatory basis, many HMOs are based on a model of primary health care. Within this model physicians and nurses may collaborate in the delivery of primary care services, intervening when their specific expertise is required. The client population is defined and limited, the clinical practice is shared, and the patients identify a physician-nurse team as their health care provider.

PRIMARY NURSING AND PRIMARY CARE

Primary nursing and primary care may be contrasted in terms of definition, identified provider as care-giver, and setting in which that care is delivered. The requirements established by the Department of Health, Education and Welfare for the Nurse Practitioner Program Grant define primary care in terms of broad-based health care delivery:

"Primary Health Care" means care which may be initiated by the client or provider in a variety of settings and which consists of a broad range of personal health care services including: (1) promotion and maintenance of health, (2) prevention of illness and disability, (3) basic care during acute and chronic phases of illness, (4) guidance and counseling of individuals and families, and (5) referral to other health care providers and community resources when appropriate. In providing such services (1) the physical, emotional, social, and economic status, as well as the cultural and environmental background of individuals, families, and communities (where applicable) are considered; (2) the client is provided access to the health care system; and (3) a single provider or team of providers, along with the client, is responsible for the continuing coordination and management of all aspects of basic health services needed for individual and family care (*Federal Register*, 1977, pp. 60880-60884).

According to this definition, primary care differs from primary nursing in operational terms, not in philosophy. A primary care provider may be a physician, a nurse, or both, but a primary nurse is always a nurse. A primary care provider may have initial contact with the patient when the patient is well, during an acute illness, or during a stable or unstable phase of a chronic illness. A primary nurse in an inpatient setting always has the intial interaction with the patient during the crisis of an illness. The primary care nurse may have the chance to get to know the patient and collect data during a noncrisis period when the patient is coping normally, a luxury that the primary nurse does not have.

The nurse-patient relationship in primary care is nondependent, because patients are free to remain or leave according to how well their needs are met. Patients actually select and directly pay the primary care provider which allows for freedom of choice and the ability to change their minds if the relationship does not work. Thus, primary care nurses must understand and address immediate and long-term patient needs in the context of the patient's normal culture and environment because the patient is in control.

The primary nurse-patient relationship, on the other hand, is a dependent one, because patients have little or no control over staying or leaving. Patients do not select and directly pay their ordinary nurse and they do not have the freedom to choose another if they are unhappy. Because primary nurses deal with crisis situations, they can only guess at the patient's normal culture and environment, and therefore end up meeting the patient needs according to the artificial hospital environment. Patients must meet the nurse on the nurse's ground and, consequently, give up control.

Although the role of the primary nurse and primary care nurse often differ operationally, conceptually the roles differ very little. The care delivered is patient centered and nurses are responsible and accountable for their actions regardless of the institutional setting in which they function.

ORGANIZATION OF NURSING

In an HMO that functions according to a primary care model where physicians and nurse practitioners collaborate in teams for the care of patients, coordination of the health care delivery system is crucial. Depending on its structure, the HMO can enhance or undermine the collaborative nature of the physician-nurse relationship. Professional roles are defined according to practice rather than function, and as such they can vary from team to team and often overlap. Role definition and problem solving take place on many different levels, depending on the nature of the problem. Each physician-nurse team is expected to practice autonomously within the system. Each team is considered an independent practice which is responsible for the delivery of care to a specific group of patients. A certain number of practices form a unit, which is the physical area where patients are seen; a group of units forms a specialty or primary care area, such as internal medicine or pediatrics; and all of these areas together form the health care delivery system.

Nursing management in all of these levels must support the autonomy of each collaborative practice, while clearly defining and maintaining the lines of organizational authority. Some decisions clearly must be made at a top management level, others at the middle management level, others at the unit level, but some decisions can only be made by the physician-nurse team. Nurses are asked to be autonomous and independent in some situations and dependent on the organization in others. Is it any wonder that there is confusion about who is responsible for solving which problems and when?

The nurse-manager serves as unit manager, administrative problem solver, and planner, as well as professional role model and parent during physician-nurse disputes. Although nursing practice is defined organizationally according to legal guidelines, the nature of each individual team is governed by the collaborative relationship of the physician and nurse. They must work out their roles within the team, such as who handles telephone calls and who gives injections, develop trust, identify strengths and weaknesses, and come to a mutual agreement about how patients will be cared for. According to Kahn et al. (1964) this process takes at least one year to complete, is affected by variables inside and outside the organization, and is often fraught with anger and disagreement. It would be much easier for the nurse-manager to intervene in physician-nurse disputes by solving problems and making decisions for them. However, this would prevent the formation of a strong collaborative relationship and would also foster dependence on the organization. Instead the nurse-manager's energy should be spent in coaching the staff on how to solve disputes among themselves and in serving as mediator as needed.

The nurse-manager is in a key position to serve as a role model for professional clinical practice as well as problem solving, thereby adding credibility to the primary care model. The nurse-manager must be an excellent clinician as well as an assertive manager, and the system's organizational structure should reflect the value of the team approach to problem solving. The nurse-manager carries a part-time clinical practice which functions as a model for other collaborative practices. Supervision and policy making on a unit level are carried out in collaboration with a physician chief and both report to the same person (see Figure 12-1). In this model, splitting nursing and medicine into discrete groups with separate lines of authority would only emphasize the differences between nurses and physicians, create barriers, and undermine the collaborative nature of the health care delivery system.

Figure 12-1 Management Structure of the Health Care Delivery System in an HMO

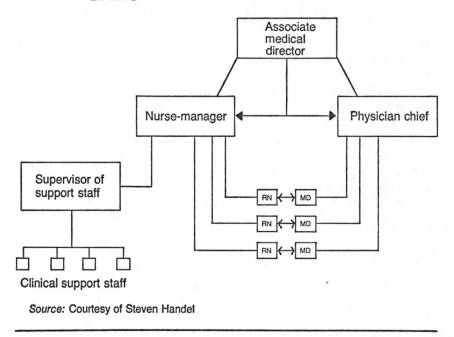

Source: Courtesy of Steven Handel

PROVIDER-PATIENT RELATIONSHIP

The collaborative practice model of primary care not only requires the commitment of the nurse and physician to the practice, but also the commitment of the team to the patients and vice versa. The length of stay with a provider team depends on how well patients feel that their needs are met and how accepted they feel. Although practices are shared, patients fall into four categories: (1) nurse patients; (2) physician patients; (3) shared patients; and (4) complex patients.

Nurse patients are those who have predominantly nursing needs that rarely require physician intervention. They may have social or environmental needs, involved teaching needs, or acute, episodic illnesses that require life style modification. They may also have chronic illness that requires regular follow-up and chronic care management through community resources which are best coordinated by the nurse. Nurses make a commitment to these patients through the nurse-patient relationship and mutual fulfillment of needs. If patients feel that their needs are being met, they are more likely to continue the relationship and to comply with the treatment and management regimen. This gives the nurse positive gratification, the relationship is maintained and commitment is enriched.

For example, acute episodic venereal disease is evaluated and treated mainly by nurse practitioners with physician intervention only for complications, such as penicillin-resistant gonorrhea or medication allergy. Patients require strict follow-up and may need concurrent psychosocial intervention. Furthermore, patients with repeated infections or difficulty complying with medical instructions require good teaching and close follow-up so that they are not lost in the system. These patients will continue this relationship with the nurse practitioner as long as they feel that their medical needs are being met.

Physician patients have diagnoses or recurrent symptomatology that go beyond the expertise of nurses. These are patients who, the nurse and physician agree, require physician intervention almost exclusively. The nurse interacts around specific questions or acute problems, but does not have major responsibility for patient management. Although the nurse's involvement with these patients is minimal, the nurse is still identified as the patient's primary care nurse. For instance, a patient with chronic renal failure is likely to be monitored solely by the physician for most medical care. However, the patient may interact with the nurse in the physician's absence or for a nonmedical reason such as family planning.

Shared patients require the expertise of both team members. They may have involved medical histories and concurrent social, family, or environmental problems complicating their management. The nurse and physician may alternate visits with the patient, or they may see the patient together, and contribute equally to care. The plan of care is often arrived at mutually, and the commitment to the patient is shared.

This shared commitment is frequently found in the prenatal care of obstetrical patients. The physician and nurse determine a plan of care and the patient alternates visits with each provider. The physician usually handles the physical exam, assessment for labor and delivery, and monitors physical signs, while the nurse does nutritional counseling, teaching, assessment of the family situation, and psychosocial intervention when necessary.

Problem patients pose a unique dilemma that is aggravated rather than minimized by the physician-nurse team approach. These patients have complex medical, social, and psychological needs that are so intertwined, it is necessary to address all areas in order to influence one. Problem patients have so many needs that they tend to take up an inordinate amount of provider time with little problem resolution. In this no-win situation providers must give more and more but get less and less, until they give up from guilt and frustration. Providers are reluctant to make commitments to problem patients, because they rarely get any rewards from the relationship. The collaborative practice model makes it possible to avoid commitment by passing the problem patient back and forth. Although this prevents the physician and nurse from becoming overwhelmed and burned out, the lack of commitment may increase the patient's problems because it does not provide a stable provider-patient relationship within which limits can be set. Furthermore, the patient lacks a stable patient advocate to intervene with social and community agencies.

An example of this type of patient is the nudnik or hypochondriac who appears several times a week with a grocery list of symptoms. Although the symptoms may be real and very important to the patient, the physician and nurse become easily exasperated, because the lists never seem to end and the complaints are often trivial. These patients are often passed back and forth, and at times they are even referred out of the practice to a specialist or another primary care team. Occasionally, they are referred to the mental health department after the patience of the primary care team has been exhausted. In one such case it was found that several of the patient's friends had died within the past two years and that the patient's fears and loneliness had been translated into insignificant physical symptoms. After the patient dealt with the grief, the symptoms disappeared.

Sometimes the nurse-patient relationship becomes so important that nurses are extremely possessive and have difficulty letting go of a patient. While some possessiveness is necessary, too much is destructive. When nurses derive basic satisfactions from patient rather than peer relationships, professional objectivity is lost. Deriving satisfaction for needs such as status, nurturing, respect, and personal reward from patients makes the stakes too high, because when patients do not comply with the management regimen or miss an appointment, it is a personal failure for the nurse. It also becomes impossible to relinquish the patient to another provider or institution, even when it is necessary to do so. Although this example may seem extreme, possessiveness and loss of objectivity occur to varying degrees in many nurse-patient relationships. It is the responsibility of the nurse-manager to help nurses meet these basic professional and personal needs outside of the nurse-patient relationship, thereby protecting the professional integrity of the relationship.

GUARANTEEING GOOD PRIMARY NURSING

The nurse-manager is in a position to guarantee good primary care nursing by influencing the organization in four ways: (1) selection of nurses; (2) development of the knowledge and attitudes of nurses; (3) organization's response to the needs of nurses; and (4) setting standards for care.

Selection of Nurses

Through the hiring process, the nurse-manager influences which nurses enter the system by seeking qualities in nursing candidates that will enhance the collaborative nursing role. These qualities include excellent clinical skills, independence in clinical decision making, ability to collaborate, commitment, problem-solving skills, and ability to function as part of a team. Most of these can be identified by a skilled interviewer and from verbal and written references. Consistent experience, preferably in a collaborative role with other health professionals but definitely in a role requiring independent decision making, is vital in order to ensure teamwork, problem solving, and responsibility to patients and the organization. Nurses who change jobs every six months without good reason have some obvious difficulty making a commitment and are probably not viable candidates. This can be assessed easily in the interview and initial screening process.

Some qualities, however, should not be assessed by the nurse-manager alone, but must include the collaborating physician and the unit. While the nurse-manager reserves the final hiring decision, the opinions of those who will work closely with the nurse must have some influence. Final candidates should spend at least one day in the clinical unit, preferably seeing patients, before the final decision to hire is made. This allows the nurse-manager to evaluate clinical competence more clearly, and it gives the unit staff and the candidate a chance to decide if they can work together.

The importance of the hiring process in guaranteeing good primary care nursing cannot be overemphasized. The nurse-manager must assure that nurses entering the organization meet the standards of clinical competence for the practice and share the values upon which the nursing structure is based.

Knowledge and Attitude Development

The nurse-manager influences the knowledge and attitudes of nurses through orientation and continuing education programs that will support the positive aspects of the nursing role. Orientation programs include administrative information unique to the HMO, introduction to patient support systems such as the computerized medical record (Gluck, 1979), and precepted clinical practice. Precepting should be conducted by the collaborating physician during the orientation and probationary periods. However, the nurse-manager must be available to serve as nurse preceptor and role model.

Once the orientation and probationary periods are over, a program of continuing education is necessary to address the instructional needs of nurses in all areas of practice. The program should be flexible enough to encourage nurses to grow and should enrich perception of the nursing role and professional identity. In an organization that breaks with tradition by emphasizing professional collaboration, the professional identity of physicians and nurses can become obscured, and reinforcement is imperative.

A weekly continuing education program provides the chance to meet as a group to discuss issues common to nursing and the collaborative role. The most common educational issues dealt with include clinical skills involving the assessment, management, and indications for consultations and specialty referral of specific problems, physician-nurse-patient relationships, and protocol writing for nursing diagnoses. Professional identity is addressed through discussion of state and federal political issues, the political process, and national nursing organizations. Continuing education programs that are well planned, organized, and approved by the state nursing organization also meet at least a portion of the continuing education requirements for relicensure in many states.

Not all educational needs can or should be met through in-house continuing education programs. Going outside of the organization provides an opportunity for new and creative views of common problems and prevents the development of too narrow a perspective on patient care. The nurse-manager should provide information about available programs, professional conventions, and seminars and should encourage the staff to take advantage of outside educational opportunities in order to share information with colleagues.

Organization's Response

The nurse-manager can influence the organization to meet the needs of nurses for status, respect, and recognition. The organization through the nurse-manager recognizes and rewards nurses in a variety of ways, including public recognition of special achievements, merit reviews, monetary rewards, professional activities such as continuing education, and inclusion of nurses in policy decisions directly affecting them. As long as the goals of nursing do not conflict with the goals of the organization, this process functions smoothly and the nurse-manager need not intervene. However, when the goals of nursing do conflict with the goals of the organization, such as in a growth period when resources may be tied up, nursing priorities are at risk. A nurse-manager who has already established a relationship of authority and respect may be able to influence the organization to maintain nursing priorities even when others take precedence.

Whatever influence the nurse-manager has results from strong management skills, not exclusively from the position in the organization. In order to have a voice in organizational policy, nursing must have something to say, be able to say it clearly and constructively, and be prepared to make compromises. A nurse-manager who does not have strong management skills and a clearly established position in the organization will be lost in the shuffle of conflicting priorities. Status and respect must be earned and then used to show the organization the value of nurses at all levels. The nurse-manager must be willing to compromise lesser issues in order to ensure recognition of more important ones. For example, the nurse-manager in an HMO which is phasing in the primary care nurse practitioner role may want a certain number of hours of physician time each week to precept nurses. Because precepting is costly in terms of physician time and decreases the physician's patient load during preceptive sessions, the nurse-manager must be willing to compromise less important issues to win this one. This is a negotiation process at the management level.

The nurse-manager must not only be a strong manager within the nursing department, but must also be willing to invest energy as a member of the organizational management team. Nurse-managers who have established themselves often become involved in management decisions which do not directly affect nursing, but in which their opinion is valued. Nurse-managers who are willing to offer their management expertise outside of their departments will find that the organization is more responsive to nursing needs as they arise.

Setting Standards

Finally, the nurse-manager guarantees good primary care nursing by setting standards of excellence for patient care which are monitored through merit evaluations, auditing nursing documentation, and quality assurance. These standards may be set by the organization through productivity standards for cost effectiveness, by the physician-nurse group through quality assurance programs and nurse practitioner guidelines, or by the nurse-manager through merit evaluations. Nurse practitioners in the Harvard Community Health Plan (Note 1) are evaluated according to the following standards:

1. Physical assessment and patient management skills
2. Ability to collaborate
3. Quality of work, including establishing and evaluating clinical outcome criteria and continuity of care
4. Skill at problem-solving in patient care, practice management, and colleague relationships
5. Productivity
6. Responsibility and accountability
7. Professional growth and development
8. Professional commitment

The evaluation process provides for variability in achieving these standards by assessing performance as outstanding, average, minimally acceptable, or unacceptable. Unlike systems that only provide for acceptable or unacceptable responses, this variability allows nurses to grow professionally in order to achieve a higher merit rating and gives the nurse-manager some flexibility in assessing performance.

COLLABORATION IN AN HMO

The *American Heritage Dictionary* defines collaboration as working together, "especially in a joint intellectual effort" and as cooperating "treasonably, as with an enemy occupying one's country." When discussing nurse-physician collaboration, there is often innuendo of the second definition among physicians and nurses alike. Health care professionals on many levels in many settings still consider professional collaboration as a means of coercing nurses to do a physician's work or as a usurpation of a physician's territory. It is noteworthy that after physicians and nurses have worked in a collaborative practice, many find it difficult to return to separate roles and, consequently, find positions that allow them to practice collaboratively.

Primary care nurses in an HMO collaborate with a variety of health care professionals for a variety of reasons, depending on the patients' needs. Nurses and physicians practicing in primary care collaborate for help and direction in patient care, for legal reasons, because a patient's problem is not a nursing diagnosis, and for continuity. Primary care nurses also collaborate with nurses in other specialties such as, the primary nurse in a hospital to which a patient has been admitted, physicians in other specialties, as well as other health professionals, such as psychologists, social workers, and nutritionists.

For the collaborative process to be productive physicians and nurses must be clear about what they are asking each other in a consultation and what they expect as the outcome. There is always the risk that if expectations are not fulfilled, the result will be conflict between the nurse and physician that may also involve the patient. For example, a primary care nurse may spend a great deal of energy reviewing and studying the management of angina pectoris in order to manage some of the more stable patients in the practice. The next day the nurse evaluates a patient with acute substernal chest pain and starts the workup for uncomplicated angina. The nurse expects to present the patient to the physician and subsequently to be responsible for managing the patient, informing the physician about progress and changes in physical status. However, the nurse had not discussed this with the physician ahead of time and did not state the goal for the patient at the time of the consultation. Although the patient presentation was clear, concise, and complete, the physician was not specifically aware of the nurse's intent. The physician expected to see the patient to recheck certain physical findings, to discuss the possible diagnosis and medication, and to arrange for further evaluation and follow-up. The nurse expected the physician to see the patient to recheck the questionable physical findings and then to allow the nurse to take over management. As a result both providers were confused and angry, and they left the patient with a potentially serious diagnosis and no clear idea of which provider was responsible for follow-up care.

This situation could have been avoided if the nurse had stated the reason for the consultation and the expected outcomes clearly. The physician probably would have agreed to the nurse managing the patient with a system worked out for physician intervention if it became necessary. If the physician were not agreeable to this, the time to discuss it would have been before the consultation, when all the issues could be fully and leisurely discussed. It is important to set aside time with no interruptions to discuss difficult issues as well as general items pertaining to patient care. This way conflicts can be settled outside of the clinical area where patient care is not adversely affected.

Conflict of expectations can also arise from physicians' actions, again with the risk of involving the patient. A physician who was not comfortable with the accurate fitting of diaphragms or the teaching involved was asked to fit a diaphragm during a pelvic exam. Rather than rescheduling the patient or referring her directly to the primary care nurse, the physician asked the nurse to assist with the pelvic exam. The physician expected to have the nurse do the diaphragm fitting after the pelvic exam. The nurse expected to spend a short time chaperoning the exam, and then to return to another patient who had been waiting for several minutes. Because the physician did not make the expectation clear to the nurse at the time of consultation, the conflict surfaced during the exam in front of and at the expense of the patient. This situation could have been avoided if both parties had made their needs known to each other.

Primary care nurses collaborate with primary nurses when patients change settings. When patients enter the hospital, the responsibility for care shifts to the primary nurse in the inpatient setting. Upon discharge, it shifts back to the primary care nurse. In order to ensure continuity of care, it is imperative that the nurses who are responsible for the patient collaborate not only upon admission and discharge but throughout hospitalization, sharing information about such things as the patient's perception of illness, family and social relationships, patient teaching, and discharge planning.

Ms. B had been treated by the same physician-nurse team for five years. She had a long history of asthma, chronic obstructive lung disease, hypertension, and coronary artery disease complicated by being 40 pounds overweight, smoking two packs of cigarettes a day, and having numerous social and economic problems. Ms. B was very close to her physician-nurse team, and they had stabilized her asthma, chronic lung disease, and hypertension with minimal medication and regular follow-up appointments. Although she did not lose weight or quit smoking, she was able to work and take care of her home for two years without a major asthma attack. However, then her physician left and she became a member of another physician-nurse team. Ms. B missed several appointments, did not seek treatments for upper respiratory infections, and became lax about taking her medications. Her condition quickly deteriorated until she finally suffered acute respiratory distress. She was evaluated by her physician-nurse team, but when her asthma did not clear despite medication, she was admitted to the hospital.

It was clear to the physician-nurse team that the deterioration of Ms. B's condition was due in part to the loss of her original physician-nurse team and it would be difficult to stabilize her condition until she had come to terms with the end of the first team relationship and formed a new one with her new team. Through constant dialogue the primary care nurse and the primary nurse in the hospital helped Ms. B to do this. The primary nurse supported Ms. B through her sadness and helped to reinforce the relationship with the new primary care providers. The nurses collaborated in writing the patient care plan, teaching plan, and discharge plan, and the primary care nurse participated in much of the patient teaching while Ms. B was in the hospital to develop the nurse-patient relationship prior to discharge. By working together both nurses responsible for Ms. B's care were able to address not only the illness but some of the issues responsible for the illness, making it possible to stabilize the patient.

WHAT NEXT?

Nursing roles are not as conceptually distant as might be thought. Although many roles are operationally quite different, accountability and responsibility to patients and to the profession are common to all. Thus, colleagueship is the wave of the future with other health professionals as well as fellow nurses. If nurses continue to jealously guard their nursing role, any new found autonomy and accountability will fail to positively affect the future of professional nursing. Barriers must come down and professional sharing replace them, both within the profession and between nursing and other related professions. Only when collaboration replaces separatism can the positive future of nursing be realized.

REFERENCE NOTE

1. Harvard Community Health Plan. *Criteria for performance levels in merit review: Nurse in expanded role,* Department of Nursing, Boston, May 1978.

REFERENCES

Gluck, J. Computerized medical record system: The challenge for nursing. *Journal of Nursing Administration,* December 1979, *IX*(12).

Haendel, A., Sinclair, L., & D'Erasmo, M. Health maintenance organizations. *Nurse Practitioner,* November-December 1978, *3*(6), p. 25.

Department of Health, Education and Welfare, *Federal Register:* Nurse Practitioner Programs-Grants, November 29, 1977, *42*(229), 60880-60884.

Kahn, R., Wolfe, D., Quinn, R., Snoek, J., & Rosenthal, R. *Organizational stress.* New York: John Wiley & Sons, 1964.

Part IV

"I Will Use My Experience with You to Evaluate the Consequences of Primary Nursing"

Chapter 13

First Experience as a Primary Nurse

by Dolores Bournazos

Mrs. Ruth C was an 86-year-old Protestant woman admitted to the general medicine service about two weeks after primary nursing had been initiated on our floor. She had been widowed for ten years and lived alone in a large house. Prior to her admission Mrs. C had been active in community affairs, had many friends, and was quite independent. She had one married daughter, Mary, to whom she was very close. Mrs. C was brought to the hospital by Mary, who for the week before her mother's admission, had noticed a change in her mental status: forgetfulness, untidiness, urinary incontinence, left hemiparesis, nausea, vomiting, and complaints of abdominal pain. The physical exam showed an enlarged liver and ascites, and laboratory results showed electrolyte imbalance and anemia.

Mrs. C was admitted with a diagnosis of right cerebral vascular accident and also to rule out cancer. When I introduced myself to Mrs. C as her primary nurse who would be responsible for her nursing care while she was in the hospital, she seemed pleased. She informed me that she had come to the hospital reluctantly and if it were her time to go, she would rather die at home than in a hospital bed. As the primary nurse I did the initial patient assessment, began the master problem list, and initiated the care plan. I addressed myself to Mrs. C's problems of abdominal pain, nausea and vomiting, nutrition, fluid and electrolyte imbalance, and her feelings of isolation from significant others and familiar surroundings. I also included her fear of a lonely, painful death.

For her nausea and vomiting, I consulted with the physicians, who ordered Compazine one-half hour before each meal and a liquid diet with supplements recommended by the dietitian. I also found it helpful if Mary fed Mrs. C because she had a better appetite at these times. Around-the-clock pain medication was arranged for comfort, and fluids and electrolyte replacements were ordered.

As the primary nurse, I tried to spend as much time as possible listening to Mrs. C verbalize her realistic fears and offering as much support as possible to her and her daughter. The intern and I explained to Mrs. C the tests and procedures she would be going through, such as blood work every morning and abdominal and liver scans. Reluctantly Mrs. C agreed to these tests. However, in her second week in the hospital, after having a liver scan which increased the suspicion of cancer, Mrs. C announced that she would have no further treatment and that she wished to be left alone. This decision greatly upset Mary, who had difficulty accepting her mother's terminal illness.

At this time the intern and I felt it was necessary to meet with Mrs. C and Mary to redefine some goals. We spoke with Mary about the fact that her mother had cancer, but refused further tests and wished to leave the hospital. It was decided by Mrs. C and Mary to consider nursing home placement. This was difficult for the patient, who wanted to go home but was too ill and required too much physical care. I tried to spend time talking with Mrs. C and offering emotional support, allowing her to express her need to be independent and her fear about being placed in a chronic nursing care facility.

I also understood that Mary had guilt feelings about not taking her mother home. I tried to point out that since she worked full-time, had a family, and her mother was so ill, this would not be feasible. I also discouraged her from taking time off from work to visit each day. Instead I arranged to be in Mrs. C's room around 10:00 a.m. when Mary called so that I could answer her questions and reassure her. This way Mary could limit her visiting hours to the evening but could still feel secure because she could call the nursing staff at any time.

About two and a half weeks after her admission, Mrs. C became increasingly disoriented, the ascites increased, she became weaker, and apparently had reached the end stages of her terminal illness. At this time Mrs. C was very withdrawn and wanted only the company of her daughter.

At this time the psychiatric nurse consultant met with the nursing staff to help us explore our feelings of helplessness and to suggest what we could do to allow Mrs. C to die with dignity. Unfortunately, I was leaving the floor for a vacation. I explained this to Mrs. C and Mary and spoke to another nurse about assuming the care of this patient while I was gone.

Several days later I learned that Mrs. C had died a peaceful death. Later I made contact with Mary, who was able to talk about her mother's life before she died. She felt that her mother had received good care and that at least now she was not suffering any more.

Primary nursing works well for several reasons. In this instance, family, patient, and the hospital staff worked together to set goals for the patient. Because of this, Mrs. C really had some control over what her hospitalization would mean to her. Primary nursing is especially beneficial for work with dying patients and their families. For example, during her hospitalization Mrs. C withdrew from people and wanted only her daughter close by. This was one way in which she was preparing for death. Therefore, having a primary nurse who knew her well and cared for her each day worked better for Mrs. C than having to deal with many different staff members. Primary nursing also benefited Mrs. C's daughter. Mary knew that I was Mrs. C's nurse and felt that she had a person on the staff whom she could always seek out.

As a primary nurse, documentation was much easier simply because of the continuity of following the same patient day by day, and it was easier to detect changes and to follow progress. Documentation was also more meaningful to me and to others who read what I wrote. Primary nursing makes it easier to coordinate care and utilize other members of the health team. Dietary, continuing care, and clergy were all consulted and all were able to communicate directly with the primary nurse. Therefore, care was not fragmented and communication was more personalized.

Aides, nursing technicians and off-shift nurses were important in my role as a primary nurse because they kept lines of communication open. When I was not on duty, they carried out the care plan that I had formulated. This was especially true of the evening nurses: Mrs. C's daughter usually got out of work at 2:30 and would appear on the floor at 3:30, as I was leaving. I was able to spend some time speaking to her, but the evening nurses also spent time with her. This way Mary knew her mother would usually have the same two people caring for her on days and evenings. She was reassured and eventually able to feel comfortable shortening her visiting hours. Also, the evening nurse could communicate directly with me, and together we could change or revise Mrs. C's care plan.

At times Mrs. C was disoriented, and it helped her to have the same staff members care for her because they knew her routine. This was more effective than reporting to a team leader who perhaps cared for a patient only two or three times a week and who did not have the continuing, personalized contact that primary nursing provides.

The nurse-manager helped me to assert myself as a primary nurse. At the time I was taking care of Mrs. C primary nursing was just beginning on our floor. Physicians were still going to the nurse-manager instead of the primary nurse to discuss their patients' care. I think that the best thing the nurse-manager did was to listen to the physicians, take note of what they said, and then refer them to the primary nurse. In this way the nurse-manager always knew what was going on, but allowed the primary nurses to assert their independence. However, I always knew that the nurse-manager was available and willing to be a resource person to all the primary nurses.

Aides, nursing technicians, and LPNs also helped to carry out certain parts of the care plan. The nurse on days is usually assigned to four patients and covers an aide, technician, or LPN who usually also has four patients. Mrs. C required a great deal of physical care as well as emotional support. This included frequent bed changes, skin care, lifting, turning, and being fed. The ancillary staff working with me always helped me a great deal with these aspects of Mrs. C's care and also made valuable suggestions. Many of them commented that most of the nurses spent more time at the patient's bedside and less time at the desk doing paper work after primary nursing was initiated.

There have been many rewarding aspects of primary nursing as well as difficulties. Since we instituted primary nursing, care on our floor has become more personalized. For example, when I chose Mrs. C as a primary, I knew her nursing care would be mainly my responsibility from admission to discharge, or in her case until death. I knew that her hospital experience depended greatly on how well I planned, coordinated, and provided care. I was able to develop a one-to-one relationship with my patient, to spend more time with her, and to get much more satisfaction than with the more fragmented, task-oriented, team leader approach, where in many instances the patient is everyone's responsibility but no one's responsibility—something which can be frustrating to staff and patient.

With primary nursing I have more opportunity to put nursing theory and knowledge into practice, and there is more sharing of knowledge among staff members. For example, each week we have a conference where nurses take turns presenting the case of one of their primary patients. Here knowledge and suggestions are exchanged. I am also developing a more personalized plan of care for my patients and not just depending on doctors' orders. Because of the clearer definition and control of nursing care, I can better evaluate the effectiveness of my work with individual patients.

One of the most difficult things at first was accepting the responsibilities of being a primary nurse without feeling overwhelmed—to realize that I was the nurse accountable for these particular patients! It took quite some time before I felt comfortable going into a patient's room and saying "I am your primary nurse. I'll be responsible for your nursing care while you're in the hospital." That requires a commitment!

Another problem is getting physicians to recognize the role of the primary nurse. There are still physicians and medical students who go straight to the nurse-manager or charge nurse instead of seeking out the primary nurse. I have learned that to really feel like the colleague of the medical team it is necessary to stress that you are the patient's primary nurse. You must assert yourself and take the initiative in order to be recognized. It also helps to have a supportive nurse-manager who allows primary nurses to assert themselves but does not reject them when they need assistance.

I have also encountered difficulty with losing contact with my primary patient, such as on rotation to nights for a week. Usually on nights there is one nurse with two or three ancillary staff members for 25 patients. It is usually impossible to spend much time with any one patient. We are reviewing staffing patterns and priorities which will allow nurses more contact with their primary patients in such circumstances.

There is also a tendency for many nurses to want primary patients they like and not the more difficult patients. We have tried to combat this by putting up a list of patients who need primaries. Patients who are not chosen after 24 hours are assigned to a nurse by the nurse-manager.

Since the introduction of primary nursing, nurses have been able to use their knowledge and skills to a greater degree, and they have begun to develop a more personalized, comprehensive system of patient care which is more satisfying to both nurses and patients.

Managing the Transition to Primary Nursing

Primary nursing has wide appeal in that it presents a considerable challenge to nurses on every level of an organization. Indeed, primary nursing involves many rewards and frustrations.

Primary nurses and nursing leaders need to study the experiences of adept, caring primary nurses to determine guidelines and recommendations for prospective primary nursing units and agencies. Thus, what has been gleaned from the past years of operationalizing the primary nursing concept can serve to help new generations of primary nurses and their managers.

> Changing roles is very much like negotiating a treaty between nations. There is a conflict between the traditional and the non-traditional, the past and the future.
>
> Most of us never provoke radical change in our lives, nor, for that matter do we adamantly refuse to modify our behavior, values and traditions. We are card-carrying members of neither the vanguard nor the rear guard. We don't live at either end of the corridor of change (innovation or resistance), but rather we live in that vast territory called the middleground.
>
> But in a time of transition even the middleground is not necessarily a place where people can be protected from buffeting. In many ways the people in the middleground have the most ambivalent feelings about change. They try to keep some traditional values while acquiring some non-traditional values. They try to embrace those changes that offer growth and rebuff those that threaten loss.
>
> They, like most of us, seek their own place at their own pace. Change becomes a process of resolving the most painful kinds of ambivalence. Most of us seek a resolution that will bring us to a more peaceful plateau (Goodman, 1979, p. 24).

Managing the transition to primary nursing requires skill, responsiveness, and courage. It cannot be done too quickly or too slowly. It must be done with wisdom and patience.

Said even better, *"You can't take away a comfortable role [task-defined nursing] and replace it with a concept [primary nursing]"* (Etheredge, Note 1). How then can the concept of primary nursing be implemented? There are many opinions, but certain strategies are more successful than others. These strategies are presented here in an overview of primary nursing implementation, along with the necessary organizational development that follows official implementation.

OVERVIEW OF IMPLEMENTATION

Many nurses are taught the ideal of being agents of change; however, few of us are as willing to be recipients of change. Implementing an organizational change as major as primary nursing demands that every nurse at all levels of the department be both agent and recipient of change. Therefore, the implementation of primary nursing must be well planned, gradual, and responsive to the needs of each level of nurses. The idea of transition, which connotes gradations of changes in actions, attitudes, and knowledge, is more useful than the idea of implementation, which implies force, impact, and aftershock (Wermuth, Note 2).

No matter how an agency chooses to make the transition to primary nursing, good primary nursing must be the long-range goal, not the means to an end. Primary nursing in itself does not solve chronic institutional problems, but the real determinant of its success is the positive energies and thoughtfulness of the people involved in primary nursing.

The impetus to begin primary nursing can come from any level of a nursing department, staff nurse to administrator. Once the idea has emerged, all sectors must be involved in active discussion and evaluation of primary nursing. All subgroups of the nursing hierarchy should be included in dissemination and sharing of information (Wolff, 1977). Once the idea has filtered through the department, more definitive steps must be taken by the nursing administration to help ease, though not totally resolve, the ambivalence of the majority of nurses who will probably be in the middle ground.

Changing to Primary Nursing

Primary nursing cannot be implemented on a trial or pilot basis. It must be made at the top nursing departmental level and followed through with consistency in words and actions. Primary nursing is not merely a reorganization of tasks; it is a redefinition of professional functioning. Thus, it should be a vehicle for fulfilling the philosophy and objectives of the department.

To begin changing an organization to the primary nursing modality, specific people and groups should be chosen to evaluate the existing nursing department. These people and groups may be a cross-representation of the department who are coordinated by an administrator, in-service education person, or an organizational development person. A primary nursing committee should be formed if it has not been already. Committee membership should represent the department with any majority leaning toward staff nurses. The size is not as important as having a chairman who can lead problem-solving discussions. Frequent meetings, such as weekly or biweekly, are crucial, and meeting reports should be written and distributed to the department's leadership group. The function of the primary nursing committee will evolve as the stages of transition pass. Although the committee may begin by spreading information, conducting transition classes, or developing role descriptions, after the initial implementation period it may oversee organizational development relating to primary nursing. There are innumerable situations that arise as primary nurses become increasingly efficient in their roles.

Outside consultation may also be used at any phase of transition and should be a justifiable priority in terms of time and money. The two main reasons for using outside consultation usually are the consultant's relative objectivity in the analytic, planning, and evaluative processes and experience as a primary nurse or manager of an effective primary nursing system.

Analysis of the Nursing Department

Evaluation of certain factors in the existing nursing department must be made as honestly as possible. A thorough understanding of the present system provides the framework for an analysis of the possibilities and limitations of change. Factors that should be evaluated include:

- administrative track record for change
- administrative support for the primary nursing committee and the possible consequences for the change
- department stability measured by the turnover in staff and management groups and status of the budget
- strength of nurse-managers and existence of management training
- understanding and enactment of the nursing process by staff nurses
- nursing documentation for indication of nursing process use and value to audit results
- staff education programs including orientation and continuing education
- support systems such as psychiatric nurse consultants, unit coordinators, and interdisciplinary committees
- acceptance or resistance to primary nursing in the department
- mechanisms for research and evaluation, such as patient classification tools and formal performance evaluation tools

There is a variety of tools that can be used to evaluate a department, such as readiness checklists, force field analysis, knowledge/attitude questionnaires, and more formal analysis through research. However, the actual diagnostic method is not as important as the process that an organization goes through in evaluating itself.

The best indicators of success for future primary nursing are those that show a stable but flexible nursing department. Some of these predictors are:

- decentralization of the nursing department in which those making changes, especially in the nurse-manager position, have the power to make decisions, control variables, and recommend new organizational policies
- participative management, including regular, frequent staff meetings at all levels and active standing committees
- departmental ability to plan ahead about staffing, programs, and professional practice and development
- departmental ability to send and receive accurate information
- clinical specialists who were primary nurses before and carry administrative responsibility for clinical areas
- collaborative relationship with physicians
- creative freedom (O'Leary, 1977) balanced by the willingness to reinforce a workable primary nursing structure
- business knowledge about budget, staffing ratios, and cost effectiveness
- willingness to evaluate changes through research

Although primary nursing is not in itself more expensive to operate (Marram, 1976), there is a staffing level of RNs that is necessary to operationalize primary nursing. The factors that matter the most in a financial assessment of the department are the ratios of nurses to aides, to patients, and to each shift and the cost-effective utilization of all levels of staff. Staffing patterns should meet acceptable standards, and plans should be made for future staffing goals (Ciske, 1977). Some of these goals may be to equalize staffing between days, evenings, and weekends, to phase out LPNs, and to fill some aide positions with nurses when vacancies occur. Other goals may be to decrease sick calls by the staff and to revise recruitment programs for new staff. On the other hand, methods such as districting are not cost effective and should not be used as a staffing option. It is better to hire an assistant nurse-manager or an evening clinical specialist than to divide the unit into mini-units. Most important, staffing must be realistic. A staff of all nurses is not mandatory in primary nursing, but a nurse-manager is. So decisions will have to be made carefully and adjusted with new input at each stage of the transition.

Decision to Make the Transition

Once the analysis is made, the department is halfway to its goal of primary nursing. At this juncture a definite decision must be made to convert from the existing system. A commitment must be made:

- to develop a management plan that includes objectives, actions, target dates, and key people to move the department towards its goals (Swansburg, 1978)
- to stick with the plan and iron out the snags that result from changes
- to help all levels of the department adjust to the loss of former areas of emotional comfort and to provide new areas of security and praise

Although many nursing departments choose to experiment with primary nursing in one or two pilot units, this is awkward and ultimately unworkable. Pilot units have near optimal conditions regarding personnel support systems and administrative attention and hence do not reflect the feasibility of primary nursing on an institutionwide basis.

Therefore, the transition to primary nursing should be made for a whole department, and individual units can announce their achievement of this goal whenever they meet the predetermined criteria for the change. Consequently, the most important decision is not that primary nursing will be implemented, but that the department will take the steps necessary to make a smooth transition.

Transition to Primary Nursing

The transition to primary nursing may take several months to several years, depending on how close the department is to the elements that make primary nursing work. These elements result from sound management: an operational definition, a professional commitment, expertise in clinical practice, accountability for clinical practice, a professional milieu, collaboration of energies, and professional growth and development. Nursing administrations will have to rely on their feedback mechanisms to help formulate plans for the transition. It may be comforting to know that "there is no particular mystique involved in the change to the primary nursing system. The same planning process that has made other projects successful can be implemented to facilitate the change to primary nursing. These steps should not differ drastically from other concepts of the change process" (Marram, 1977, pp. 22-23).

A great deal has been written about the process of change. The most important thing is to ensure that each step toward the larger goal is solidly in place before another step is introduced. If the department's goal is to stabilize staffing, smaller goals may be to decrease sick calls, turnover, and interunit floating. Each smaller goal should have its own plan for achievement, and each achievement needs to be firmly established before a new one is attempted. However, achievements can be made toward several larger goals at the same time. For instance, requiring the nurse-manager to conduct weekly staff meetings at the unit level can occur simultaneously while instituting a preceptorship program for orientees. In fact, one change may augment another.

In any transition to primary nursing, the position of nurse-manager is the most crucial to success. Too often, the role of the nurse-manager is overlooked as everyone in the system focuses on how the staff primary nurses are functioning. The nurse-manager has the most stressful role in the implementation process, because the position is between administration and staff nurses. The nurse-manager should never be put in the uncomfortable and untenable position of saying or doing something without administrative support.

Of course, the nurse-manager needs to feel that there will be personal benefits as well as benefits for the staff and the patients. The nurse-manager must be given assistance to resolve middle ground ambivalence. Sometimes the nurse-manager may need to help ease the ambivalence of the administration, which can arise at any phase of the change process. To create a climate for personal motivation and cooperation between sectors of a nursing department:

1. approach possible apprehension delicately,
2. encourage self-competition,
3. display confidence in subordinates,
4. provide freedom within a framework of controls,
5. encourage subordinate involvement,
6. avoid over-the-shoulder, constant supervision,
7. give praise, recognition, and credit when they are earned (Asprec, 1975, p. 21).

Workshops for nurse-managers should be held to discuss primary nursing management as it relates to their work situation. Classes outside the agency are useful, but should not replace in-house sessions. The needs of the nurse-manager cannot be neglected in the eagerness to help staff nurses to learn primary nursing. Nurse-managers as a group can probably define many of their own instructional needs, which can be integrated with the following suggestions for workshop objectives:

- define the concept of primary nursing in their own words
- present an assigned article on primary nursing to enable others to analyze its potentials and problems for their units
- identify the signs and symptoms of problem areas, of which some will be unit specific but most will be agencywide
- review skills for nursing process steps and management interventions to facilitate each

- participate with the group in detailing time scheduling, roles of aides and off-shift nurses, assignments, and mechanisms for relaying information, opinions, and problems
- identify resources to facilitate, ensure, and evaluate the change to primary nursing

Once the nurse-manager is relatively comfortable with primary nursing, the steps of the transition will be relatively smooth. The nurse-manager who decides that a unit is ready to move to the next phase must be allowed to move ahead. Every unit or clinic will always be at a different level of development from other units.

Classes for the professional nursing staff of a unit in transition are useful if timed properly. The opportunity to discuss their work together, away from the unit if possible, is perhaps more valuable than the content presented. Thus some sessions should be given by experts in primary nursing and others by those who are adept at leading discussions. The staff can be divided into numerical subgroups so that all can attend the classes with good scheduling. The nurse-manager should also attend each session. Although nurse's aides will not be interested in the discussions of primary nursing, they should be given classes that specifically address their needs. After classes are completed, the staff is theoretically prepared to begin primary nursing. However, the nurse-manager will have to determine the date on which the staff will be officially called primary nurses. It should be clear from this discussion that putting nurses' names on a bulletin board next to patients' names is tokenism unless the role is reinforced by the entire system.

One Week Later: The Critical Point

Shortly after the official transition to primary nursing, anxiety and confusion are inevitably experienced to some degree by the nursing staff:

> Feelings were not readily available at the conscious level and did not emerge until the formal aspects of change had been completed . . . . (p. 108)
> Even though teaching, explanation, and definition of the primary nurse role had been accomplished, confusion was experienced by the nurses; they had difficulty understanding the expectations of the role . . . . (pp. 110-111)
> Most of the feelings of fear and anxiety were specifically related to the change in the assignment of responsibility and accountability . . . . (Pisani, 1977, p. 110)

Although a nursing staff may be well prepared and motivated, the exhilaration of the first days and weeks levels off to a new, though not peaceful, plateau. This juncture is the test of whether primary nursing will endure.

The less that primary nursing seems like a change from the week before it was declared, the less shock occurs among the staff. However, there are always things that need managerial attention, such as:

- Who substitutes for sick primary nurses?
- Who changes a care plan?
- What happens if there need to be more nurses on the evening shift?
- Who is responsible for orienting new medical students to primary nursing?
- What happens when a family asks for a primary nurse's home phone number?
- Why don't patients remember their primary nurse's name?
- What if a patient wants a new primary nurse?
- How is a disagreement between a primary nurse and a supervisor resolved?
- What happens to nurses who find that they do not like primary nursing?
- How assertive can peers be with each other?
- What should be done if the staff wants to divide into geographic districts?

The nurse-manager will need to keep on top of the questions that arise as a result of primary nursing. There will always be some questions, and the best answers are usually found within the staff group. Eventually the structure will be clear enough for staff members to concentrate on their own development rather than survival. Hopefully, the nurse-manager will be able to rely upon organizational development mechanisms beyond the unit level for objective input and consultation.

ORGANIZATIONAL DEVELOPMENT

The transition to primary nursing is managed best by people who have expertise in organizational development. Organizational development (O.D.) is the application of the helping process at the organization and department levels by an individual skilled in group dynamics, systems analysis, management, and consultation. The O.D. person is a clinical specialist in organizational behavior whose goal is to assist the department in identifying and accomplishing its objectives.

Because of the many aspects of implementing primary nursing institutionwide, the use of a skilled person in an O.D. role is mandatory for the successful conversion to and development of primary nursing. The individual does not need to have worked with primary nursing previously, because the purpose is to help those in key leadership roles to develop the primary nursing concept themselves. In other words, the O.D. specialist is involved in the process of the decisions for change, such as clarification, evaluation, and coordination, not necessarily in the content of the change.

Positions That Promote Organizational Development

Nurses who are traditionally in O.D. roles are full-time, in-service coordinators or consultants in clinical areas who are hired by a department on a short-term basis. Either of these positions can be invaluable to the development of primary nursing if they have direct access to the director of nursing and the other nurses who hold power and influence in the department.

Institutions that want to begin or improve primary nursing should also consider two other positions: a primary nursing coordinator or an organizational development specialist. Either position should be used as advisory.

Primary Nursing Coordinators

A primary nursing coordinator focuses attention and interventions on operationalizing the primary nursing concept by working with nursing leaders to build the kind of primary nursing that the agency wants. "The chief focuses. . .are educating the nursing staff about primary nursing, supervising the actual implementation process of primary nursing, evaluating primary nursing after implementation, and providing and suggesting new tools relevant to primary nursing" (Marram, Schlegel, and Bevis, 1974, p. 87).

The primary nurse coordinator could be a staff education instructor or a specially funded position. However, the person must be free to make primary nursing a priority, because time is definitely required to work with leadership personnel and to set up the in-house programs that are requested. The coordinator should also be the chairperson of a primary nursing committee made up primarily of staff nurses. This gives the coordinator firsthand knowledge about the responses of nurses to their new, complex roles.

Organizational Development Specialist

The O.D. specialist focuses attention on the dynamics of the nursing department through a continual, systematic analysis of its strengths and weaknesses. The O.D. specialist perceives primary nursing as a concept that values certain behaviors and attitudes which become stimuli for further changes. The O.D. specialist gathers data from all levels of the organization to determine the effectiveness with which various mechanisms work, such as staffing and budget systems, transfers of patients, job descriptions and evaluations of nursing staff, roles of physician assistants, and provision of unit secretaries. The O.D. specialist also gains information from concurrent and retrospective audit reports and ideally from formal nursing research.

Because the O.D. specialist is concerned with the total work setting, an accurate plan for developing primary nursing can be made with the leadership. Thus, the right hand knows what the left hand is doing, and any changes in departmental policies and procedures should also augment primary nursing. In this way, the O.D. specialist ensures that double messages are not passed between administration, primary nurses and their managers.

Having an O.D. position provides a good guarantee that changes will be evaluated and coordinated, whether or not they are obviously connected to primary nursing. Hiring an O.D. specialist is administration's response to the operating mechanisms and the climate of the work environment.

Because primary nursing will only be successful if the leadership group is comfortable with the concept and its implications, leaders rather than staff primary nurses are the target of the O.D. specialist. A professional milieu between nursing supervisors and administrators is conducive to a professional milieu at the unit and clinic level:

> The trick is to introduce [primary nursing] in a way that enhances the ability of the group of nurses to work together to provide excellent patient care, and that minimizes the risk of separating or dividing the group so that its members can't work together. . . .
>
> For primary nursing to succeed it has to be done in an atmosphere where risk-taking and judgement making are supportive, where everything isn't done according to rules and regulations, but where a nurse is expected to use clinical judgement in this or that precise situation. Now that is the tough part in implementing primary nursing (Manthey, 1978, p. 426).

In order to be effectively involved in the development of primary nursing, the O.D. specialist needs contacts with leadership personnel, administration, and the primary nursing committee over an extended period. Therefore, the position should be half- or full-time and permanent. The O.D. specialist should make a verbal or written contract with those requesting services in order to delineate realistic expectations for the position and the institution.

Programs That Promote Organizational Development

Programs other than the initial implementation classes need to be developed to promote primary nursing from the beginning stages. Indeed, conversion to primary nursing does not end the work of administration, management, or staff education. There are no limits on how far primary nursing will grow.

Primary nurses and their managers are too involved clinically to identify and meet all of the needs that arise after the transition to primary nursing. These needs emerge for several reasons: (1) Role changes at all department levels that result from primary nursing cannot be completely anticipated ahead of time. Even if it were possible, discussing a role change before it occurs is purely theoretical. Therefore, the real anxiety, which is often experienced by new primary nurses as guilt, and the real problems must be approached after the transition. (2) Primary nursing requires a gradual but definite decentralization of the nursing department which should occur in stages as each group is adequately prepared for the responsibility. (3) Primary nurses are more aware of their learning needs when they apply the nursing process with individual patients because someone else cannot be expected to follow through on problems. (4) Primary nurses develop expertise in areas that should be recognized by the organization. (5) Technical, legal, and ethical influences are closely involved in the daily work of primary nurses. As society changes, primary nurses and their managers must adjust knowledgeably.

There are two kinds of programs that promote organizational development and hence primary nursing. Programs for the system become part of the formal structure of the department. Preceptorships for all new primary nurses is such a program. Topical programs, such as classes and seminars aimed at a specific skill or attitudes are the second kind of program. Classes in physical assessment or assertiveness training fall into this group. Both system and topical programs are needed for a department to grow. Programs that contribute to organizational development should occur when specific instructional needs are expressed, not because of pressures from nonclinical sources. For example, if primary nurses cannot set outcome goals for their patients, they should be given classes in that instead of classes in patient advocacy. This principle can be very difficult to adhere to if key people become impatient with the rate of progress. There is a tendency to push ahead to new theoretical frontiers before the groundwork has been laid. The people who oversee either type of program must strive to stimulate primary nurses without overwhelming them.

Topical Program Progression

1. Management skills for a staff nurse in charge of a shift.

2. Advanced interviewing and assessment skills, including nursing diagnosis and other innovations.

3. Refined goal-setting abilities, including contracts with patients.

4. Expanded repertoire of interventions, including patient teaching individually or in groups, value awareness, and working with the families of hospitalized primary patients.

5. Techniques in discharge planning.

6. Increased comfort with the techniques, ethics, and legalities of patient advocacy.

7. Enlarged capacity to collaborate with physicians.

8. Attention to attitude and mechanisms for giving and receiving peer support.

9. Instruction on how to present work formally.
10. Courses in how staff nurses teach staff nurses.
11. Information about nursing certification and other professional recognition.
12. Workshops on publication of primary nursing cases and information.

System Programs

Suggestions for the content of system programs are easier to make than recommendations for the timing of them. The progression should be determined from a variety of sources such as the primary nursing committee, the management group, the off-shift clinical supervisors, the in-service education staff, and audit results. The primary nursing coordinator, O.D. specialist, or in-service coordinator can synthesize input and work with the nursing administration to formulate an official program based on the standards and operation of the department.

Preceptorships are discussed at length in Chapter 3, and documentation that facilitates the role and accountability of primary nurses is discussed in Chapter 4.

Regular seminars are needed for nurse-managers. Because the nurse-managers' role undergoes the most change and because the nurse-managers need to stay one step ahead of the staff, they need their own programs for professional growth. Seminars are most effective on a monthly basis and are most helpful to nurse-managers if representatives from nursing administration are involved. The seminar group should be small enough for everyone to participate in discussions; the sessions should be long enough to cover the issues on more than a superficial level. Seminars should include topics and readings in the areas of

- motivation
- group dynamics
- management by objectives
- hiring and evaluating staff
- policy making with medical staff
- regulatory agencies
- staff development on the unit level
- legal issues
- management of staffing and budget

Primary nursing forums are programs offered to the entire nursing department on at least a semiannual basis for the purpose of platform presentations and audience participation on different aspects of primary nursing. Because staff nurses do most of the primary nursing, the forum should address their expressed interests. Enough sessions should be offered so that most of the staff can attend one. Such a program may include:

- general update on the nursing department
- case presentations by primary nurses from representative clinical areas
- papers which the primary nursing committee identifies as timely
- multidisciplinary panel discussions
- presentations of research plans and results
- staff nurses' assessment of primary nursing (see Exhibit 14-1)

By formal recognition of clinical generalists, who are primary nurses with expertise developed in several unrelated clinical areas, an agency can add to its flexibility. Clinical generalists could contract to work for a designated period of time, rotating to various clinical areas when mastery as a primary nurse in each location is gained. For instance, a primary nurse may spend a year in a general adult surgical unit learning good primary nursing and then move to a pediatric or an intensive care unit, where the nurse is again precepted until functioning autonomously. The nurse may want to work in another specialty area rather than move into a management position. An organization can benefit from primary nurses who want to increase clinical expertise rather than to be progressively promoted away from clinical practice. Increased pay is not needed for a clinical generalist program because the nurses improve their pay and benefits by virtue of longevity. However, the nursing department should devise a method to formally recognize expert nurses who have contributed to primary nursing care.

Any method by which staff nurses positively interact with each other at the unit level promotes organizational development. Peer audits, whether live or retrospective, can establish expectations for sincere and professional interaction. However, such a program should be one of the last instituted, because it requires a high level of clinical confidence and peer trust. Marram (1974) suggests live audits in which an auditor and a primary nurse review the nurse's work using the care plan and medical record. The auditor rates the primary nurse in specific areas, and results are given to the nurse and the audit committee. The atmosphere in which peer audits are conducted is the most critical aspect of these programs. If people are too critical or too fearful, a peer audit program will backfire. The goal of peer audits should be the constructive appraisal of concurrent primary nursing. Therefore, staff nurses should predetermine the criteria and be well prepared as auditors and presenters, with an emphasis on how to give and receive feedback. Peer audits should never be used as a replacement for the nurse-manager's evaluative and supportive functions with the staff. Peer evaluation should be only one of many sources of information about the work of nurses.

An organization should never stop changing and growing, especially where primary nursing is concerned. However, the direction of changes and the pathways of growth need thoughtful attention and tangible reinforcement. Organizational development requires committed, knowledgeable leaders who can provide the staff with helpful programs. If primary nurses feel that the department leadership

Exhibit 14-1 Primary Nursing Development Questionnaire

Your unit:

Your major question or concern about primary nursing:

   To what degree are the following areas difficult for primary nurses to fulfill? (Check one/write comments)

Topic	*Degree of Difficulty*		
	None	Some	Much

 1. Introducing and describing yourself to your patients as the primary nurse
 2. Documentation of:
       initiat assessment
       nursing index
       progress notes
       nursing orders
       discharge planning checklist
       patient teaching
 3. Determining immediate goals for patients
 4. Determining outcome goals with patients and families
 5. Having direct contact with your primary patients
 6. Obtaining supervision/suggestions/consultations from fellow nurses
 7. Getting support and guidance from:
       your nurse-manager
       your off-shift supervisor
       administration
       staff education
       other
 8. Coordinating nursing care with:
       peers
       associates
       physicians
       social service
       other
 9. Obtaining satisfaction from the primary nursing role
10. Orienting nurses new to the unit

Please state what you are personally planning to do to resolve your major concern about primary nursing on your unit.

has the staff's interests and development at heart, they will provide care to their patients more energetically aod expertly. "The ecstasy [primary nursing] creates and the rewards it provides are ego-sustaining. The agony encountered in attempting to fulfill one's responsibilities can be ego-depleting. The future task is to reduce the agony to a healthy challenge" (Spoth, 1977, p. 233).

Evaluating Primary Nursing

Because primary nursing involves all areas of a nursing department, it would be impossible to use one tool to measure the status or direction of primary nursing in an institution. Therefore, a combination of measuring sticks should be used to create as total a primary nursing profile as possible. The following measures can be used by units and departments to determine the extent and quality of primary nursing:

- results of retrospective audits
- results of concurrent audits
- satisfaction questionnaires of those involved
- placement on cog's ladder of group development (see Chapter 5)
- sick calls/turnover rates
- formal research on the nurse-primary patient relationship

REFERENCE NOTES

1. Etheredge, M. Comments made at the seminar Assessing Primary Nursing: A Forum for Professional Nurses, Tufts-New England Medical Center Hospital, Boston, January 1978.
2. Wermuth, M. Comments made at the seminar Assessing Primary Nursing: A Forum for Professional Nurses, Tufts-New England Medical Center Hospital, Boston, January 1978.

REFERENCES

Asprec, E. S. The process of change. *Supervisor Nurse*, October 1975, *6*(9), 15-24.

Ciske, K. Misconceptions about staffing and patient assignment in primary nursing. *Nursing Administration Quarterly*, Winter 1977, *1*(2), 61-68.

Goodman, E. I'm not a feminist, but. . . *Boston Sunday Globe*, March 18, 1979, pp. 7+.

Manthey, M. If you are instituting primary nursing. *American Journal of Nursing*, March 1978, *78*(3), 426-427.

Marram, G. The comparative costs of operating a team and primary nursing unit. *Journal of Nursing Administration*, November 1976, *6*: 21-24.

Marram, G. Principles and processes in instituting the change to primary nursing. In *Primary nursing: One nurse, one client, planning care together*. New York: National League for Nursing, 1977.

Marram, G., Schlegel, M., & Bevis, E. *Primary nursing, a model for individualized care*. St. Louis, Mo.: C.V. Mosby, 1974.

O'Leary, J. Primary nursing care: Implementing change. In *Primary nursing: One nurse, one client, planning care together.* New York: National League for Nursing, 1977.

Pisani, S. Primary nursing—Aftermath of change. *Nursing Administration Quarterly,* Winter 1977, *1*(2), 107-113.

Spoth, J. Primary nursing: The agony and the ecstasy. *Nursing Clinics of North America,* June 1977, *12*(2), 224-233.

Swansburg, R.C. Planning—A function of nursing administration Part II. *Supervisor Nurse,* May 1978, *9*(5), 76-80.

Wolff, K. Change: Implementation of primary nursing through ad hocracy. *Journal of Nursing Administration,* December 1977, 7: 24-27.

Chapter 15

Managing Toward a Viable Identity for Professional Nursing

There are as many opinions and forecasts about the nursing profession as there are nurses. Rather than add something new to the pot, the discussion here will focus on how to improve what is known about nursing by using the results gained from the implementation of primary nursing.

What is a viable identity? It is a positive, healthy attitude about someone or something. In this case, the nursing profession is the something which is made up of many someones who have a personal philosophy about the function and worth of nurses. Do they see nursing as viable, that is living, not just existing? When nurses label patients as viable, they indicate the expectation that with adequate input the patient will thrive at some point. How can nurses feel equally as hopeful about their own profession? What constructive measures will improve the outlook for nursing as a profession that not only exists but grows?

The answers should be sought only after careful consideration of what impact the profession has on individuals from the high school student considering a nursing career to the dynamic nurse executive. After this is known, attention should turn to analyzing how nurses interact with each other and their environment. Finally, some conclusions can be drawn about the direction of primary nursing.

THE INDIVIDUAL NURSE IN THE PROFESSION

Understanding why people enter nursing is less crucial than knowing how they perceive the profession and how they revise those perceptions as a result of experiences with other nurses. People of all ages are eager to be influenced and inspired, eager to master skills and interpersonal relations. Nursing offers these opportunities if there is a positive atmosphere with reliable support systems in schools and work settings. The role of the primary nurse should be the focal point

319

of professional recruitment, classroom education and clinical curricula, and clinical performance. Therefore, nursing organizations and administrations should organize their skills and attention to develop the nursing process as carried out by primary nurses.

Nurse-Mentors

Although the constant cry of nurses is more staff to share the workload, more staffing does not in itself rectify chronic problems in an agency. Furthermore, increased staffing does not always lead to a viable professional identity. More is not necessarily better. What does make a difference is the way that the staff is used and, more importantly, the way its members are treated by other nurses. In fact when asked what gives them the most satisfaction, nursing staffs identify the chance to grow professionally with the help of a good manager. Likewise, when students are asked about the positive aspects of their basic nursing program, they usually refer to a beloved or challenging teacher who helped them to master a skill or an interpersonal relationship. In both situations the chance for a one-to-one relationship with a mentor makes the difference between a requirement and a meaningful experience.

Nurses do not necessarily want more money or benefits; they want more constructive, personal mentors. The profession has spoken endlessly about role models, and that concept needs to be expanded and personalized through the idea of the mentor—an experienced nurse who works regularly with a person at any level of the nursing hierarchy during that individual's professional development. The relationship usually lasts until the nurse has outgrown the need for a mentor, that is, until the nurse's career objectives are met as far as possible.

If it is true that "burnout occurs when people stop growing professionally" (Reres, Note 1), nurses who are studying or practicing could renew and refresh themselves through association with a mentor. By using mentors, frustration, apathy, and burnout could be reduced. Mentors can help nurses to identify assets and areas for growth and can advise them on how to get through the rough spots in education or career. Mentors help alleviate or avoid the pains of self-doubt and lack of growth "which for dynamic, independent people, are worse than physical pain. We withdraw emotionally, and a career is converted into a job" (Reres, Note 1). Mentors as nonjudgmental advisers prevent burnout by helping nurses to increase control of and esteem from their careers.

Mentors can come from inside or outside the agency. Each nurse needs something different from a mentor and will need to seek out the right person. This requires exposure to many persons who have experience in the chosen clinical or administrative area. Agencies can acknowledge the need for mentors and help nurses to find and work with them. The first step is to hire experienced people who are competent clinicians and are not threatened by newer people with potential to learn and succeed. Mentors can be in any employment position, but they must have access to those seeking their guidance. Agencies can construct a more formal mentor system by implementing a preceptorship program for new orientees and leadership seminars for nurse-managers and others in relatively isolated positions. Nurses may also be exposed to mentors by allowing staff nurses time to spend with clinical specialists or directors of nursing time to learn from other directors.

Mentors cannot be assigned; they must be found. Mentors can be a powerful influence and, therefore, should be other nurses. In this way a positive professional identity can be reinforced. If an agency cannot provide a mentor, the nurse should find one elsewhere. They are not difficult to locate for someone who is open to new ideas and investment of time in a career.

Career Planning

The development of the career concept seems to be where the nursing profession needs more emphasis. Too often a nursing career is viewed as a series of different jobs used to gain more experience. However, because this attitude lacks a goal beyond the immediate objective, the nursing career lacks direction and hence personal control.

Career planning should begin before nursing school. Applicants should be told about the potentials and problems of nursing. They need a clear idea of what nursing is and what they might contribute to the profession. A high school counselor cannot be relied upon to recruit nurses. Instead, health care agencies should offer programs and open houses to inform prospective nurses about primary nursing and other positive aspects of the profession.

Career planning should not stop after applicants enter nursing school. Nursing students should have an adviser who meets often with students and helps them to make knowledgeable decisions about matters such as elective courses or identification of strengths that persist from rotation to rotation. The adviser may not be the chosen mentor, but should help students to decide on the best steps to find a first job. This requires the adviser to stay abreast of current trends in primary nursing practice. Essentially, each nursing student needs the equivalent of one primary nurse throughout the education process. This is also true in graduate education.

When nurses approach an agency for employment, they should have a clear picture of their personal strengths, skills, preferences, and goals. However, the agency would benefit by counseling prospective employees about all the positions that are available rather than funneling them into a position. Agencies may also provide an in-house career counselor to encourage restless staff nurses to become clinical generalists rather than leave the institution to get further experience. A counselor could also help nurses to plan further education on a part- or full-time basis, so that education can be part of, not a vacation from, their careers.

With the trend toward more working mothers, there need to be new career pathways in nursing. The experience of motherhood can enhance a woman's abilities as a primary nurse. Career pathways need to be developed to use the experiences of nurse mothers while making it possible for them to have the time that they need with their families. Perhaps part-time nurses could be used as preceptors or in other key positions on the staff, depending on their hours. Their need to spend more time with their families should not detract from their value as teachers, mentors, shift charge nurses, and clinicians.

Just as setting short- and long-term outcome goals for patients makes primary nurses more effective, setting and evaluating career goals give immediate purpose and eventual direction to the energies of nurses. Although life looks long and hopeful upon graduation from nursing school, career decisions made in the subsequent ten years determine a great deal about earning potential and professional satisfaction. Nurses should be encouraged and guided in long-range career planning. If they feel the agency, as represented by nursing leadership, is genuinely interested in them, most nurses will return the respect with highly motivated work.

Each nurse has the responsibility for his or her own career planning. No agency can hand a nurse a career; it must be molded from feedback about work and integrated by the nurse's personal evaluation of assets. Hopefully, the nurse will receive positive information in order to decrease self-doubt and increase the self-respect that makes a career worth caring about.

Educating New Primary Nurses

The half-life of nursing knowledge is about five years. Even the rate of half-lives has accelerated (Reres, Note 1). What are the implications of this for primary nursing? New primary nurses will need to know how to think and cope as well as how to do things. Because technical clinical knowledge is expanding and being replaced at a rapid rate, perhaps the most useful educational objective for primary nurses is to teach them how to integrate the multitude of data which are received in a clinical area into an approach that is useful to patients. Consequently, the primary nursing process should be the framework on which all curricula and clinical rotations are based.

Undergraduate Education

There are specific tools that primary nurses will need in order to develop critical thinking (see Chapter 3), to cope with the pressures of the daily clinical setting, and to integrate interventions with process. Some areas of knowledge that future primary nurses will need in their repertoires are:

- How to Think:
  primary nursing process
  problem-solving techniques
  logic
  creative thinking
  decision making
  priority setting
- How to Cope:
  personal assertiveness
  dynamics of group membership
  personal time management
  use of consultation
  techniques of collaboration, negotiation, and compromise
  peer support techniques
  role theory
  systems theory and organizational behavior
  change theory, as agent and recipient
  ways to increase validation and decrease self-doubt
  personal career planning
  personal health maintenance
- How to Do:
  establish an alliance with patients
  patient education
  patient advocacy
  working with ancillary personnel
  contract setting with patients and families
  be a mentor for younger nursing students
  communicate through technical writing
  put concerns and questions into informal clinical research

Future primary nurses will need time to integrate instruction on all three areas. This can be provided by lengthening precepted time in the clinical area without compromising attendance at nonnursing classes. Some schools do this through work-study programs, senior year agency placements for 6 to 12 weeks, and other directed clinical studies. These arrangements offer students primary patient assignments and give a realistic perspective about the working world. Although these programs are often relegated to the senior year, they should be made available earlier.

If more time cannot be arranged, better utilization of clinical time must be made a priority. This involves structuring the clinical experience so that students can function as associates to primary nurses who are on duty. It may also require fewer rotations so that students do not have continual adjustments to new surroundings, personnel, and patients. If the objective is to teach nurses sound theory and integrated thinking, it makes the most sense to expose them to similar patients in familiar units with the same instructor.

Along these lines, perhaps the soundest instruction could be achieved if students were progressed along a clinical course which is not necessarily matched with the classroom curriculum. For example, after a basic anatomy and physiology course, give students classroom courses in how to think, cope, and do, but also provide them with a clinical instructor to teach them how to integrate their clinical knowledge with classroom instruction. In this way they can learn the details of diseases, medications, and treatments. Let them learn about diabetes when they need to—when they have a diabetic primary patient.

The concepts of nursing diagnosis may be used as a framework for clinical expectations. The school would provide students with a primary patient in each broad nursing diagnostic area before graduation. This would permit fewer rotations and more flexibility of assignments. For example, the diagnosis of immobility could be studied in a variety of clinical settings. The value of clinical generalists would also be reinforced. If student nurses were guided along a nursing diagnostic path, they would learn how to think in broader ways. Their self-definition would not be as limited, and their careers would be open to many more possibilities.

Reorganizing clinical experiences would also have an impact on educators. Reorganization aimed at expanding, consolidating, and individualizing education involves different methods of planning and structuring, and requires that instructors function as primary nurses at some point in their own careers.

There are surely many more aspects of nursing education that primary nursing will eventually challenge. Until there are more agencies that have solidly established primary nursing, it will be difficult to expose students to the role before graduation. However, they still must receive the fundamental underpinnings of the role to be able to use what they learn when primary nursing reaches their units.

Graduate Education

Nurses educated at the graduate level have an important place in the success of primary nursing. Master's level nurses can contribute in several major areas as:

- primary nurses
- clinical specialists and coordinators with line authority and accountability for units within their areas of expertise
- organizational development specialists
- researchers
- public relations and political strategists

Graduate education provides an opportunity for learning theory and techniques to promote growth in other nurses, as well as gaining advanced knowledge in a specialty. At this point, the nursing profession cannot afford to train people in advanced specialty fields only, because there is no guarantee that the wealth of a graduate education will be transmitted to other nurses. Nursing needs to learn how to replenish itself before nurses can take care of patients independently.

In a familiar example, "Private duty nurses never changed the system" (Twyon, Note 2). Similarly, clinical specialists can only change the system if they are appointed to influential and potentially powerful leadership positions within health care agencies. Only in this way will changes favorable to nursing be made. The most efficient, effective use of clinical specialists is a combined role as specialist and manager or administrator in a type of joint appointment. Thus, those who know what should be done clinically have the power to get it done administratively. This minimizes red tape and maximizes quality assurance and staff development. Because the clinical specialist is also the clinical leader, decisions are streamlined and nursing authority within the interdisciplinary organization is respected.

NURSES AND THEIR ENVIRONMENT

Primary nursing provides an effective mechanism for investigating the complex dynamics of nurses and their environment because of the specific assignment of a single primary nurse to a primary patient over time. Some areas related to primary nursing have been thoroughly studied and the study of some others would not help solve the perplexing problems that agencies face today. For example, comparing team nursing and primary nursing is not a valid indicator, because neither modality exists in a pure state in a single institution. Similarly, investigating the effectiveness of primary nurses by measuring care plans has little value, because nursing care plans have been outmoded by the results-oriented documentation.

Clinical Areas for Research

Suggestions for study areas on a clinical level are offered here as broad questions which arise whenever primary nursing is discussed.

1. How is a professional commitment measured and what influences the ability of nurses to commit themselves to patients and families?
2. Does primary nursing decrease complication rates and length of admission?
3. What are patients and families taught about primary nurses?
4. What kind of educational preparation produces the best primary nurses?

5. What kind of orientation program prepares new graduates for their primary nursing role?
6. What are the special needs of primary nurses in different clinical areas?
7. What is the nature of accountability and why do nurses shy away from it?
8. Does a staff group in the cohesive or esprit stage achieve better patient outcomes than a staff group in a less advanced stage?
9. What are the staffing patterns which are most conducive to primary nursing?
10. How do primary nurses perceive their jurisdiction in relation to other nurses and other health care providers?
11. What factors influence the complete follow-through of the patient advocacy loop in the primary nursing process?
12. Does making contracts with patients and/or families really influence the speed and quality with which those contracted outcomes are achieved?
13. What are the factors that determine patient compliance with treatment regimes?
14. Will a clinical generalist program decrease agency turnover?
15. What is the best preparation for primary nurses to move into primary care roles or management positions?
16. Does primary nursing improve the public image of nurses?

REFERENCE NOTES

1. Reres, M. *How to prevent professional burnout.* Program presented at the Beth Israel Hospital Seminar in Nursing, Boston, April 1979.
2. Twyon, S. Comments made at the Spring Nursing Forum, Tufts-New England Medical Center Hospital, Boston, April 5, 1979.

Chapter 16

The Role of Head Nurses: The Perceptions of Primary Nurses

by Joyce Bloom

Primary nursing is an important issue in nursing administration, and the implementation of the primary nursing system of delivery is a major change in the organization of nursing care in the hospital setting (Brown, 1977). As systems change, roles change. The two major roles that change when implementing primary nursing are those of the staff nurse and the head nurse. Staff nurses become primary nurses and assume a more autonomous, professionally based practice. Head nurses take the major responsibility of providing support and guidance to staff nurses who assume the increased professional demands as primary nurses.

This investigator believed it would be worth while to study head nurses' behavior in a primary nursing system of delivery since it is such a critical leadership position for the operationalization of the concepts of primary nursing.

PURPOSES OF THE STUDY

The primary purpose of the study was to examine whether or not head nurses carry out those role behaviors that are described in the literature on the primary nursing system of delivery. Since the head nurse is in the leadership role at the operational level, it is important to know how primary nurses perceive leadership behavior. Only those patterns of behavior which have been documented were explored. A secondary purpose of this study was to provide information which could be used in additional research concerning leadership roles at the operational level of nursing care delivery.

STATEMENT OF THE PROBLEM

The question addressed in this study is: Do head nurses exhibit the six general categories of role behavior that the literature on primary nursing suggests for the role of the head nurse?

Many believe that primary nursing is not just another method of organizing the delivery of nursing care, but a method which allows nurses to practice in a professional one-to-one client relationship. Manthey, Ciske, Robertson, and Harris (1970) indicate that the organizational pattern of primary nursing evolved from the idea of designing an organizational structure which "embodies an arrangement of nurse and patient that facilitates professional practice and the delivery of nursing care" (p. 65). The organizational pattern allows hospital nurses to assume a more autonomous role in planning, implementing, and coordinating the nursing care of their primary patients.

Because head nurses are the first line clinical and administrative leaders, the implementation of primary nursing will be greatly influenced by their ability to make decisions to operationalize its concepts. "The factor most critical to the success of primary nursing is the part played by the head nurse. She must be a strong leader who has earned the staff's respect, and in consequence, can exert an effective influence on their attitudes and behavior" (Manthey, 1973, pp. 86-87). Zander (1977) indicates that the key variable in the success or failure of primary nursing is the head nurse who is in the critical position of ensuring or sabotaging the development and implementation of primary nursing. According to Brown (1977), "Primary nursing will be no more than a fad that is here for a decade and gone when replaced by another organizational pattern if we do not bring to the delivery system the fullest practice of the professional role of the nurse" (editorial).

SUMMARY OF FINDINGS

The sample was taken from 15 head nurses and 68 staff nurses in two acute care teaching hospitals of over 400 beds. The findings indicate that staff primary nurses often perceived that their head nurses exhibited the following four out of six categories of behavior: (1) facilitating the primary nurse role; (2) validating and evaluating primary nurses' ability to provide nursing care; (3) encouraging primary nurses to be independent problem solvers; and (4) demonstrating leadership and administrative management abilities. In one hospital, head nurses were perceived by their staff primary nurses as exhibiting behavior which facilitates staff development sometimes too often. In the other hospital, head nurses were often perceived by their staff primary nurses as exhibiting behavior which facilitates staff development.

Clinical role model behavior was positively correlated with education, $R = 0.5390$. This was significant at the 0.01 level. Therefore, in this study, the higher the head nurses' level of education, the higher the mean score in the clinical role model category regardless of the hospital setting.

DEFINITION OF TERMS

The head nurse refers to the nurse who has the responsibility of planning the provision of nursing care for all patients on a specific unit in a general, acute hospital setting.

The primary nurse refers to the staff nurse who has the complete responsibility, accountability, and authority for the nursing care for an assigned number of patients.

Primary nursing as a system of delivery refers to a method of organizing the delivery of nursing care whereby primary nurses are given the complete responsibility, accountability, and authority for planning, implementing, and coordinating the nursing care of their primary patients from admission through completed discharge.

A role refers to one or more recurrent activities which are made up of behavioral cycles. These behavioral activities in combination produce organizational output and are held in the form of expectations by some members of a role set (Katz & Kahn, 1966).

CATEGORIES OF ROLE BEHAVIOR

A literature review was conducted to determine the role of the head nurse and the specific behaviors that the head nurse assumes. The six role behaviors that were identified and the sources in which they were located are given below:

1. *Clinical role model:* Anderson, 1976; Elpern, 1977; Esposito, 1977; Garber, 1977; Guilianelli, 1977; Law, 1977; Marram et al., 1974

2. *Validator and evaluator:* Manthey et al., 1970; Marram et al., 1974; McCarthy & Schifalacqua, 1978; Page, 1974; Zander, 1977

3. *Facilitator of the primary role of the primary nurse:* Anderson, 1976; Logsdon, 1973; Manthey, 1973; Manthey & Kramer, 1970; Manthey et al., 1970; McCarthy & Schifalacqua, 1978; Zander, 1977

4. *Facilitator of staff development:* Ciske, 1974; Esposito, 1977; Manthey & Kramer, 1970; Manthey et al., 1970; Marram et al., 1974; Zander, 1977

5. *Leadership skills and administrative management:* Esposito, 1977; Manthey, 1973; Marram et al., 1974

6. *Encourages independent problem solving and decision making:* Manthey et al., 1970; Marram et al., 1974; Page, 1974; Zander, 1977

GENERAL METHODOLOGY

This study was conducted in two acute care teaching hospitals, both over 400 beds, which utilized primary nursing in the northeastern United States. A study proposal was submitted to both hospitals requesting permission to seek the participation of ten of the most experienced head nurses and their primary staff nurses in a study that would involve the completion of a questionnaire. Permission was obtained from both hospitals and a consent form was signed by each participating nurse. The data collection method used provided for confidentiality of information.

Two questionnaires were developed. A head nurse questionnaire was used to collect data on demographic characteristics of the head nurse, including nursing education, length of experience as a head nurse in team and primary nursing, and formalized preparation for the role as head nurse in primary nursing. This information was used to determine if there is any relationship between demographic characteristics of head nurses and the perceptions of staff primary nurses. A questionnaire was also developed to collect information about how primary nurses perceived the role behaviors of their head nurses.

DEVELOPMENT OF STAFF NURSE QUESTIONNAIRE

To ensure content validity of the questionnaire, a review of the literature was used. The questionnaire contained 49 behavioral statements of role behaviors for the head nurse in primary nursing which were derived from the review. The questionnaire was tested several times using nursing administration students and nurse educators. During pretesting five items were eliminated.

The questionnaire, which was designed to be given to staff nurses in the primary nurse role, asked nurses to indicate those behaviors that most closely fit their perception of how their head nurse carries out the responsibilities of the position. The questionnaire also asked for information about the primary nurse's length of experience in the nursing unit and the length of time since graduation from nursing school. The questionnaire was based on a five point Likert rating scale for behaviors as follows: 1 = never, 2 = seldom, 3 = sometimes, 4 = often, 5 = always. A panel of nurse judges assisted in categorizing the remaining 44 behavioral statements into the six categories of behavior. Statements that presented difficulty were categorized by general consensus of the judges or using statements from the literature. Before analyzing the data in each of the six behavioral categories, the 44 behavioral statements were examined for reliability (internal consistency) by obtaining satisfactory alpha coefficients.

Statements used include:

- The head nurse assigns him/herself to be a primary nurse for a patient.
- The head nurse teaches patients.
- The head nurse reviews my nursing notes.
- The head nurse and I make joint nursing care rounds on my primary patients.
- If my primary patients' physicians have any questions, the head nurse directs them to me.
- The head nurse provides for or keeps me aware of educational programs which will enhance my professional growth.
- The head nurse promotes an atmosphere whereby nursing care conferences are conducive to problem solving sessions.
- The head nurse offers me support and guidance to find my own solution to problems rather than giving me "his/her" solution.

SCOPE AND DESIGN

This study was limited to the primary nurses' perception of their head nurses' role behavior, and therefore, only nurses who were designated as primary nurses participated. Because the study did not seek to answer how head nurses saw their own role behavior, their perception of their own role behavior could not be compared with the primary nursing staffs' perception. The criterion that was used to select head nurses was the level of experience. Validation of behavior was based on the document studies of head nurses working in a primary nursing system. Since questionnaires were used for data collection, the types of data were limited.

Since the Likert scale can be assumed to be an interval measurement scale, some basic assumptions regarding the design of the questionnaire for primary nurses and its relationship to data analysis were made: (1) equal weighting for each of the 44 behavioral items in the primary staff nurse questionnaire; and (2) always, often, sometimes, seldom, and never, had the same meaning for all members of the sample population. The analysis of variance (ANOVA) model was used because it detects small differences. Assumptions of this model are: (1) homogeneity of variance within groups and (2) Gaussian distribution of error.

Every head nurse received a score for each of the six general categories of role behavior that was derived by calculating the mean score of the head nurse's primary nursing staff who responded to the questionnaire. These mean scores indicated the primary nursing staff's perception of how frequently their head nurse exhibits the six general categories of role behavior. An analysis of variance was performed to detect the differences in mean scores between the head nurses in each agency. The null hypotheses were:

1. The mean score for head nurses in hospitals A and B will be equal in category one: "The head nurse is a clinical role model."

2. The mean score for head nurses in hospitals A and B will be equal in category two: "The head nurse is a validator and evaluator of the primary nurses' abilities to carry out their nursing care responsibilities."

3. The mean score for head nurses in hospitals A and B will be equal in category three: "The head nurse facilitates and encourages primary nurses to be the 'primary' communicator, coordinator, and planner of nursing care for their patients."

4. The mean score for head nurses in hospitals A and B will be equal in category four: "The head nurse facilitates and encourages professional staff development."

5. The mean score for head nurses in hospitals A and B will be equal in category five: "The head nurse utilizes leadership skills and is the nursing administrative manager of nursing care of all the patients on the unit."

6. The mean score for head nurses in hospitals A and B will be equal in category six: "The head nurse encourages primary staff nurses to be independent problem solvers who will feel free to learn, to risk, and who will seek guidance when it is necessary." The acceptance of a significant difference was set at the 0.05 level.

Pearson correlation coefficients were calculated on the behavioral scales to analyze the relationships between the mean score and the demographic data obtained from the head nurses. The null hypotheses were tested for each of the Pearson correlation coefficients. Again the 0.05 level of significance was chosen for determining if correlations were significantly different from zero.

RESPONSE AND RESULTS

Questionnaires were distributed to 20 head nurses and 200 staff primary nurses, and 16 head nurses and 68 staff nurses responded. One head nurse was eliminated, because no staff nurses responded.

Clinical Role Model Behavior (Table 16-1)

In hospital A the head nurse mean score on clinical role model behavior was 26.054 with a standard deviation of 4.916. This indicated that the staff nurses perceived their head nurses as sometimes exhibiting clinical role model behaviors. In hospital B the head nurse mean score was 31.348 with a standard deviation of 5.288. This indicated that the staff nurses often perceived their head nurses as exhibiting clinical role model behaviors.

There was a significant difference in the head nurse mean scores between hospitals A and B. An F of 15.5227 with P at the 0.01 level of significance was obtained by ANOVA. Pearson correlation coefficients were obtained for the head

Table 16-1 Clinical Role Model Behavior

Hospital	Head nurse	No. of respondents*	Mean score	Standard deviation	Sum of square
A	1	4	25.250	2.500	
	2	5	19.800	5.215	
	3	10	30.300	1.767	
	4	4	29.750	3.594	
	5	3	24.333	5.132	
	6	2	27.500	2.121	
	7	4	26.750	2.986	
	8	5	21.400	2.967	
B	9	3	22.000	7.071	
	10	4	33.250	2.217	
	11	3	36.667	3.512	
	12	5	30.714	3.639	
	13	2	34.500	2.121	
	14	3	31.333	3.512	
	15	3	28.000	9.899	
A		37	26.054	4.916	869.902
B		23	31.348	5.288	615.223

Analysis of variance:

	SS	DF	MS	F-test
between groups	397.4687	1	397.4687	15.5227
within groups	1485.1250		25.6056	

Level of significance = 0.01.

Highest obtainable score = 40. Possible score range: 40 = always; 32 = often; 24 = sometimes; 16 = seldom; and 8 = never.

*The total number of responses in this category was 60. There were eight who did not respond.

nurse demographic data and the clinical role model behaviors. When controlling for agency, a positive correlation between the level of education and the role model behaviors resulted in $R = 0.5390$. This was significant at the 0.01 level. To control for variation in education level between agencies, the mean education level for each agency was subtracted from each head nurse's education level. In this study, the higher the head nurse's level of education, the higher the score on clinical role model behavior regardless of the hospital setting. The following data on educational level were obtained from the head nurse demographic questionnaire:

Type of program	Hospital A (N)	Hospital B (N)	Total population (N)
Diploma	6	2	8
Associate degree	0	1	1
Baccalaureate degree	2	4	6
	8	7	15

Validation and Evaluation Behavior (Table 16-2)

In hospital A the head nurse mean score for validation and evaluation was 33.839 with a standard deviation of 6.089. In hospital B the head nurse mean score was 36.481 with a standard deviation of 5.740. These results indicate that the staff nurses in each agency perceived their head nurses as often exhibiting validation and evaluation behaviors.

Behavior Facilitating the Primary Nurse Role (Table 16-3)

In hospital A the head nurse mean score for facilitating the primary nurse role was 23.457 with a standard deviation of 4.871. In hospital B the head nurse mean score was 24.148 with a standard deviation of 4.713. These mean scores indicate that the staff nurses in both hospitals often perceived their head nurses as exhibiting behaviors which facilitate the primary nurse role.

Behavior in Facilitating Staff Development (Table 16-4)

In hospital A the head nurse mean score for facilitating staff development was 24.412 with a standard deviation of 5.100. This score indicates that head nurses in that agency were perceived as exhibiting behaviors which facilitate staff development between the sometimes and often range of frequency.

Table 16-2 Validation and Evaluation Behavior

Hospital	Head nurse	No. of respondents*	Mean score	Standard deviation	Sum of square
A	1	3	37.667	2.310	
	2	4	24.250	2.363	
	3	9	36.556	6.729	
	4	2	32.500	6.364	
	5	3	35.667	2.082	
	6	2	32.000	1.414	
	7	3	29.667	3.215	
	8	5	37.000	3.536	
B	9	2	36.000	1.414	
	10	5	39.600	4.336	
	11	3	38.333	4.163	
	12	6	35.667	2.503	
	13	6	35.333	2.733	
	14	3	38.667	3.786	
	15	2	29.000	21.213	
A		31	33.839	6.089	1112.207
B		27	36.481	5.740	856.750

Analysis of variance:

	SS	DF	MS	F-test
between groups	100.7930	1	100.7930	2.8667
within groups	1968.9570		35.1599	

Not at significant level.

Highest obtainable score = 45. Possible score range: 45 = always; 36 = often; 27 = sometimes; 18 = seldom; and 9 = never.

*The total number of responses in this category was 58. There were ten who did not respond.

Table 16-3 Behavior in Facilitating the Primary Nurse Role ("Primary" Communicator, Coordinator, and Planner of Nursing Care)

Hospital	Head nurse	No. of respondents*	Mean score	Standard deviation	Sum of square
A	1	4	26.250	2.872	
	2	4	20.500	4.203	
	3	7	22.111	5.061	
	4	4	20.500	4.123	
	5	3	23.667	4.163	
	6	4	25.000	0.0	
	7	4	22.500	7.594	
	8	5	28.400	2.074	
B	9	3	27.000	1.732	
	10	4	26.333	3.215	
	11	3	22.000	2.000	
	12	7	25.429	2.226	
	13	5	23.167	8.994	
	14	3	24.333	4.163	
	15	2	18.000	16.971	
A		35	23.457	4.871	806.691
B		27	24.148	4.713	577.410

Analysis of variance:

	SS	DF	MS	F-test
between groups	7.2812	1	7.2812	0.3156
within groups	1384.1016		23.0684	

Not at significant level.

Highest obtainable score = 30. Possible score range: 30 = always; 24 = often; 18 = sometimes; 12 = seldom; and 6 = never.

*The total number of responses in this category was 62. There were 6 who did not respond.

Table 16-4 Behavior in Facilitating Staff Development

Hospital	Head nurse	No. of respondents*	Mean score	Standard deviation	Sum of square
A	1	3	25.000	7.550	
	2	4	18.750	1.893	
	3	9	25.000	5.172	
	4	4	21.000	2.944	
	5	5	24.667	4.509	
	6	2	27.000	5.657	
	7	4	25.000	5.354	
	8	3	28.000	3.647	
B	9	1	25.000	0.0	
	10	5	28.400	3.362	
	11	3	30.000	4.163	
	12	6	25.333	4.885	
	13	5	25.000	5.874	
	14	3	25.000	7.550	
	15	1	34.000	0.0	
A		34	24.412	5.100	858.242
B		24	26.833	5.088	595.340

Analysis of variance

	SS	DF	MS	F-test
between groups	82.4961	1	82.4961	3.1782
within groups	1453.5820		25.9568	

Not at significant level.

Highest obtainable score = 35. Possible score range: 35 = always; 28 = often; 21 = sometimes; 14 = seldom; and 7 = never.

*The total number of responses in this category was 58. There were ten who did not respond.

In hospital B the head nurse mean score in facilitating staff development was 26.833 with a standard deviation of 5.088 indicating that the staff nurses in that agency often perceived their head nurse as exhibiting behaviors which facilitate staff development. There were no significant differences between the head nurse scores in hospitals A and B.

Leadership and Administrative Management Behavior (Table 16-5)

In hospital A the head nurse mean score for leadership and administrative management behevior was 37.300 with a standard deviation of 5.559. In Hospital B the head nurse mean score was 38.500 with a standard deviation of 4.694. These scores indicate that the staff nurses in both agencies often perceived their head nurses as exhibiting leadership and administrative behaviors.

Behavior in Encouraging Independent Problem Solving (Table 16-6)

In hospital A the head nurse mean score for encouraging independent problem solving was 21.243 with a standard deviation of 3.419. In hospital B the head nurse mean score was 21.300 with a standard deviation of 3.087. These mean scores indicate that the staff nurses in both agencies often perceived their head nurses as exhibiting behaviors which encourage independent problem solving.

CONCLUSIONS

The purpose of this study was to determine whether or not head nurses exhibit those behaviors which were documented in the literature for the role of the head nurse in primary nursing. The findings indicate that staff primary nurses often perceived their head nurses as exhibiting the following four out of six categories of behavior: (1) facilitating the primary nurse role; (2) validating and evaluating primary nurses' ability to provide nursing care; (3) encouraging primary nurses to be independent problem solvers; and (4) demonstrating leadership and administrative management abilities.

In hospital A head nurses were perceived by their staff primary nurses as exhibiting behavior which facilitates staff development in the sometimes to often range. In hospital B head nurses were often perceived by their staff primary nurses as exhibiting behavior which facilitates staff development.

Clinical role model behavior was positively correlated with education, $R = 0.5390$. This was significant at the 0.01 level. In this study, the higher the head nurses' level of education, the higher the mean score in the clinical role model category regardless of the hospital setting.

Table 16-5 Leadership and Nursing Administrative Management Behavior

Hospital	Head nurse	No. of respondents*	Mean score	Standard deviation	Sum of square
A	1	4	40.250	2.986	
	2	3	28.667	0.578	
	3	7	40.857	3.625	
	4	5	30.500	4.203	
	5	3	37.333	4.163	
	6	2	42.500	0.707	
	7	3	36.750	4.992	
	8	3	40.000	3.000	
B	9	3	36.333	3.005	
	10	4	42.500	2.646	
	11	3	41.667	2.887	
	12	7	36.286	3.592	
	13	7	39.000	5.132	
	14	2	36.000	5.657	
	15	2	37.000	10.607	
A		30	37.300	5.559	896.316
B		28	38.500	4.694	595.000

Analysis of variance:

	SS	DF	MS	*F*-test
between groups	20.8711	1	20.8711	0.7837
within groups	1491.3164		26.6306	

Not at significant level.

Highest obtainable score = 45. Possible score range: 45 = always; 36 = often; 27 = sometimes; 18 = seldom; and 9 = never.

*The total number of responses in this category was 58. There were ten who did not respond.

Table 16-6 Behavior in Encouraging Independent Problem Solving (Facilitates the Freedom to Learn, Risk, and Seek Guidance)

Hospitals	Head nurse	No. of respondents*	Mean score	Standard deviation	Sum of square
A	1	4	22.000	2.160	
	2	5	18.200	5.070	
	3	10	22.500	2.915	
	4	4	17.250	1.708	
	5	3	22.333	3.055	
	6	2	24.000	0.0	
	7	4	21.000	2.582	
	8	5	22.800	2.800	
B	9	3	19.000	2.646	
	10	6	22.400	1.949	
	11	3	22.333	2.517	
	12	7	21.571	2.760	
	13	6	22.000	2.309	
	14	3	18.667	6.110	
	15	2	21.000	5.657	
A		37	21.243	3.419	420.816
B		30	21.300	3.087	276.309

Analysis of variance:

	SS	DF	MS	F-test
between groups	0.0547	1	0.0547	0.0051
within groups	697.1250			

Not at significant level.

Highest obtainable score = 25. Possible score range: 25 = always; 20 = often; 15 = sometimes; 10 = seldom; and 5 = never.

*The total number of responses in this category was 67. There was one who did not respond.

DISCUSSION

When analyzing the data in all six categories of role behavior, the mean scores for head nurses in hospitals A and B were generally equal. The mean scores for head nurses in hospital B were slightly and consistently higher than those obtained in hospital A; however, the idfference was not significant. The only correlation between head nurse demographic data and results on the perceived role behaviors was the head nurses' level of education and the mean score on the clinical role model behavior. This correlation may reflect the trend in higher education to emphasize that head nurses are clinical role models who guide and teach staff nurses by direct patient and family contact.

In general, the staff nurses often perceived their head nurses as exhibiting the role behaviors that were presented in the literature on the role of head nurses in primary nursing. However, the size of the population, 15 head nurses, limits generalizations. Also for each head nurse, the staff nurse response rate was small. Even though confidentiality was assured, staff nurses may have been more inclined to participate if they had a favorable impression of the head nurse than if the reverse were true. The size of the staff nurse response rate may also have been related to the time of the year that data were collected. Summer months tend to be periods of nurse turnover, and staff nurses may have been in a state of flux that influenced their decision not to participate in the study.

The results of the study may have been influenced by the fact that it was not a random population of head nurses and that both hospitals have had primary nursing implemented on some of their nursing units for several years.

RECOMMENDATIONS

It is hoped that the study can be repeated with a larger population using a questionnaire that elicits information not only about the primary nurses' perception of their head nurses' role behavior, but also about the head nurses' perception of how they carry out the responsibilities of their positions. The questionnaire items should be refined and retested for their reliability. Since a Likert scale poses limitations when analyzing data, the study might be replicated with a structured interview guide to get more comprehensive data of the primary nurses' perception of their head nurse and the head nurses' perception of their role.

AREAS FOR RESEARCH

Since primary nursing is a major management and organizational change in the delivery of nursing care, other areas of study should be pursued. A study could be developed to explore issues which the head nurses perceive as important to their role. Some questions to be addressed could be: What administrative support systems are most helpful in assisting the head nurse to function in the role? What type of job descriptions, performance evaluation tools, and reward systems has the head nurse found to be effective in promoting the growth and development of staff nurses? What type of selection process has the head nurse found to be effective in hiring primary nurses who are successful in the role? What educational programs can in-service education provide to assist the head nurse in performing the functions associated with the head nurse role? What type of interdepartmental policies and procedures are supportive for operationalizing primary nursing? What are the most difficult aspects of the supervisor/consultant function associated with the head nurse role? How are patient care outcomes affected by the role functions of the head nurse?

At the executive level of management, a study could be developed to explore some of the following issues: What type of selection process is effective for hiring head nurses to function in a primary nursing unit? What are the key elements to address when establishing an organizational milieu which supports the implementation of primary nursing? What type of administrative data are being collected in the nursing organization to evaluate the effectiveness of primary nursing? Does the type of service affect the implementation of primary nursing? What methods of implementation were found to be most effective, total organizational change or pilot project? Are there lower absenteeism and turnover rates in units which have established primary nursing? If we are to evaluate the administrative effectiveness of primary nursing, many of these issues need to be objectively addressed and explored.

REFERENCES

Anderson, M. Primary nursing in day-by-day practice. *American Journal of Nursing*, May 1976, *76*(5).

Brown, B. (Ed.). *Nursing Administration Quarterly: Primary Nursing*, Winter 1977, *1*(2), editorial.

Ciske, K.L. Primary nursing: An organization that promotes professional practice. *Journal of Nursing Administration*, January-February 1974, *4*(1), 30.

Elpern E.H. Structural and organizational supports for primary nursing. *Nursing Clinics of North America*, June 1977, *12*(2).

Katz, F., & Kahn, R. *The social psychology of organizations*. New York: John Wiley and Sons, 1966.

Logsdon, A. Why primary nursing? *Nursing Clinics of North America*, June 1973, *8*(2).

Manthey, M. Primary nursing is alive and well in the hospital. *American Journal of Nursing*, January 1973, *73*(1).

Manthey, M., Ciske, K., Robertson, P., & Harris, I. Primary nursing. *Nursing Forum*, 1970, *9*(1), 65.

McCarthy, D., & Schifalacqua, M.M. Primary nursing: Its implementation and six month outcome. *Journal of Nursing Administration*, *8*(5), May 1978.

Page, M. Perceptions of a head nurse. *American Journal of Nursing*, August 1974, *74*(8).

Zander, K.S. Primary nursing won't work unless the head nurse lets it. *Journal of Nursing Administration*, October 1977, *7*(8), 19.

Chapter 17

After Primary Nursing?

If primary nursing continues to evolve as indicated by the results of implementation, each change will generate the need for new changes. Once primary nursing takes hold nothing remains static! The direction of primary nursing will be strongly influenced by decisions made at all levels of society, particularly those involving money. Nurses should have a firm grasp of financial matters in order to exercise some control over them.

For the role of nurses to change in relation to emerging patterns of delivery of health care services, nurses' perception of their role will need to evolve. As the business of health care grows—hospitals are one of the largest industries in the country—nurses must see themselves as a necessary and contributing part of the system in a business and an organizational sense. To participate as planners as well as providers of care, nurses must combine their sensitivity and specialized assessment and treatment skills with some knowledge of business and management.

Nurses should be educated as generalists more than ever before. Upon graduation they should know at least the nature of delivery systems and the basic issues that systems deal with, such as finances, politics, marketing, organizational hierarchies, residency training priorities, research grants, computers, and regulatory agencies. Idealism must be tempered with knowledge of the practicalities of day-to-day functioning. The only way to see nursing ideals come close to reality is to be able to function within the system. Schools of nursing should structure the learning experience to include instruction on the functions of delivery systems. For instance, schools should require a course in business administration and management which covers material about organizations and their dynamics, budgeting, personnel policies and management, unions, and decision making. This could well cover organizations other than hospitals and be the general course offered for all university students.

Student nurses should be exposed to health care issues, including health care insurance mechanisms. Nurses in private practice or positions of authority in

343

agencies and clinics need to handle financial data, as well as the legal issues that arise when dealing in public service. The nature of such issues should be emphasized in undergraduate education to keep nurses aware of and able to cope with the realities of health care settings.

Developing a business consciousness does not detract or devalue the humanitarian approach of nursing care. The most well-intentioned nurse may not have any patients to help if the clinic closes down or third party payments do not cover comprehensive nursing care. Business skills will not only make the planning and provision of health services possible, but may also improve them. For instance, viewing psychiatric patients as customers with spoken and unspoken desires, as A. Lazar (Note 1) suggests, helps in the evaluation process and in negotiating for treatment. In Lazar's setting of a walk-in clinic, treating the patient as a customer increased the individualization of care and probably the speed at which the patients received treatment.

Budget and treatment programs go hand in hand, so the person who knows where the money comes from and where it is going has a certain amount of control, especially in hiring and decision making. Nurse-managers should be intimately involved in budget discussions about staffing. Interviewing and hiring privileges also influence the type of teamwork and the quality of nursing care in a unit. These management responsibilities take time and energy but should be expected by every nurse-manager above the staff level.

Separation of nursing charges from hospital room rates is necessary so that nurses are aware of how they fit into the total hospital picture. Fee for service can certainly reinforce a strong professional image. A business sense also is important on a personal level in order to be able to get the kind of job desired. Questions about salary, responsibility, and benefits must be dealt with, and state nursing associations cannot be substituted for individual negotiating. Generally, nurses are quick to sell themselves as bodies and hands rather than as productive thinkers.

No matter what direction health care delivery systems take and no matter which functions and skills nurses wish to call their own, an appreciation and knowledge of business management will help the nursing profession to grow and to give the kind of care it deems best. Nurses must not shy away from math figures or administrative complexities. They must take an active interest in procedures and policies and must learn what makes organizations run smoothly, just as they do for people's bodies. With these attitudes nurses will be able to take an active part in determining the type of health care given to the public.

Figure 17-1 depicts some of the levels on which decisions that affect the direction of primary nursing are made. Each level has its own pressures and problems, so it is difficult to say what may evolve after primary nursing. Weisensee (1979) cautions:

Figure 17-1 Levels of Decisions That Influence Primary Nursing

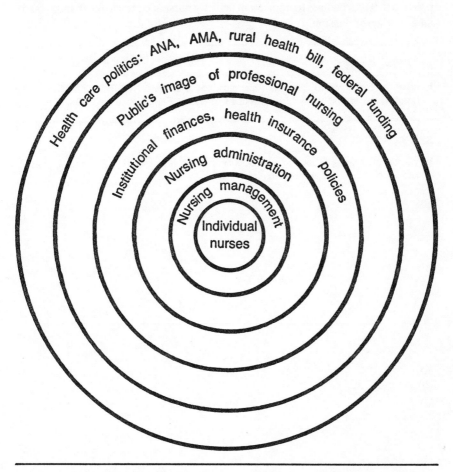

If nursing is to survive as a viable helping profession, it must first help itself through a peaceful settlement as to the role and purposes it desires to achieve rather than through an attempt to be all things to all people and doing a haphazard job at all of them. If the energy that was spent on infighting over trivial matters could be eliminated, there would be time and energy for accomplishing the bigger and better things that are waiting to be done (p. 77).

If competent and confident nurses are not ready to respond to the dynamics of health care delivery, other groups will provide the necessary services. Primary nursing in itself does not guarantee a viable identity for the nursing profession.

However, the changes in attitudes, administration, management, and clinical practice that are required to implement primary nursing generate the foundation for an enduring profession.

REFERENCE NOTE

1. Lazar, A. *The patient as customer.* Paper presented at the Tufts-New England Medical Center Hospital, Department of Psychiatry, Ziskind Conference, Boston, February 1972.

REFERENCE

Weisensee, M. Nursing's future role. In D. Kjervik and I. Martinson (Eds.). *Women in stress: A nursing perspective.* New York: Appleton-Century-Crofts, 1979.

Index

About the Author

Since 1970 Ms. Zander has served in various positions at Tufts-New England Medical Center, Boston. She is currently serving as nurse leader (clinical specialist) for the psychiatric inpatient and day hospital service and also as the organizational development specialist for the Department of Nursing. She has had extensive experience in the use of the group modality. She has been a primary nurse, a manager of a primary nursing staff, and a staff education instructor. Since 1977 Ms. Zander has been chairman of the Primary Nursing Committee, chairman of the Documentation Committee, and member of the Retrospective Audit Committee. She coordinates management training seminars and special projects.

Ms. Zander received her bachelor of science in nursing at Illinois Wesleyan University and her master of science in nursing in the psychiatric-mental health specialty at Boston University. Presently, Ms. Zander is an assistant clinical professor for Adelphi University's School of Nursing and a graduate program preceptor for Boston University's School of Nursing. She has also been on the faculty of Tufts Medical School. In addition to freelance consultation and workshops, Ms. Zander maintains a private practice in psychotherapy in the Boston area and is an active member of NURS (Nurses United for Reimbursement of Services). She also belongs to the American Nurses Association.

Her publications include "Primary Nursing Won't Work . . . Unless the Head Nurse Lets It," (*Journal of Nursing Administration,* 1977) and *Practical Manual for Patient-teaching* (1978), which she co-edited with Bower, Foster, Towson, Wermuth, and Woldum.